Methods in Pharmacology and Toxicology

Series Editor
Y. James Kang
Department of Pharmacology & Toxicology
University of Louisville, Louisville
Kentucky, USA

For further volumes:
http://www.springer.com/series/7653

Lyophilization of Pharmaceuticals and Biologicals

New Technologies and Approaches

Edited by

Kevin R. Ward

Biopharma Process Systems Ltd., Winchester, UK

Paul Matejtschuk

National Institute for Biological Standards & Control (NIBSC), Potters Bar, Hertfordshire, UK

Humana Press

Editors
Kevin R. Ward
Biopharma Process Systems Ltd.
Winchester, UK

Paul Matejtschuk
National Institute for Biological Standards & Control
(NIBSC)
Potters Bar, Hertfordshire, UK

ISSN 1557-2153 ISSN 1940-6053 (electronic)
Methods in Pharmacology and Toxicology
ISBN 978-1-4939-8927-0 ISBN 978-1-4939-8928-7 (eBook)
https://doi.org/10.1007/978-1-4939-8928-7

Library of Congress Control Number: 2018962406

This Humana Press imprint is published by the registered company Springer Science+Business Media, LLC, part of Springer Nature.
The registered company address is: 233 Spring Street, New York, NY 10013, U.S.A.

Dedication

This book is dedicated to the memories of Alan P. MacKenzie and Michael J. Pikal, who contributed so much to the world of lyophilization.

Preface

So why another book on freeze-drying?

Lyophilization (freeze-drying) has been employed since the early twentieth century in the medical field. While the principles of the process and the laws of physics governing it remain unchanged, advances in technology and changes in the regulatory framework have meant that the equipment has continued to evolve. Approaches to the development and manufacturing processes have undergone a paradigm shift from a largely empirical trial-and-error approach to one based upon initial determination of intrinsic physicochemical properties, followed by a more methodical approach to both formulation, process development and monitoring. As editors who have between them over fifty years of working experience in this field, we have witnessed these changes firsthand and so are delighted to be able to bring together insightful contributions from many who are also actively involved in delivering freeze-drying solutions at both laboratory and industrial scales.

The stabilization of active materials is a fundamental requirement across a range of products, not limited to small drug molecules and biological materials, but also veterinary products, advanced therapy medicines, and molecular diagnostics. Recent trends in the pharmaceutical market alone have seen the rise to prominence of biopharmaceutical therapeutics [1] and the majority of these are lyophilized to ensure adequate stability and competitive shelf life. Similarly, the rise in the use of molecular diagnostics and the power of technologies such as polymerase chain reaction (PCR) assays mean that many of the essential reagents contained within these assays kits must be lyophilized to ensure ease of delivery.

There have been numerous texts and review articles devoted to the principles and practicalities of lyophilization in the last 70 years, so this volume is not designed to rehash what has previously been documented perfectly adequately elsewhere [2–5], nor indeed to cover one specific aspect of lyophilization in detail, but rather, it seeks to highlight areas of recent developments and technological advances in the field. In the present work, we have drawn together experts in the particular facets of the lyophilization challenge in order to update the reader with latest trends in each aspect. Advances in technology and improvements in the way data are handled and presented have contributed to where we are today. Developing freeze-drying knowledge in-house and purchasing one's own equipment rather than relying solely on external organizations or consultants are now the order of the day.

From providing initially an outline of the principles of effective product formulation and analytical characterization of the physicochemical properties of the materials to be dried, we progress to the discussion of one of the most widely impacting new developments in industrial freeze-drying—that of controlled ice nucleation. Across two chapters, different authors present and evaluate the full range of potential solutions, both those already commercialized technologies and also the more developmental approaches.

Possibly one of the greatest changes we have witnessed in our careers is the move from a trial-and-error-based approach to one that relies on prior understanding of the physicochemical aspects of a formulation before attempting to load the freeze-dryer. While some analytical technologies had been developed prior to the twenty-first century [6, 7], they were not necessarily widely applied in lyophilization due to the lack of understanding of the methods, the data interpretation, and how it could be applied in a real-life freeze-drying cycle, especially in the days when chamber pressure and shelf temperature were themselves not necessarily controlled or measured accurately.

The regulatory drivers have encouraged the increasing adoption of risk-based approaches such as Quality by Design. This is addressed in this volume in a seminal contribution from both former and present regulatory experts. These regulatory and technological factors combine to present us with fresh challenges and new opportunities in delivering freeze-drying solutions to stabilization problems. The principles and technologies that have developed as a result of these drivers have application beyond the narrow specialty of pharmaceutical parenteral delivery and impact the development and manufacture of in vitro diagnostics, novel therapeutics, and new-format vaccines right through to nutraceuticals and foodstuffs.

Process Analytical Technology has become mainstream in the pharma industry and so its presence is also increasingly felt within pharmaceutical freeze-drying. Three chapters are therefore devoted to descriptions of both established and emerging technologies and how they can be used practically within process development and the all-important scale up.

Developments in associated areas, such as the vital role of primary packaging, containment, and automation of industrial lyophilization, are also presented.

The demand for new high-dose therapeutic biologicals has led to specific challenges in terms of both processing and freeze-drying of such drugs. These are reviewed in a dedicated chapter on the aspects of delivering high concentration biotherapeutics at industrial scale.

The quality attributes of lyophilized products have also experienced a marked paradigm shift over the past decade. Critical Quality Attributes are key to developing and consistently manufacturing a licensed therapeutic and so with increasing pressure to define attributes quantitatively rather than qualitatively, new technologies are emerging. The appearance and structure of lyophiles is one such area, with time-consuming and subjective visual inspection being supplanted by precise metrics such as cake resistance and robustness and the advent of 100% inspection of such properties by increasingly automated methodologies.

In this volume, we have aimed to bring together leading practitioners in the freeze-drying community to address recent progress, not only in new analytical tools and application of the data derived in cycle design but also in the manufacturing of lyophilized products in the healthcare sector—whether these be therapeutics, vaccines, or diagnostic products—and indeed the equipment to deliver this scale of freeze-drying.

Some of the contributions in this volume and the areas they cover are highlighted in the following sections:

Analytical and Formulation Issues:

- New techniques for determination of critical formulation physicochemical parameters and using multiple methods rather than a single one to arrive at consensus values—*Ward and Matejtschuk* (Chap. 1)
- Steps to address subjectivity in interpretation of freeze-drying microscopy results—*Ward and Matejtschuk* (Chap. 1)
- Traditional and Design of Experiment (DoE) approaches to formulation of complex products are covered by *Matejtschuk et al.* (Chap. 2)
- Application of noninvasive testing methods for integrity of containers and moisture content—*Matejtschuk et al.* (Chap. 2)

- Challenges of understanding the interaction of multicomponent formulations and strategies for handling complex biological samples (e.g., viruses)—*Matejtschuk et al.* (Chap. 2)

Process Monitoring and Control:

- Review and assessment of Controlled Nucleation (CN) methods (technological advances) are covered by *Luoma et al.* (Chap. 3) and *Pisano* (Chap. 4), illustrating the variety of methods and the different underlying principles, status of commercialization and scalability, and impact on quality and consistency
- Use of specific Process Analytical Technology (PAT) equipment and methods is described in detail by *Kessler and Gong* (Chap. 5) and *Smith and Polygalov* (Chap. 11), while the role of statistical data in process understanding and scale-up is illustrated by *Bourlès et al.* (Chap. 10)
- Regulatory aspects of freeze-drying, and the application of a Quality by Design approach in this context, are covered by *Awotwe-Atoo and Khan* (Chap. 8)
- Understanding the impact of primary packaging (glass, closures, etc.) on the dried product—still fundamental to long-term storage—is portrayed by *McAndrew et al.* (Chap. 9)
- The need to control and contain the product during processing forms the basis of the contribution by *Cherry* (Chap. 6) who also presents a novel approach to primary packaging, while the automated handling technologies often used at large-scale manufacture are highlighted by *Guttzeit et al.* (Chap. 7)
- The special challenges posed by highly concentrated protein products and their impact on filling and lyophilization are discussed by *Garidel and Presser* (Chap. 12)

Post-lyophilization Analysis:

- Analysis of the structural and mechanical properties of lyophilized products and an emerging technique to assess the Young's modulus and strength of freeze-dried materials are described by *Hedberg et al.* (Chap. 13)
- Solid-state Hydrogen-Deuterium Exchange Mass Spectrometry and molecular labeling are novel and powerful technologies for the detailed analysis of freeze-dried proteins, the impact on structure, and their interactions with excipients—this is presented by *Balakrishna Chandrababu et al.* (Chap. 14).

Inevitably, this is a snapshot only of the areas of progress within the field of lyophilization toward the end of the second decade of the twenty-first century, and doubtless it will have been to some degree influenced by the interests of the editors, both of whom come to the field from a developmental perspective. However, as we have highlighted above, this area has perhaps been the one which has developed most rapidly over the past decade. Also, it is the rising clinical importance of these lyophilized materials that has driven the demand for better and more robust process and product characterization.

We are indebted to all of the authors for their excellent contributions to this work and recommend it to those seeking an update in this rapidly changing field. Finally, we thank David C. Casey and all the team at Springer for their enthusiasm for the work and guidance during its compilation.

We hope the readers will share our enthusiasm for these topics as they are expounded by the respective authors and find inspiration and encouragement to pursue their own interests in the field of freeze-drying.

Winchester, UK *Kevin R. Ward*
Potters Bar, Hertfordshire, UK *Paul Matejtschuk*

References

1. Seymour P, Ecker DM (2017) Global biomanufacturing trends, capacity, and technology drivers: industry biomanufacturing capacity overview. Am Pharmaceut Rev 20(4). Accessed from https://dialog.proquest.com/professional/docview/1920294549
2. Hua T-C, Liu B-L, Zhang H (2010) Freeze-drying of pharmaceutical and food products. CRC Press/Woodhead Publishing Ltd, Oxford
3. Haseley P, Oetjen G-W (2018) Freeze drying, 3rd edn. Wiley-VCH, Weinheim
4. Franks F, Auffret A (2008) Freeze drying of pharmaceuticals & biopharmaceuticals. Royal Society of Chemistry, Cambridge
5. Rey L, May JC (eds) (2010) Freeze drying/lyophilization of pharmaceutical and biological products, 3rd edn. Informa, New York, NY
6. Rey L (2010) Glimpses into the realm of freeze drying: classical issues and new ventures. In: Rey L, May JC (eds) Freeze-drying/lyophilization of pharmaceutical and biological products, 3rd edn. Informa, New York, NY, pp 1–28
7. Ward K, Matejtschuk P (2010) The use of microscopy, thermal analysis and impedance measurements to establish critical formulation parameters for freeze-drying cycle development. In: Rey L, May J (eds) Freeze-drying/lyophilization of pharmaceuticals and biological products, 3rd edn. Informa Healthcare, New York, NY; London, pp 112–135

Contents

Contributors

DAVID AWOTWE-OTOO • *Division of Post Marketing Activities II, Office of Pharmaceutical Quality, Center for Drug Evaluation and Research, Food and Drug Administration, Silver Spring, MD, USA*

KARTHIK BALAKRISHNA CHANDRABABU • *Department of Industrial and Physical Pharmacy, Purdue University, West Lafayette, IN, USA*

THOMAS BEUTLER • *GEA Lyophil GmbH, Hürth, North Rhine-Westphalia, Germany*

ERWAN BOURLÈS • *GSK Vaccines, Rixensart, Belgium*

YUAN CHEN • *Department of Industrial and Physical Pharmacy, Purdue University, West Lafayette, IN, USA*

CHRIS CHERRY • *PDR, Cardiff Met University, Cardiff, UK*

GAEL DE LANNOY • *GSK Vaccines, Rixensart, Belgium*

FRANCES L. DEGRAZIO • *West Pharmaceutical Services, Inc., Exton, PA, USA*

SHARMILA DEVI • *Surfaces and Particle Engineering Group, Department of Chemical Engineering, Imperial College London, London, UK*

ARNOLD DURALLIU • *Surfaces and Particle Engineering Group, Department of Chemical Engineering, Imperial College London, London, UK*

CHINWE DURU • *Standardisation Science, National Institute for Biological Standards and Control (NIBSC), Potters Bar, Herts, UK*

FERNANDA FONSECA • *UMR GMPA, AgroParisTech, INRA, Université Paris Saclay, Thiverval-Grignon, France*

PATRICK GARIDEL • *Corporate Division Biopharmaceuticals, Process Science, Protein Science, Boehringer Ingelheim Pharma GmbH & Co. KG, Biberach an der Riss, Germany*

EMILY GONG • *Physical Sciences Inc., Andover, MA, USA*

MAIK GUTTZEIT • *GEA Lyophil GmbH, Hürth, North Rhine-Westphalia, Germany*

SARAH H. M. HEDBERG • *Surfaces and Particle Engineering Group, Department of Chemical Engineering, Imperial College London, London, UK*

DOUGLAS HOSTETLER • *West Pharmaceutical Services, Inc., Exton, PA, USA*

RAJASHEKAR KAMMARI • *Department of Industrial and Physical Pharmacy, Purdue University, West Lafayette, IN, USA*

WILLIAM J. KESSLER • *Physical Sciences Inc., Andover, MA, USA*

MANSOOR KHAN • *Irma Lerma Rangel College of Pharmacy, Texas A&M Health Science Center, College Station, TX, USA*

LOKESH KUMAR • *Genentech, Inc., South San Francisco, CA, USA*

JACOB LUOMA • *Genentech, Inc., South San Francisco, CA, USA*

GRAHAM MAGILL • *Genentech, Inc., South San Francisco, CA, USA*

KIRAN MALIK • *Standardisation Science, National Institute for Biological Standards and Control (NIBSC), Potters Bar, Herts, UK*

PAUL MATEJTSCHUK • *National Institute for Biological Standards and Control (NIBSC), Potters Bar, Hertfordshire, UK*

T. PAGE MCANDREW • *Scientific Communications, Scientific Affairs and Technical Services, West Pharmaceutical Services, Inc., Exton, PA, USA*

STEPHANIE PASSOT • *UMR GMPA, AgroParisTech, INRA, Université Paris Saclay, Thiverval-Grignon, France*

ROBERTO PISANO • *Department of Applied Science and Technology, Molecular Engineering Laboratory, Politeccnico di Torino, Torino, Italy*
EVGENY POLYGALOV • *Pharmaceutical Technologies, Leicester School of Pharmacy, De Montfort University, Leicester, UK*
INGO PRESSER • *Corporate Division Biopharmaceuticals, Process Science, Protein Science, Boehringer Ingelheim Pharma GmbH & Co. KG, Biberach an der Riss, Germany*
BERNADETTE SCUTELLÀ • *GSK Vaccines, Rixensart, Belgium*
JOHANNES SELCH • *GEA Lyophil GmbH, Hürth, North Rhine-Westphalia, Germany*
GEOFF SMITH • *Pharmaceutical Technologies, Leicester School of Pharmacy, De Montfort University, Leicester, UK*
ELIZABETH M. TOPP • *Department of Industrial and Physical Pharmacy, Purdue University, West Lafayette, IN, USA*
IOAN CRISTIAN TRELEA • *UMR GMPA, AgroParisTech, INRA, Université Paris Saclay, Thiverval-Grignon, France*
KEVIN R. WARD • *Biopharma Process Systems Ltd, Winchester, UK*
DARYL R. WILLIAMS • *Surfaces and Particle Engineering Group, Department of Chemical Engineering, Imperial College London, London, UK*
CAROLIN WOLF • *GEA Lyophil GmbH, Hürth, North Rhine-Westphalia, Germany*
ZAKARIA YUSOFF • *SP Scientific, Warminster, PA, USA*

Chapter 1

Characterization of Formulations for Freeze-Drying

Kevin R. Ward and Paul Matejtschuk

Abstract

One of the most wide-reaching changes in freeze-drying over the past 20 years has been the commercial availability of a range of discriminating analytical methods to identify critical temperatures in formulations to be freeze dried. Here, we briefly describe the development of these techniques from the earlier bespoke methods, setting their rise in a historical context. We then review techniques such as freeze-drying microscopy, differential scanning calorimetry, and less widely applied alternative technologies. Practical examples of the results obtained with these techniques are discussed and upcoming new trends and troubleshooting problems are addressed.

Key words Freeze-drying microscopy, Differential scanning calorimetry, Dynamic mechanical analysis, Thermal analysis, Impedance, TASC, Optical coherence tomography

1 The Basis for Formulation Analysis

1.1 Introduction

Given their prominence in modern publications on freeze-drying, it is perhaps surprising to realize that the use of modern thermal analysis and techniques such as freeze-drying microscopy (FDM) in formulation development was for the most part neglected until the start of the twenty-first century. These technologies were developed by freeze-drying pioneers such as the late Prof Louis Rey [30] and Alan MacKenzie [20] but were yet to be commercially exploited. Although widely described as early as the 1960s such techniques were very much the domain of the specialist laboratory and many undertaking freeze-drying in academic or even industrial laboratories relied upon a trial-and-error approach to cycle development, sometimes supplemented by home-built simple analyzers. For instance, at NIBSC in the late 1990s, there was a home-built differential thermal analyzer built in conjunction with Brunel University, results from which went by the rather lengthy term of "solid-liquid transition temperature" and this was calibrated with isotonic saline, much as used with current thermal analyzers. To its advantage, it required only 0.2 mL of sample; however, the results

Kevin R. Ward and Paul Matejtschuk (eds.), *Lyophilization of Pharmaceuticals and Biologicals: New Technologies and Approaches*, Methods in Pharmacology and Toxicology, https://doi.org/10.1007/978-1-4939-8928-7_1,

were plotted on graph paper—a far cry from modern technology. Quite common at the time was freeze-drying formulation based solely upon trial-and-error experiments (see [22]) without any formulation analytical characterization and these time-consuming studies meant that formulation was often developed slowly with "one factor at a time" (OFAT) approaches. This seems a long way from the modern analytical laboratory where thermal and optical methods vie for predominance and analytical characterization is a prerequisite to anything being loaded into a freeze dryer!

The history of these developments and of others which still remain the domain of the specialist laboratory have been previously described by Rey [32, 33]. In this chapter, we will review the common technologies used for formulation characterization to optimize freeze-drying and also highlight some of the newer technologies that have recently come to the market place.

1.2 History of Using Analytical Formulation

As stated previously, the development of these technologies has been reviewed by some of those who initially developed them [33]. Smith has also reviewed the history of one area of such technology—that of impedance technology (see Chap. 11 in this volume). The first such techniques were recommended by Rey [30, 31] and Lachman et al. [18]. MacKenzie [20, 21] and also Rey [31] described bespoke freeze-drying microscopes. The technology of freeze-drying itself was reviewed on several occasions by the *Developments in Biologicals* series [4, 23].

The disadvantage of thermal analyzers is that they respond best with salty ionic solutions, but these formulants are not the best for optimizing freeze-drying. Although largely applied to aqueous samples, analysis of mixed organic phases can also be analyzed [16].

1.3 Advantages of Pre-lyophilization Analysis

The advantages of performing thorough pre-lyophilization analysis of samples intended for drying are quite easily appreciated. The amounts of material required are small compared to that needed for a reproducible freeze-drying run, and the time taken even for slow scan runs is orders of magnitude shorter than a freeze-drying run (minutes rather than tens of hours). In addition, by combining several techniques, a comprehensive analysis of the spectrum of thermal and rheological properties can be accumulated within a comparatively short time. This will then make a significant saving in terms of the number of freeze-drying trials which will be needed before arriving at a viable scalable lyophilization cycle. This must be offset against the cost of the analytical equipment, which is not insignificant, in the range of \$25K–\$100K per item. Some of these techniques are highly specific, such as a freeze-drying microscope; however, other techniques (e.g., DSC, DMA) can be applied in other areas of pharmaceutical development and so the effective cost may be offset in organizations with a broader formulation remit than just a freeze-dried format.

2 Techniques Used to Characterize Formulations

2.1 Electrical Impedance (Zsinφ) Analysis

The premise of using electrical properties to identify changes in frozen solutions prior to (and even during) lyophilization was discussed by Rey in 1960; however, the idea was never widely commercialized, possibly because electrical resistance (or resistivity) analysis seemed to display little sensitivity to solutions containing much lower levels of ionic or polar species. This was often the case with many biopharmaceutical and biological products where buffers or other salts would typically be significantly lower than in traditional injectable drug molecules (or sometimes absent altogether) and even in the liquid state, the electrical resistance would sometimes not be zero.

Rey demonstrated in 2004 that examining impedance (and in particular, a function of impedance known as "Zsinφ") rather than simple resistance would typically give a much clearer signal of mobility changes occurring in the frozen state. Indeed, for a number of different solutions, plotting the value of Zsinφ (in Ohms) against temperature during cooling and warming often gave an obvious indication of a softening event, even when such events could not be easily detected by traditional thermal methods such as DSC. After examining Zsinφ at a series of input frequencies between 300 and 3000 Hz for a range of aqueous solutions, it was concluded that a frequency of 1000 Hz gave the most acceptable balance between amplitude of signal and clarity of event. An industrial collaboration with Biopharma Process Systems enabled Rey to commercialize the technology in the form of the Lyotherm2 instrument in 2005. We have employed this form of analysis very widely in our own laboratories at BPS and NIBSC since that time, particularly after much of the early data indicated that for more complex formulations, there can be marked changes in mobility at temperatures far lower than appear to translate to an obvious visible change in the material when observed using freeze-drying microscopy (FDM) [39]. The thermogram containing the Zsinφ and DTA profiles for a human plasma reference sample is shown in Fig. 1.

2.2 Differential Thermal Analysis (DTA)

Differential Thermal Analysis (DTA) is a means of analyzing endothermic and exothermic events in a sample by comparing its thermal behavior with that of a suitable reference material—in the case of a liquid formulation, the reference material would typically be the solvent (such as water). Being a relatively simplistic method, it has largely been superseded by DSC (see later in this chapter) for dry state analysis, due to the enhanced accuracy and sophistication of the latter [17]. However, DTA does remain in use today in lyophilization R&D, particularly for analysis of liquid samples pre-lyophilization, where, for example, in modern instruments such as

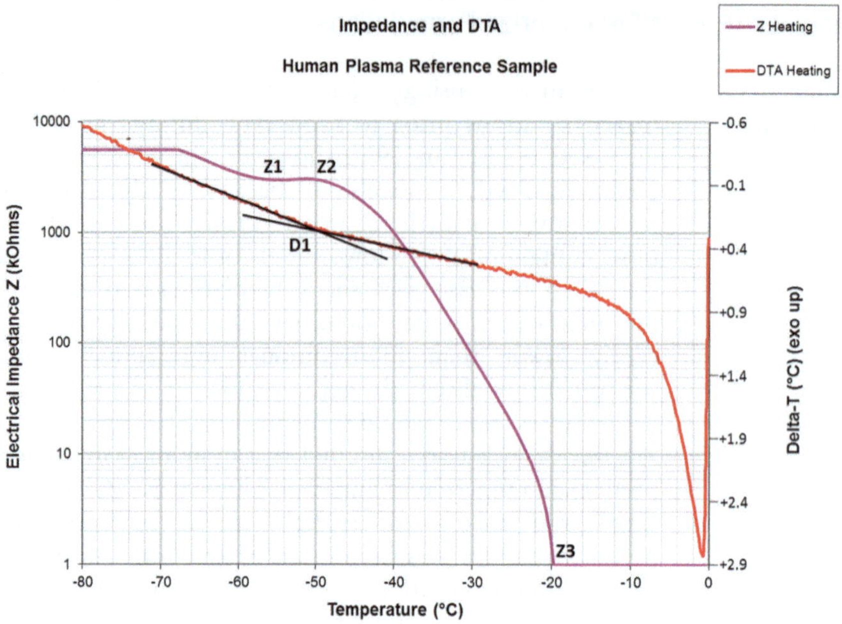

Fig. 1 Lyotherm Impedance and DTA profile for a human plasma reference sample. On the impedance (pink) curve, the flattening at point Z1 indicates a stabilization within the structure upon warming, which ties in with the minor thermal event at D1 in the DTA curve. The increase in downward gradient at point Z2 represents an increase in molecular mobility within the frozen formulation, culminating in minimum impedance being reached at −20 °C (Z3), which coincides with the temperature of total collapse reported for plasma

the Lyotherm3 (where it can run simultaneously alongside Zsinφ analysis, as shown in Fig. 1), the relatively large sample size (3 mL) can help overcome the traditional issues with lack of signal strength often observed for the analysis of dilute aqueous solutions where the relatively high energy thermal events associated with the water itself tend to dominate the profile.

2.3 Freeze-Drying Microscopy (FDM)

Even the first designs of FDM apparatus focused on the use of thin samples sandwiched between cover slips, in order to minimize any sublimation cooling effects, since the temperature of the sample itself was not measured directly and by minimizing such effects, the sample temperature and the measured temperature could then be assumed to be near-identical. Resulting data could be validated against standard solutions—usually crystallizing solutions such as sodium chloride, which would have a known eutectic melting temperature and would visibly melt over a very narrow temperature range when warmed sufficiently slowly. The same principle is still employed today, but with various incremental improvements in the accuracy of measurement, the precision of control and the optical quality.

A typical FDM experiment involves cooling the liquid sample until it appears to be completely frozen, then applying a vacuum and observing the structure immediately behind the drying front (sublimation interface). If the structure remains visibly intact, then the temperature is raised until the point is reached where defects are evident in the structure; if, on the other hand, the structure is poor or there is no drying structure visible at all when sublimation commences, then the temperature is lowered in order to determine whether evidence of drying structure can be obtained. Examples of lyophilization-related events that can be identified using FDM are discussed in the sections below.

2.3.1 Collapse

The term "collapse" is often used generically to describe any visible loss of structure in a material undergoing freeze-drying; however, strictly speaking, it refers to viscous flow in an amorphous—or partially amorphous—material, as distinct from an eutectic melt that would occur in a crystalline sample (or crystalline phase of a "mixed system"). Ultimately, either form of event may be considered to produce a process defect in a product, although the manifestation of collapse and melting can be visibly different and may have differing consequences on the product, process, and equipment. An example of this is that a crystalline sample having undergone an eutectic melt (meaning there will be eutectic liquid between the solvent crystals) may then see the liquid component boil under the levels of vacuum employed during the sublimation process, which may also lead to a loss of pressure control; on the other hand, an amorphous sample undergoing collapse will become more resistant to vapor flow (Rp increases) due to pores closing down and surface area reducing, and therefore will not tend to lead to loss of pressure control.

Since virtually all formulations of pharmaceuticals, biopharmaceuticals, vaccines, and medical/environmental diagnostics are at least partially amorphous (with most being completely amorphous apart from those containing small drug molecules and/or crystalline excipients such as mannitol), collapse is an event that is relevant to most products [26]. Therefore, for most freeze-drying scientists, the primary function of FDM is to determine the collapse temperature of a formulation. After gaining some experience of working with lyo-formulations, it may be possible to predict what the collapse temperature may be, although this can be somewhat challenging for formulations containing a mixture of crystallizing and amorphous components, since the latter may inhibit (or even prevent) the crystallization of the former, and this will also be dependent on the ratios of the components, and often also on the freezing conditions employed.

In our laboratories, we often carry out FDM analysis on a sample multiple times, and as a minimum, for samples that display low collapse temperatures when initially analyzed in the absence of an annealing step, analysis will be repeated with the inclusion of an annealing step, in order to determine whether this may have a positive impact on the thermodynamic stability of the material. This is discussed further later in this chapter. Additionally, it may be advisable to run thermal/impedance analysis prior to FDM in order to enable a suitable temperature to be selected for the annealing step in FDM.

Figure 2 shows images of sucrose solutions during FDM analysis. If the sample is warmed slowly, or the temperature setpoint increased in small steps (e.g., 0.1 °C) after a period of holding in each step, then the determination of the onset of the collapse event should be possible to within a fraction of a degree. This is enabled by the acquisition of images at short intervals (often taken as frequently as every 5 s during certain steps of the analysis), which allows for retrospective analysis of images where the aim is to find two consecutive images in the resulting gallery, one of which shows the sample to have perfect appearance and the subsequent one showing the first signs of imperfection. The ability to pinpoint the precise onset of collapse may be enhanced through the use of an analyzer collar and tint plate assembly; visualizing a sample with polarized light and a first order red filter enables in-depth analysis of crystal structures in the frozen material, while the false color also allows for easier identification of critical events.

2.3.2 Microcollapse

Microcollapse has been an identifiable phenomenon in its own right for a number of years, as discussed by Wang [38] and Liu et al. [19] and is one that we have frequently observed in our laboratories in formulations containing a mixture of crystalline and amorphous components (which may be excipients and/or the active ingredient). For example, a solution containing 2% mannitol and 1% glucose where the mannitol crystallizes during freeze-drying (either as a controlled event during a deliberate annealing step, or perhaps in a less controlled manner during sublimation) would be expected to comprise separate phases in the frozen (and drying) structure where mannitol exhibits a Teu of −1.4 °C but glucose undergoes viscous flow around −41 °C, thus microcollapsing onto the scaffold of crystalline mannitol (see Fig. 3). In this case, a conservative estimate of the critical temperature might be considered to be −41 °C, and indeed, some defects in the freeze-drying structure are clear at this temperature when viewed by FDM (Fig. 4), although we have observed that in such a mixture, total loss of structure at the macroscopic level often does not occur until above −20 °C. This is still significantly lower than the eutectic temperature of crystalline mannitol alone; whether this is attributable to significant levels of viscous flow in the amorphous glucose phase at this temperature that was able to counter the mechanical strength afforded by crystalline mannitol, or whether indeed some of the mannitol persisted in the amorphous phase due to the presence of amorphous glucose and/or the thermal history of the

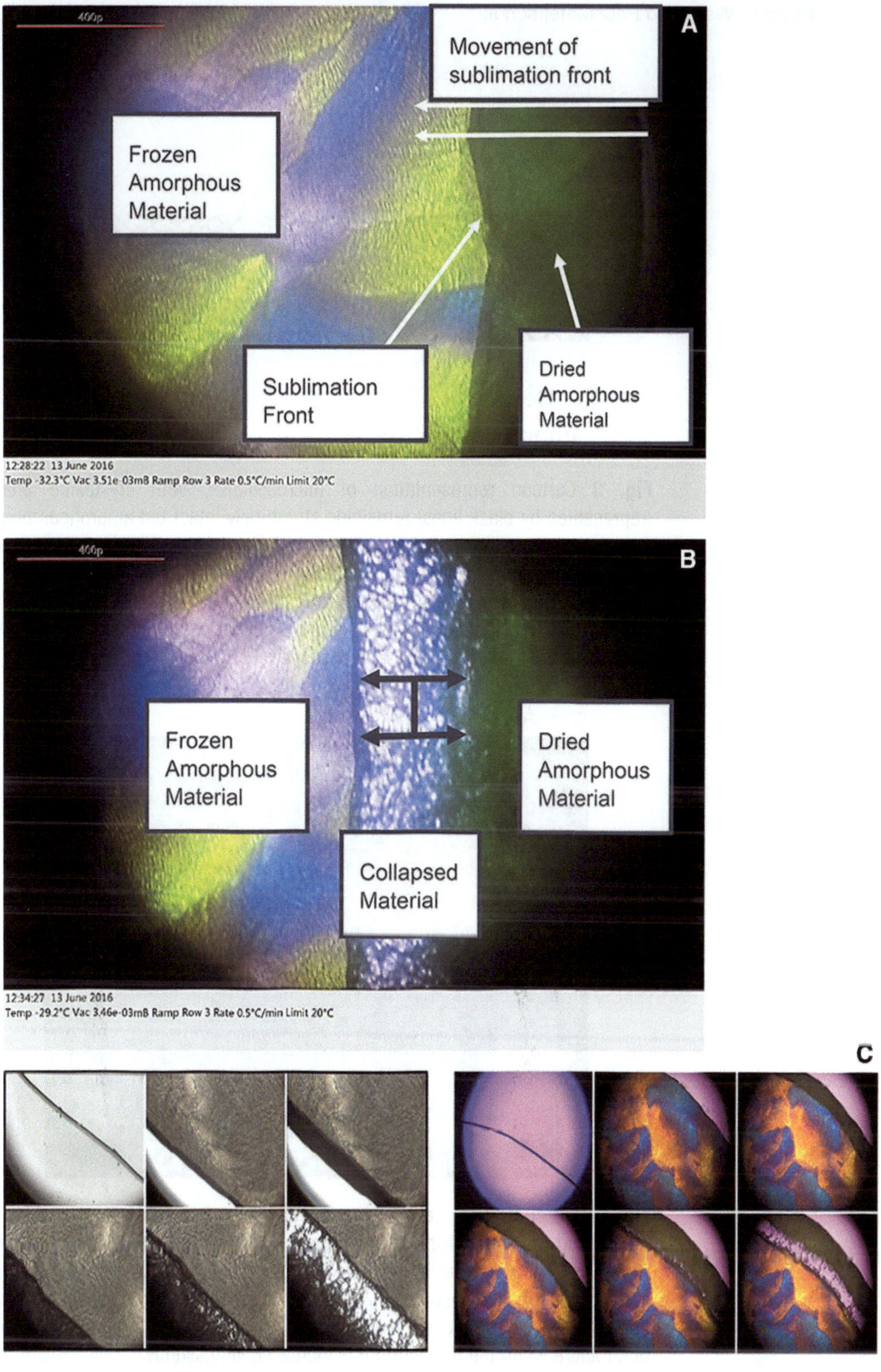

Fig. 2 Examples of FDM images taken at various key points during the analysis of disaccharide samples, in each case frozen to −40.0 °C initially, then once vacuum applied, gradually warmed until loss of structure observed: (**A**) sample immediately before onset of collapse occurs, (**B**) the same sample 6 min later, having been warmed to the point of complete collapse, and (**C**) demonstrating the visual effect of using a polarizer and first order red filter (right) compared with using no filters or polarization (left) throughout FDM analysis

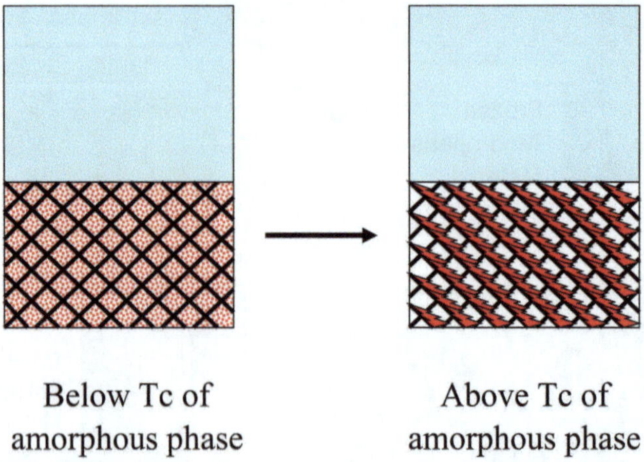

Fig. 3 Cartoon representation of microcollapse, with crystalline phase (represented by black lines) remaining structurally intact but amorphous phase (shown in red) collapsing when the sublimation interface temperature exceeds the Tc of this phase during primary drying. Micro-melting, as defined by us previously [39], would be analogous to microcollapse but with the amorphous phase remaining structurally intact and crystalline phase undergoing eutectic melt when the Teu of this phase is exceeded

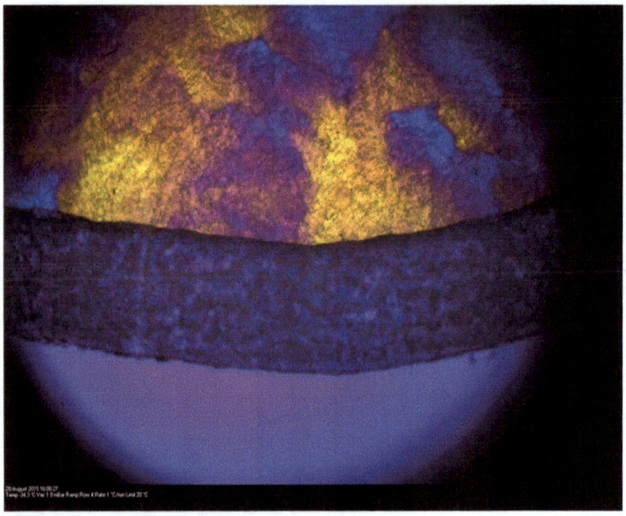

Fig. 4 Typical FDM image showing microcollapse in a real sample, which is manifested in a "multi-layer" semi-opaque appearance with the crystalline phase retaining its structure but the amorphous phase collapsing onto it. Evidence of this observation as being microcollapse (as opposed to the onset of a classic collapse event) may be confirmed if there is no further loss of structure when the temperature is increased very slightly

sample, was not clear. This example illustrates the point that combining crystalline and amorphous components does not always give a single critical temperature that can be predicted from the behavior of the individual components, and that exceeding a particular ratio could lead to step changes in critical temperature with respect to the macroscopic structure due to phase/state changes in one or more of the components, which may also be a function of thermal history. Similar observations were made by Adams and Irons [1] for mixtures of sodium chloride and lactose.

Conceivably, in mixtures where the collapse temperature of the amorphous phase is higher than the eutectic temperature of the separate but coexistent crystalline phase could lead to an analogous phenomenon that we have notionally termed "micromelting" [39], where a crystalline formulation component (or combination of such components) with a low eutectic temperature melts onto the "backbone" of a rigid amorphous phase within the material. An example of this that has been observed in our laboratories is that of a biological product containing a small amount of calcium chloride as part of a buffer system; in this case, while macroscopic collapse was not observed until temperatures above −30 °C (by FDM, unpublished data), the use of other methods suggested significant mobility changes around −53 °C, the eutectic temperature of calcium chloride. When the formulation was freeze-dried above −53 °C, no shrinkage was observed at the macroscopic level, although there was evidence of heterogeneity in the form of small visible "spots" on the base of the cake.

2.3.3 Eutectic Melting

For samples that are largely or wholly crystalline, the eutectic melting temperature will be the critical temperature above which defects will occur in lyophilization. This phenomenon can be easily identified using a number of analytical methods, including FDM. Figure 5 shows a sample of sodium chloride solution drying below and above its eutectic temperature, illustrating the fact that the eutectic temperature can be identified very clearly using FDM, due to the marked visible change in sample appearance that occurs at Teu. This includes the previously frozen part of the sample appearing visibly as a "partial liquid" and also the contraction of this part of the sample which then recedes away from the previously dried material.

2.3.4 The Effect of Annealing

The technique of annealing (also called heat-annealing or tempering) as part of the thermal treatment segment of a lyophilization cycle has been well established as a means of influencing the ice structure and/or encouraging crystallization—or polymorphic changes—in solutes. It is outside the remit of this chapter to discuss the physicochemical theory and basic principles of the processes occurring in annealing, which have been covered previously in

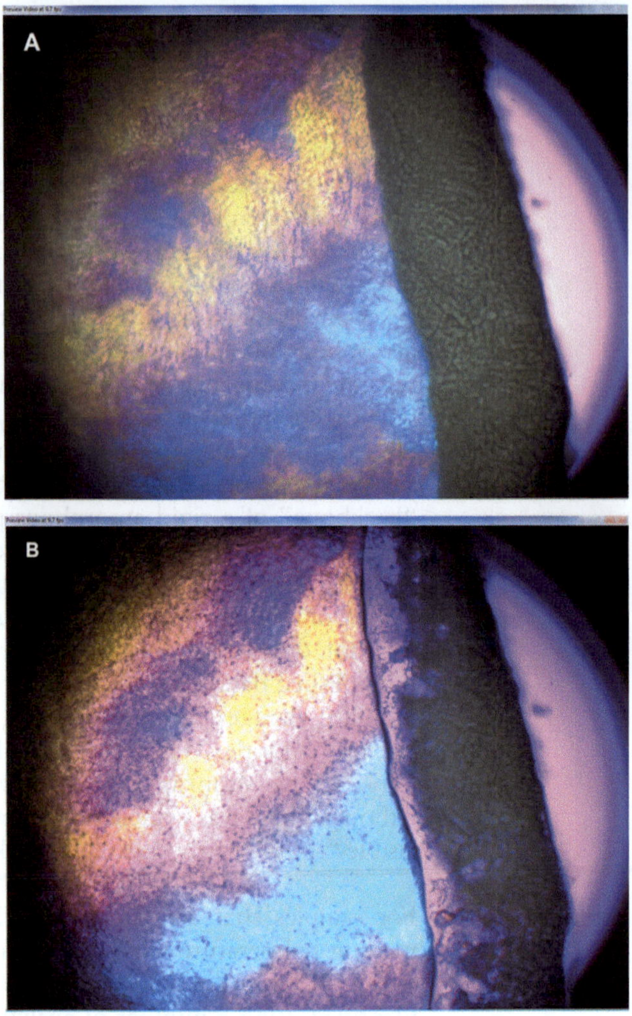

Fig. 5 FDM images showing a frozen solution of sodium chloride drying (**A**) below and (**B**) slightly above its eutectic temperature

other texts, but to highlight the information regarding the practical effects of the annealing process that can be observed for real formulations using FDM.

Figure 6 shows the visual effect of annealing a sample of frozen formulation (initially frozen to −40 °C) at −10 °C for 10 min. While in this example it is not possible to quantify the extent and speed of ice crystal growth, FDM experiments employing different conditions (temperatures and holding times) can be carried out and the relative differences established, in order to direct the user toward the selection of the most suitable or effective annealing conditions in a real lyophilization scenario.

Figure 7 illustrates the fact that following the initial nucleation and ice crystal growth phase, it is not necessarily possible to

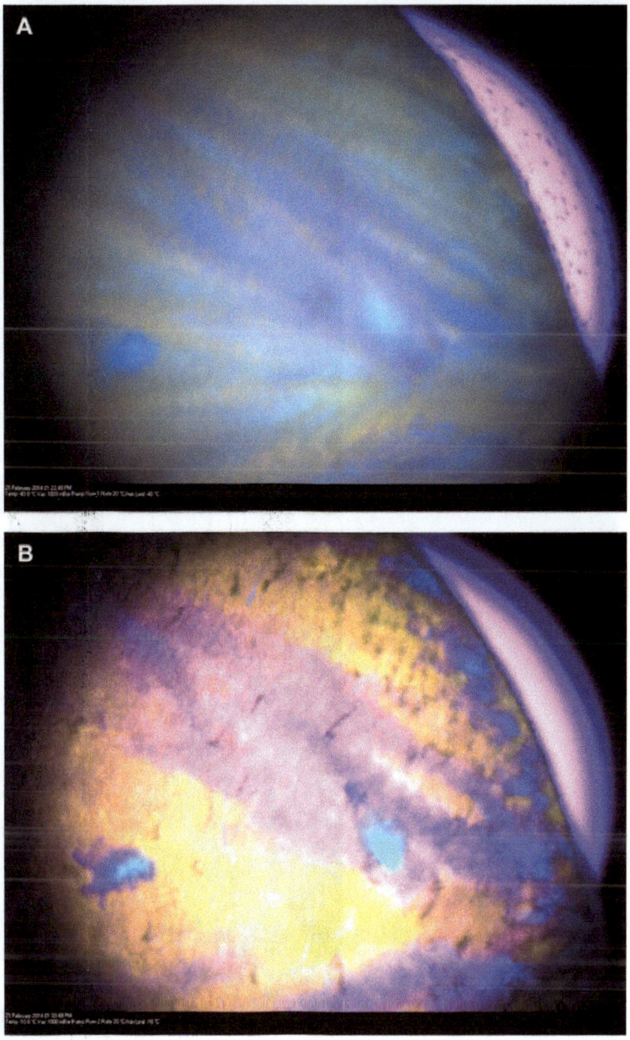

Fig. 6 FDM images of a frozen sample immediately prior to (**A**) and after 10 min of (**B**) annealing at $-10\ ^{\circ}C$, depicting the visible change in appearance, related to increasing ice crystal size and networking. Light level and focus remained unchanged during this time

determine whether the solute has crystallized, but that upon holding the sample for an extended period, solute crystallization may be confirmed by the observation of a second freezing event—in this case, the appearance of a "crystallization front" that sweeps through the amorphous solute. A similar effect may be observed more quickly by the use of annealing, with the general rule of thumb that this is accelerated considerably when the amorphous material is held above its characteristic glass transition temperature (Tg′), which may be identified using thermal methods as discussed in other sections of this chapter.

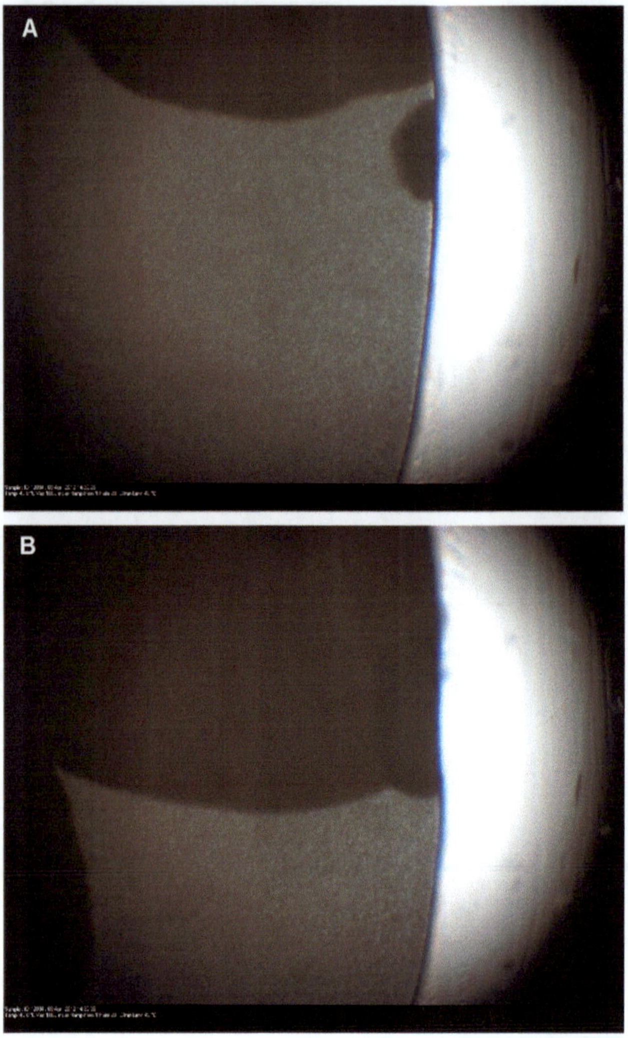

Fig. 7 Extended holding of a sample at −40 °C eventually leads to the appearance of a crystallization front (**A**) which then moves slowly through the frozen amorphous material (**B**)

2.3.5 Formulations Containing Organic Solvents

There are many drug products on the market that are freeze-dried from organic solvents or co-solvent mixtures (usually mixtures of water + an organic solvent). The lyophilization of such formulations brings its own challenges, not least in achieving complete freezing and avoiding phase separation, the control of the sublimation process and establishing whether the co-solvents behave as azeotropic or zeotropic mixtures, residual solvent levels allowable in the final product, and the safety and environmental issues of handling, condensing, and reclaiming the organic solvents themselves. A comprehensive review of such challenges was provided by Teagarden et al. [36] and it is not the intention of this chapter to reiterate these points here, but again to highlight how the use of

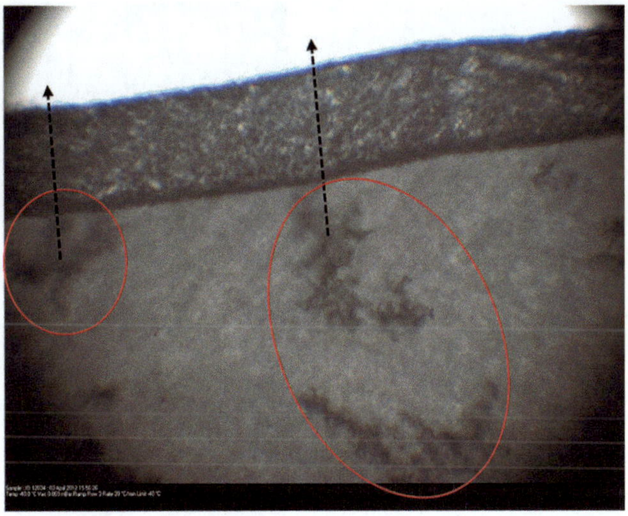

Fig. 8 FDM image of a co-solvent-based formulation following freezing and the application of vacuum, showing evidence of egress of the (more volatile) organic solvent from certain areas (examples highlighted by red circles, with direction of solvent vapor movement indicated by dashed arrows)

FDM can provide information as to the practical aspects of freeze-drying a formulation containing multiple solvents. Figure 8 shows a sample undergoing sublimation during FDM analysis where the organic solvent is visibly being removed via its own network of channels, while the frozen aqueous component dries from the edge of the sample in the same way as if it were a purely aqueous-based sample. This observation suggests that phase separation of the two solvents has taken place, which may indicate that there may be an opportunity to remove the two solvents sequentially (especially if the vapor pressures are sufficiently different), although care should be taken if the solutes have partitioned into the different solvent phases, as this may lead to microcollapse or micromelting within the structure.

2.3.6 Formulations Susceptible to Skin/Crust Formation

It has been noted that certain formulations are particularly susceptible to forming a surface skin (crust) on freezing, which will subsequently impede the sublimation process or even prevent drying altogether. Since none of the traditional thermal methods is able to pick up on the potential for this phenomenon to occur, it is rarely noticed until post-lyophilization inspection of the product appearance. However, FDM can sometimes highlight such behavior, as was the case for the sample shown in Fig. 9. Samples exhibiting a particular propensity to form a skin or crust tend to be dilute solutions, where ostensibly the viscosity of the liquid formulation at the moment of ice nucleation is very low and consequently, the physical action of ice crystal growth results in the solute

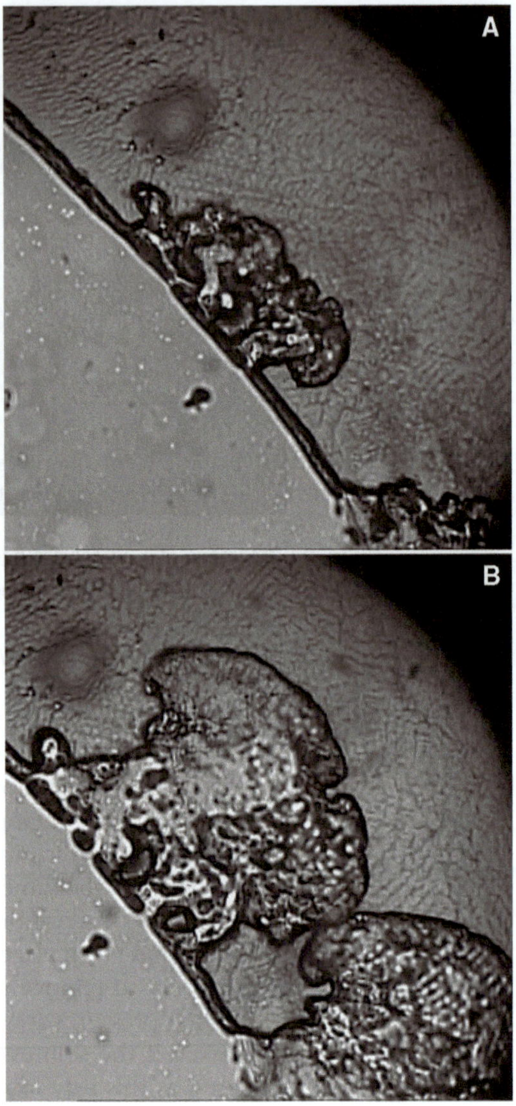

Fig. 9 Example of skin (crust) formation during freezing, resulting in a dense concentrated wall of solute at the edge of the sample and reluctance to dry until the skin ruptures (**A**), whereupon the action of sublimation results in further breakup of the skin, allowing drying to progress more quickly but with an uneven sublimation front (**B**)

being forced to the edge (or surface) of the liquid as it solidifies. This phenomenon can also be commonly observed when freezing solutions containing particular proportions of certain salts and sugars, such as a solution of 1% lactose + 1% sodium chloride. Skin or crust formation can sometimes be avoided by altering the total solute concentration, varying the proportions of components or using a controlled nucleation method to instigate "top down" freezing (as discussed in Chaps. 3 and 4 of this volume). If the phenomenon cannot be avoided altogether, then it may be possible to increase the porosity in the skin or crust by including an annealing step, if indeed annealing is compatible with the formulation in question. Alternatively, heterogeneity may be reduced by using rapid initial cooling during the freezing process, which although is likely to give smaller ice crystals and thus increased product resistance (Rp) to vapor flow, the value of Rp may still be lower in this case than the equivalent value in the presence of the skin or crust.

2.3.7 Formulations Containing Glycerol

One of the more recent challenges we have faced is in the lyophilization of formulations that contain glycerol, such as with some PCR (polymerase chain reaction) reagents. The PCR-based method of detection in In Vitro Diagnostics (IVDs) is becoming the method of choice in many applications compared with enzyme- or antibody-based detection systems. Historically, the standard storage conditions for PCR reagents have been at low temperatures (often −80 °C) but typically after the addition of glycerol to act as somewhat of an "antifreeze," thus arguably reducing the risks associated with the process of freeze-concentration, but at the same time, minimizing degradation rates by the use of low temperatures, as defined by Arrhenius kinetics. Naturally, any antifreeze effect gives such formulations an obvious lack of compatibility with the lyophilization process! We have observed this to be possible in some cases in our laboratories when the glycerol content is sufficiently low (typically less than 0.2% but also depends on the proportion of glycerol to other components). However, what often happens is that even when ice is able to form, the glycerol remains unfrozen and becomes forced toward the edges of the sample, as shown in the FDM images in Fig. 10. In the classical lyophilization situation where ice tends to form at the base of a solution (or suspension), this would translate to the glycerol being pushed to the surface of the frozen mass, where it will persist as an "oily" liquid that obstructs the sublimation process. Controlled nucleation systems may offer an opportunity to circumvent this issue, but the evidence for this remains yet to be seen.

2.3.8 Reducing Subjectivity in FDM Experiments: The Use of TASC

While operators can gain experience and confidence quite rapidly with modern FDM systems, there is still the desire to have a means of independent verification of collapse events in order to minimize subjectivity as far as is possible in such a patently optical method; it was this need for reduced levels of subjectivity that has led to the development of TASC—Thermal Analysis by Structural Characterization.

TASC works by analyzing a sequence of images and tracking the changes from one to another. First, the operator selects the range of the analytical run and clicks on the TASC option, as shown in Fig. 11.

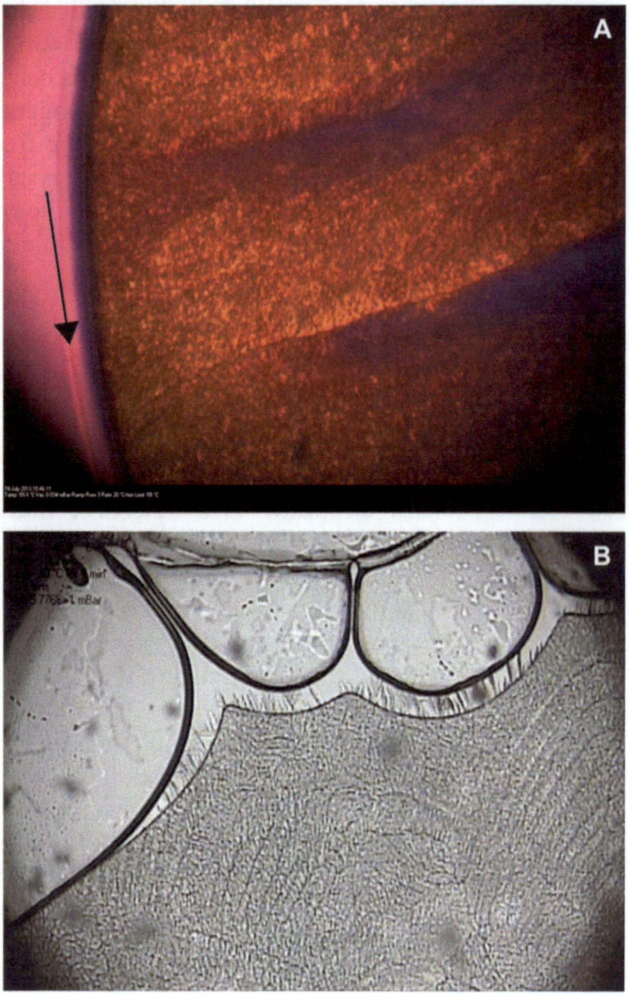

Fig. 10 Evidence of an excluded layer of glycerol on the edges of frozen samples, preventing drying from occurring in both cases. In (**A**), the liquid is indicated by the arrow, while in (**B**) the liquid layer is more obviously visible, with further evidence of ice or solute crystal growth extending into the glycerol layer

Second, a "region of interest" is selected (shown in red in Fig. 12). This area will be the part that is tracked and covers the sublimation front and the material to be dried ahead of it. Third, the "region to be scanned" is selected (shown in blue in Fig. 12). Scan size should be kept relatively small to minimize processing time, but TASC analysis typically takes less than 5 min.

The output of the analysis is a graphical plot, as shown in Fig. 13, which illustrates how the images at each TASC transition can be viewed by clicking on the associated image (1) to see how they are relevant. The two points of interest, in this case, are where the gradient of the line changes (2) and the maximum (3). Images during this analysis were captured every 5 s at a heating rate of

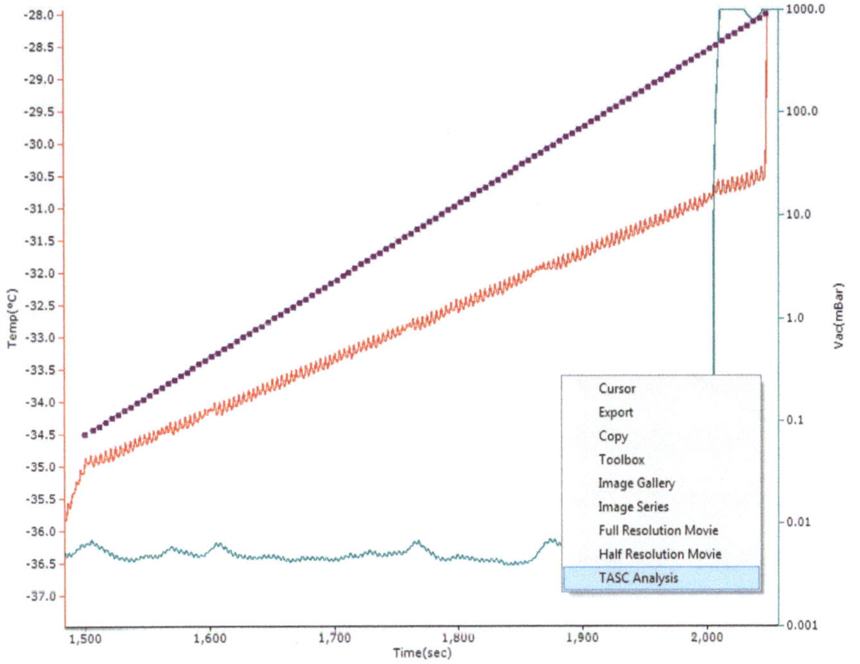

Fig. 11 Selection of TASC Analysis option for a section of an analytical run

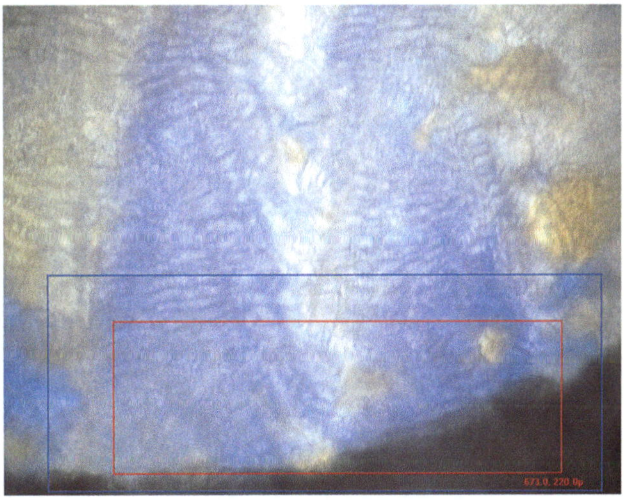

Fig. 12 Selection of areas within FDM image for TASC analysis

0.5 °C min^{-1} (2.4 images every 0.1 °C), which typically allows for a small margin of error (±0.1 °C sensitivity). Figure 14 depicts the images that coincide with these two points of interest on the TASC graph.

In order to assess the user-friendliness of TASC and to establish whether it would provide Tc (onset) values that are representative of those determined by experienced FDM operators, a "subjectivity

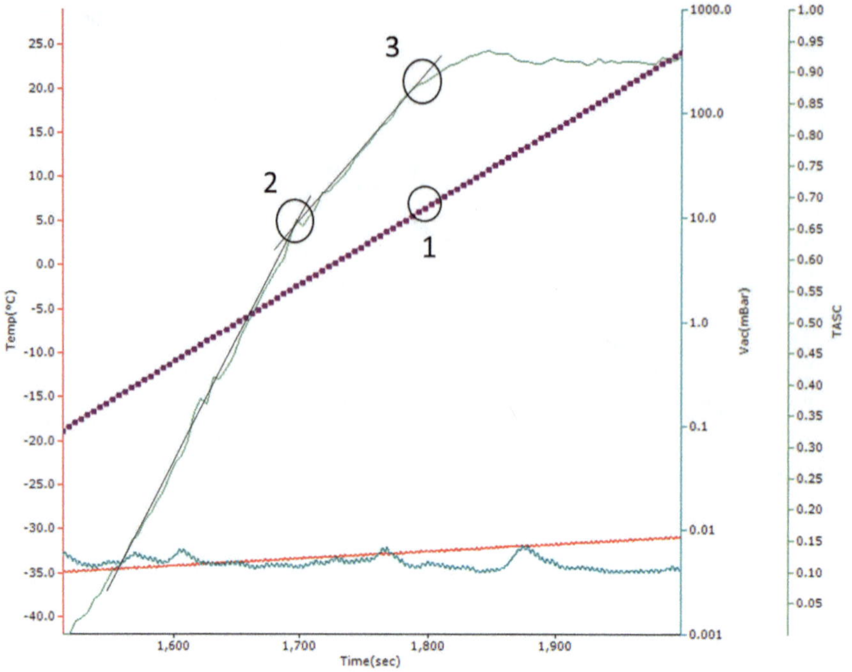

Fig. 13 Graphical plot output from TASC analysis

experiment" was conducted in our laboratories where four experienced operators were given a series of FDM images (typically taken at 5 s intervals during analysis) and asked to determine which image in the series contained the first sign of evidence of a visible microscopic defect such as collapse or eutectic melting. This was carried out for four different samples, each of which had been analyzed in duplicate; therefore, each operator viewed eight analytical runs in all. Each series of images was then subjected to similar analysis by TASC, which would determine the onset of collapse or eutectic melting via optical analysis. The results of the subjectivity experiment are shown in Table 1.

It can be seen from the data in Table 1 that the differences between mean values determined by the average experienced operator and mean values determined by TASC were similar for each sample, and no statistical difference was detected between operators ($p = 0.749$).

2.4 Variations on FDM

Two of the criticisms often leveled at conventional FDM are that (1) it is a somewhat subjective method of analysis, requiring expertise in image interpretation, and (2) the behavior of such a small sample is surely not representative of what would happen in a real lyophilizer. It is perhaps easy to see why these criticisms might be perceived to be legitimate, but in fact, it could be argued that they are largely academic, particularly when compared to the other

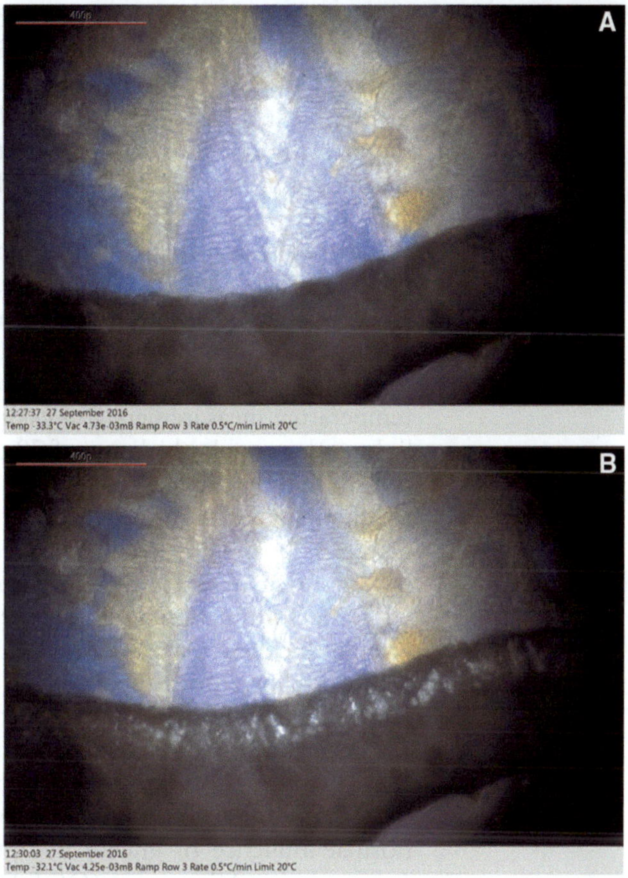

Fig. 14 Images identified by TASC as coinciding with (**A**) the onset of collapse of sucrose at −33.3 °C, and (**B**) full collapse occurring at −32.1 °C

Table 1
Results of subjectivity experiment comparing trained operator interpretation of critical temperatures for four reference solutions to that of the TASC result

Sample	Operator interpretation of onset temperature (°C)	TASC interpretation of onset temperature (°C)	Difference (°C)
Dextran 10 kDa	−9.06 (±0.13)	−9.05 (±0.15)	0.01
Sodium chloride	−21.60 (±0.19)	−21.50 (±0.10)	0.10
Sucrose	−33.54 (±0.53)	−33.80 (±0.20)	0.26
Calcium chloride	−53.34 (±0.11)	−53.10 (±0.30)	0.24

Individual results were determined to the nearest 0.1 °C in duplicate by four operators. Mean and standard deviation values are expressed to nearest 0.01 °C for illustrative purposes only methods available. First, all methods require some degree of data interpretation, and even if this is by instrument software (for example, in identification of small glass transitions in DSC, or the region of interest in FDM for TASC, as illustrated above), this typically requires the operator to first select the region of interest in the thermogram. Second, right from the first designs by MacKenzie and Rey who built their own systems, up to present day commercially-available systems (such as the Lyostat5 FDM, Biopharma Process Systems, Winchester, UK), FDM has deliberately employed thin sections of sample sandwiched between cover slips, in order to maximize the opportunity to observe detail and minimize the effect of sublimation cooling for accuracy of sample temperature measurement (for example, Lyostat5 uses transmitted light and a sample thickness of 70 μm). While this setup is clearly not the same as in a real product container, it is specifically designed to eliminate as many extraneous (formulation-unrelated) parameters as possible, such as the effects of radiative and convective heat transfer, in order that the intrinsic critical events associated with the formulation itself can be identified. Having a defined sample thickness that is the same from experiment to experiment can also allow the comparison of other parameters such as the relative speed of drying, as demonstrated by Zhai et al. [41].

A relatively recent development that has been made to offer greater information about the collapse event itself, and the dynamics of viscous flow in the container (vial) of interest while under the normal influence of gravity is Optical Coherence Tomography-Freeze-drying Microscopy (OCT-FDM), as has been described by Mujat et al. [27]. OCT is used in order to create a 3D image of the sample in real time, which provides an understanding of the ice network and any physical changes in morphology of the material during the lyophilization process. Sample temperature is typically monitored in the base of the vial, which means the sublimation interface temperature is not being measured directly, but the premise is that there is a built-in "safety margin" as the sublimation interface temperature will always be cooler than the base temperature being measured, and that the temperature difference between the two may actually be quite representative of the situation in a real lyophilizer. Here, it might be helpful for clarity to use the same terminology as in the SMART® software from SP Scientific (Gardiner, NY, USA), which refers to Tb as the product temperature measured at the base of the (inside of the) vial and Tp as the temperature of the sublimation interface. For amorphous products, it could be argued that Tb is largely irrelevant, as it is only the sublimation interface where collapse will occur at any point during the lyophilization process, since the base of the sample is not exposed to vacuum until the end of primary drying; in contrast, for a crystalline product, Tb is relevant because when the eutectic melting temperature is reached, the solute melt event will take place

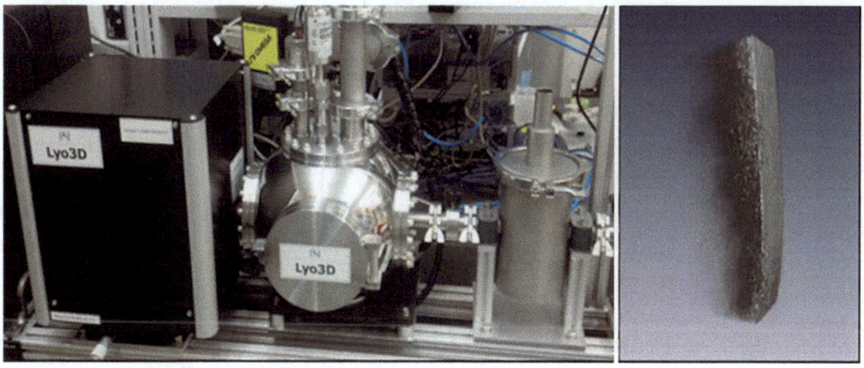

Fig. 15 OCT-FDM by Physical Sciences Inc. (Andover, MA, USA) showing prototype instrument (left) and 3D image generated for a section of freeze-dried material (right)

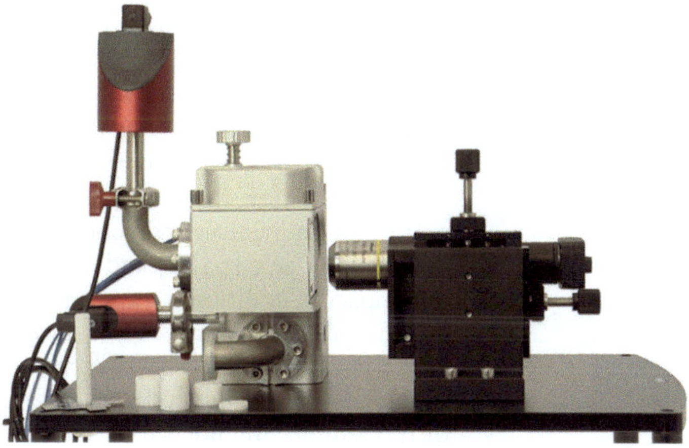

Fig. 16 Freeze-Drying Vial System (FDVS) by Linkam Scientific (Tadworth, UK)

throughout the entire frozen phase, exposing a network of eutectic liquid to the vacuum, whereupon it is likely to boil. Figure 15 shows a prototype OCT-FDM instrument and an example of a 3D image generated for a lyophilized material.

Related to OCT-FDM but using light in the visible spectrum to observe the entire height of a sample drying in a vial in real time is the Freeze-Drying Vial System (FDVS) developed by Linkam Scientific (Tadworth, UK), as shown in Fig. 16. Freeze-drying takes place in an insulated chamber containing a temperature-controlled shelf that can accommodate at least seven DIN2R vials. Time-lapse photography is used to construct a video file that shows the change in sample morphology as sublimation proceeds in one of the vials, while a number of miniaturized thermometers can be placed in either one vial at different depths, or indeed in a number of different vials in various locations on the shelf, in order to gain an understanding of "edge effects" within the chamber while running a realistic lyophilization cycle with pressure control.

2.5 Differential Scanning Calorimetry (DSC)

Differential scanning calorimetry is widely used in pharmaceutical analysis and much has been published on its utility in characterizing amorphous and crystalline states in frozen liquid and solid samples [9, 10]. Its application in the analysis of formulations destined for freeze-drying has been reviewed by Kett et al. [17] and also by Meister and Gieseler [25].

DSC is a thermal method whereby the enthalpic changes in a sample are determined by measuring the differential heat required to increase the temperature of a panned sample compared to an empty reference pan. It was introduced to chemistry in the early 1960s and is widely used in pharmaceutical analysis and in materials science. However, in modulated DSC (mDSC), a sinusoidal modulation (oscillation) is overlaid on the conventional linear heating ramp to enable weak energetic events (such as the glass transition of an amorphous material) to be resolved.

Modulated DSC is well suited to subambient thermal analysis such as that applicable to defining the properties of solutions for lyophilization. DSC has also been used to study the vitrification of water and cryopreserving solutions so has found a place in low temperature biology [3]. In the 1990s, Hatley and Franks advocated the use of DSC in freeze-drying formulation analysis [13].

Tables listing the glass transition and eutectic crystallization points for individual excipients used in freeze-drying have been published widely [5, 37] and although these are useful to predict the impact of additions to a complex formulation of a "real world" product (either pharmaceutical, biopharmaceutical, or diagnostic), they will not give the relevant temperature from which to derive a suitable freeze-drying cycle. Therefore, some experimental analysis of the samples intended for freeze-drying must be undertaken. A useful illustrative example is given in Fig. 17.

DSC even without modulation or hyper scan rates can readily detect the critical temperatures of some freeze-drying excipients, especially when these are tested at high concentrations. However, when present at the (typically much lower) formulation-defined concentrations, and especially when present in combination, such transitions may be much less readily detected by DSC and so analysis by mDSC especially can be very helpful (see Fig. 18). Often by zooming into weak events such as Tg′, these developments can allow critical temperatures to be detected.

2.5.1 DSC of Complex Formulations

Where complex formulations are analyzed, crystallization/eutectic events are energetically large and are easily seen, but weaker (yet often more relevant) glass transition events may be more difficult to separate out, especially where they occur on the edge of a strong eutectic, or for instance the ice melt endotherm, which can conceal Tg′ for polymer components such as proteins, at values of −10 °C or higher. Figure 19 illustrates how multiple thermal events can be revealed in a single warming run.

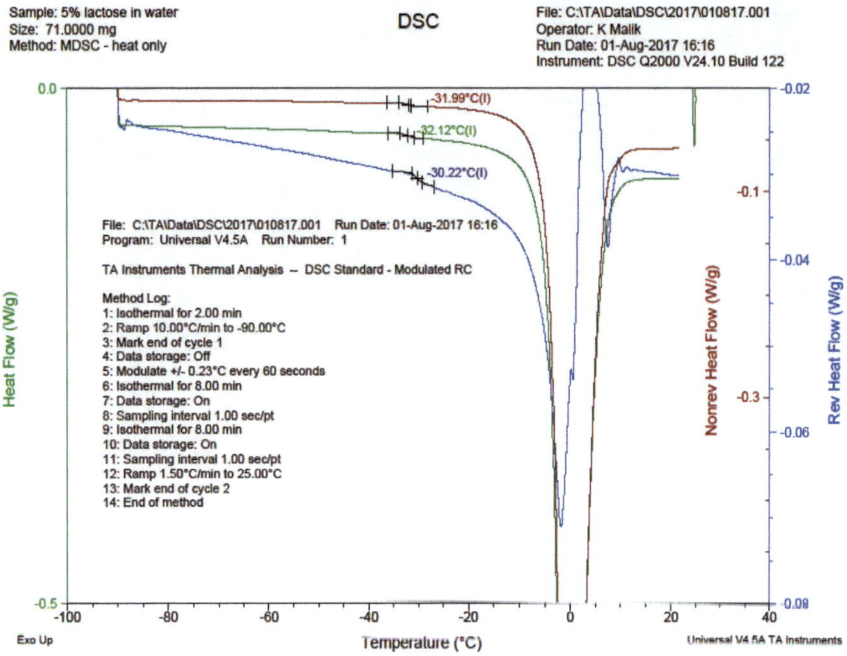

Fig. 17 DSC of typical excipient—5% lactose in water, showing Tg′ in range −30 to −32 °C

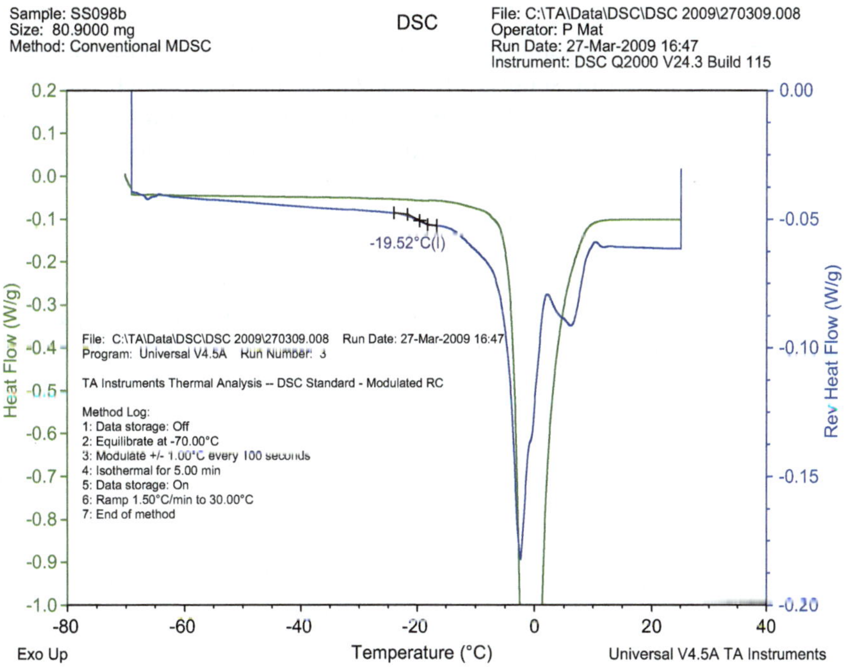

Fig. 18 Reversing heat profile showing a Tg′ (blue line) whereas total heat flow (green line) did not reveal such a transition

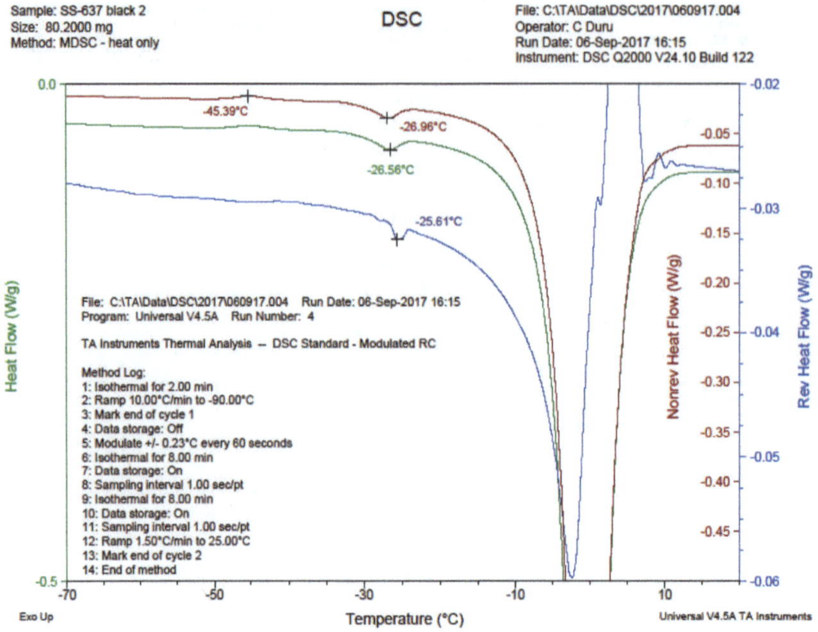

Fig. 19 Complex biologic formulation showing predominantly an eutectic melt (endotherm) at −25 °C and a weak exothermic event at −45 °C

2.5.2 Crystallization Events

The crystallization of some excipients is by no means certain during freezing stages of lyophilization and where such crystallization has not occurred (as for instance with mannitol) then spontaneous crystallization in the dry state can be deleterious [24].

In such cases thermal tempering or annealing added into the freezing protocol can induce solute crystallization. This leads to the question of what temperature is required for annealing for crystallization to occur. DSC can provide a convenient way of determining a suitable annealing temperature in such instances, as illustrated in Fig. 20 where (in Fig. 20A) the thermogram of a non-annealed solution of mannitol exhibits a detectable crystallization exotherm, whereas analysis of the same sample when an annealing cycle is included in the freezing stage of the cycle (Fig. 20B) shows no such crystallization because the material has already crystallized during the annealing step.

2.5.3 Interaction Between Excipients

Given general recommendations that high levels of salts should be avoided, where such salts have to be included they may actually contribute to the structure of the lyophilized cake. For instance, Duru et al. [8] showed that crystallization of isotonic sodium chloride in a formulation resulted in well-formed cakes, but that doubling the content of amorphous stabilizers such as sucrose or trehalose in the formulation led to the inhibition of such crystallization (as revealed by DSC), and a marked deterioration in the

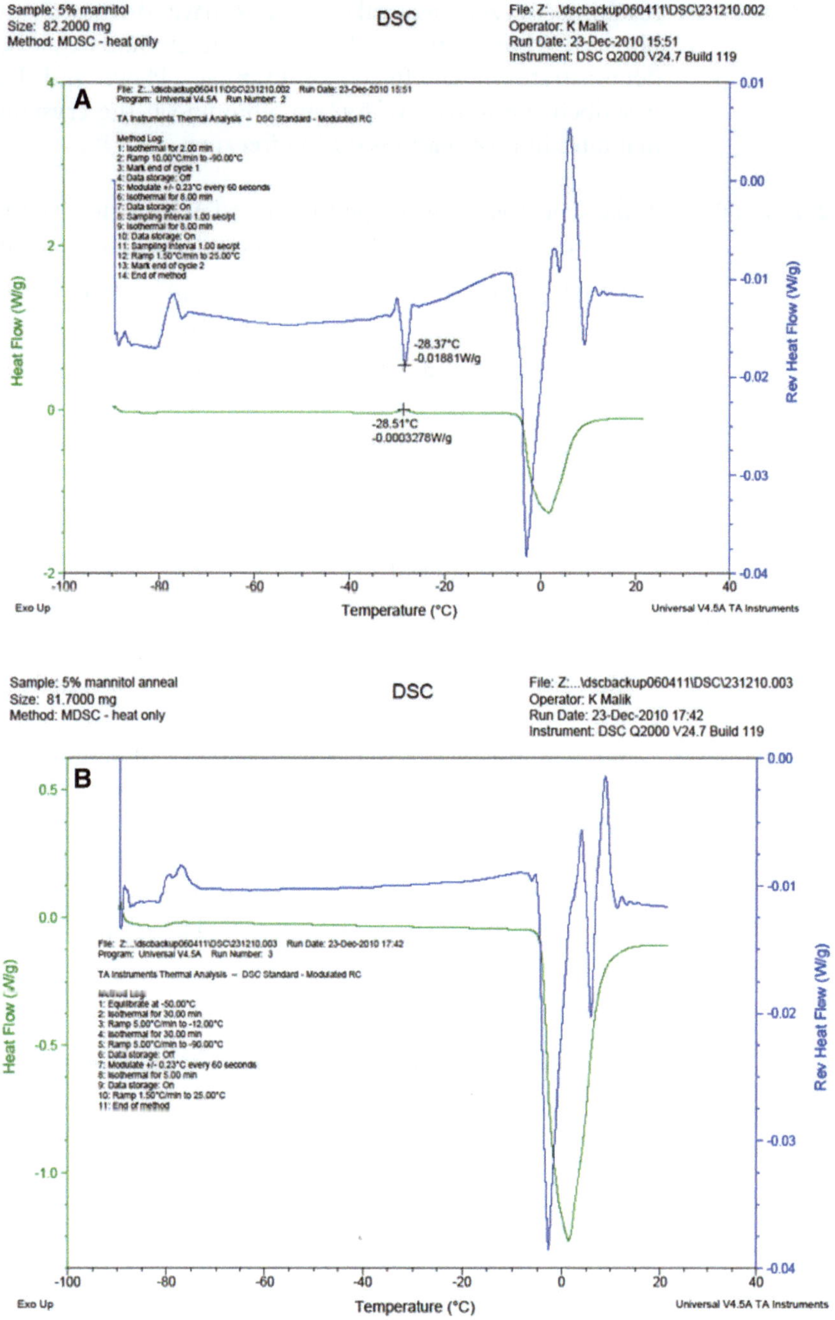

Fig. 20 (**A**) Mannitol solution frozen and warmed without annealing step—crystallization of amorphous mannitol occurs. (**B**) Mannitol solution, frozen and then annealed at −12 °C, re-cooled and warmed no crystallization event as mannitol already crystallized during annealing

resulting freeze-dried cake. Others have discussed interactions between formulants and how thermal methods can be used to demonstrate these effects for example. Hawe and Friess [14] described the impact of human albumin on the crystallization of mannitol in formulations during freezing.

2.5.4 Sub-ambient DSC Protocol

Typical protocol (developed for the TA Instruments Q2000 but could be adapted to work on any modulated DSC instrument)

- Weigh an empty DSC pan and lid to sub-milligram accuracy.
- Carefully pipette a small aliquot (30–80 μL) of the liquid sample into an appropriate DSC pan avoiding the introduction of air bubbles.
- Crimp the pan with a suitable lid. Prepare an identical empty pan.
- Place the sample and reference pans into the calorimeter.
- Freeze the samples to at least −50 °C or ideally lower using a rapid freezing rate (e.g., 5–10 °C min^{-1}).
- Start data capture.
- Run an isothermal step to allow the heat flow signal to stabilize.
- Set up a slow heating rate 1–5 °C min^{-1} (the thermal events will be determined in the heating profile) and apply a modulation (heating oscillation) pattern such that 3–6 full cycles are obtained across a weak thermal event such as a Tg. Typically, a heating rate of 3 °C min^{-1} and a modulation of 1 °C min^{-1} has been a good starting point in our experience.
- Heat the sample back to ambient (25 °C) and then stop data capture.
- Analyze the resultant profile using the manufacturer's software.

Samples should be analyzed at least in duplicate and the system should be suitably calibrated (indium with a melt of 156.6 °C is routinely used for DSC calibration but chemicals with a low temperature thermal event may also be used [29]).

2.5.5 Dry State DSC

DSC also has applicability not only in sub-ambient glass transition determination but also in the measurement of thermal events occurring in the dry state. In lyophilized samples, the glass transition value of a formulation can correlate to storage stability [6] and therefore DSC is a useful tool in screening different formulations. However, Tg will be affected by residual water content, with a higher residual moisture content resulting in a lower Tg for the same formulation (see Fig. 21), and as such, dry state DSC is also a good indicator of what constitutes an acceptably low residual moisture content for a particular product.

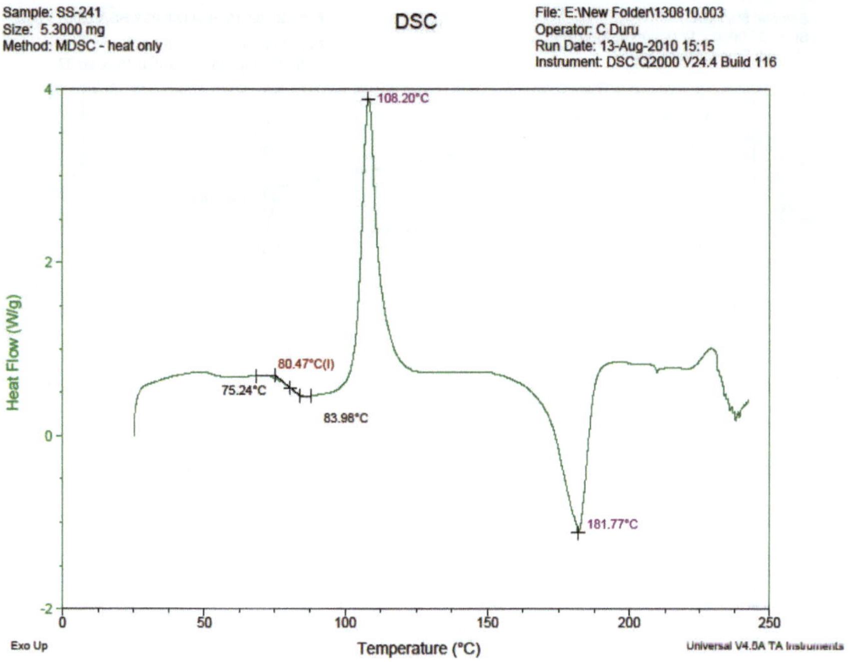

Fig. 21 Thermogram of lyophilized sucrose sample showing Tg (80.5 °C), crystallization (108 °C), and decomposition (182 °C)

It is critical to pan such lyophilized powders in a dry environment as otherwise atmospheric water vapor will be taken up by the sample. A good option would be use of a dry box or dry bag (e.g., Cole Parmer, St Neots, UK) set up with a relative humidity below 10% RH. Material should then be packed into a DSC pan using a spatula and a suitable lid crimped on before the pan is removed from the controlled environment.

Dry state DSC analysis can also enable detection of the crystallization of metastable formulants such as mannitol [40] and possible thermal decomposition [2] using much higher scan speeds than in conventional DSC.

2.6 Dynamic Mechanical Analysis

Dynamic mechanical analysis (DMA) is a rheological technique, which assesses the strain response of a material to stress force applied to a sample and so is ideally suited to measuring the forces that may be critical when considering the structural stability and hence susceptibility to collapse in a freeze-dried cake. The sensitivity for detecting a glass transition is also far higher for DMA than for DSC and so it is a valuable alternative technology when characterizing the critical temperatures for freeze-drying.

The principles of DMA for detecting Tg have been well described (see, for instance, the chapter by Duncan [7]). The use of DMA in determining Tg in food materials is perhaps more widely used than in pharmaceutical applications. However, the

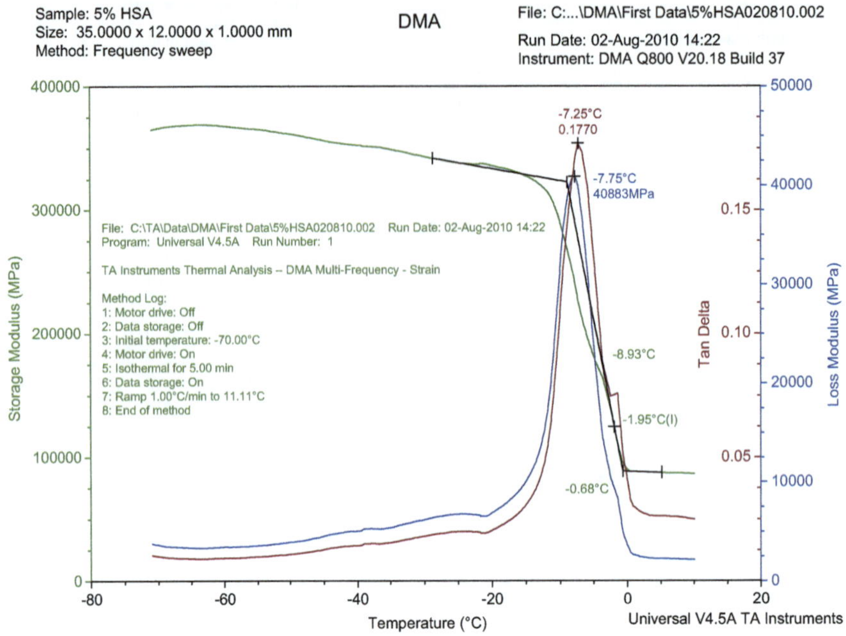

Fig. 22 DMA of 5% human serum albumin showing a clear Tg′ with Tan delta value of −7.3 °C

application to pharmaceutical challenges has been reported [15] and also its use in freeze-drying situations [11]. Samples of liquid can be applied in a steel tray or folded thin steel pocket, dependent upon the DMA system used, and multiple frequency stressing studies carried out. Dry state Tg determinations are also possible [35] and indeed the use of a steel mesh permits the impact of increasing relative humidity on the Tg of dried materials to be determined.

Values quoted for Tg derived by DMA can often be deemed to be higher than for DSC [11]; however, this question has been addressed in a number of publications [12, 34] and similar values can be derived where frequency is expressed at 1 Hz or when Tonset is considered as well as Tan delta for the start of the thermal event. Figure 22 shows the Tg′ event for a 5% human serum albumin (HSA) solution, which would be completely unresolved by conventional mDSC.

One drawback is that automation of DMA is not practical due to the nature of the sample application method, resulting in quite a user-intensive method. However, the combination of controlled variable relative humidity and the loading format with a steel mesh sample holder allows analysis of the change of Tg with changing environmental conditions (Fig. 23).

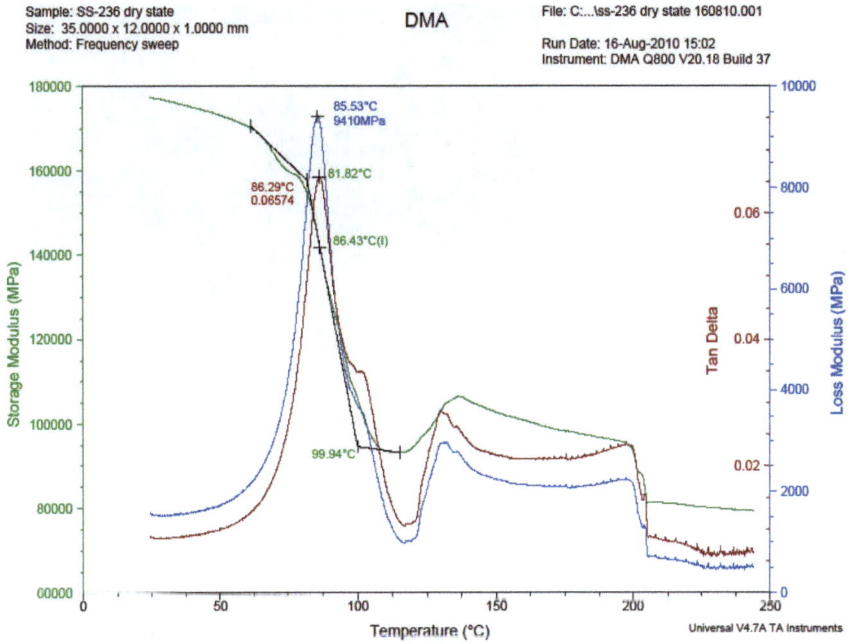

Fig. 23 Dry state DMA analysis—freeze-dried sucrose with Tg of 86 °C (analysis performed at 0% RH)

3 New Developments

One recent development in the characterization of freeze-dried materials is the advent of Optical DSC, which combines DSC with optical microscopy. Here, a similar optical setup is employed as in FDM (described in the sections above) but instead of the analysis being carried out using transmitted light (i.e., the light passes through the sample), Optical DSC is performed in reflected light mode, with an additional light source fitted to the imaging station in the form of an LED light ring surrounding the objective lens, as shown in Fig. 24. The system employs the same control modules as the FDM described above, meaning that it can offer a relatively low-cost DSC option for laboratories that currently have an FDM system. It also shares the same software, which means that TASC can be employed for identification of visible changes in the sample that can then be assigned to the endothermic or exothermic events appearing on the DSC thermogram.

4 Conclusions

We have reviewed the common thermal and optical methods used to establish the critical processing temperatures for solutions to be subjected to freeze-drying and for the analysis of the glass transition values of the dry state lyophilized materials. The use of these

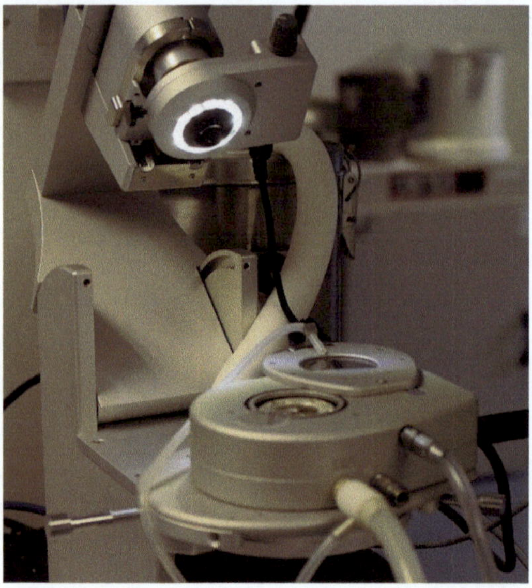

Fig. 24 Optical DSC stage showing light collar assembly around the objective lens on the purpose-built Imaging Station, for use in reflected light mode

techniques has transformed the development process for freeze-drying from largely empirical trial and error to a rapid developmental analytical stage leading to fewer freeze-drying runs with a high degree of confidence of a successful outcome. The emerging technologies highlighted above are also likely to increase the degree of confidence further.

More recently, we have seen progression for some of these methods from the bench to technologies which can be incorporated into the freeze-dryer to deliver in-line real-time analysis and ultimately influence process control [28].

Acknowledgments

We thank Kiran Malik and Chinwe Duru (NIBSC) for performing many of the thermal analyses included in the figures, Thomas Codd (BPS) for compiling many of the FDM and TASC images, and Jason Hockley (Biostatistician at NIBSC) for statistical analysis of the raw data from the TASC subjectivity study.

References

1. Adams GDJ, Irons LI (1993) Some implications of structural collapse during freeze-drying using *Erwinia caratovora* l-asparaginase as a model. J Chem Technol Biotechnol 58:71–76
2. Te Booy MPWM, de Ruiter RA, de Meere ALJ (1992) Evaluation of the physical stability of freeze-dried sucrose-containing formulations by differential scanning calorimetry. Pharm Res 9(1):109–114

3. Bryant G (1995) DSC measurement of cell suspensions during successive freezing runs: implications for the mechanisms of intracellular ice formation. Cryobiology 32(2):114–128
4. Cabasso VJ, Regamy RH (eds) (1977) Freeze drying of biological products. Developments in biologicals, vol 34. Karger, Basel
5. Costantino H (2004) Thermal analysis of lyophilized pharmaceutical peptide and protein formulations. In: Costantino H, Pikal MJ (eds) Lyophilization of biopharmaceuticals. AAPS Press, Arlington VA, pp 271–235
6. Duddu SP, Dal Monte PR (1997) Effect of glass transition temperature on the stability of lyophilized formulations containing a chimeric therapeutic monoclonal antibody. Pharm Res 14(5):591–595
7. Duncan J (2008) Principles and applications of thermal mechanical analysis. In: Gabbott P (ed) Principles and applications of thermal analysis. Blackwell, Oxford, pp 119–163
8. Duru C, Swann C, Dunleavy U, Mulloy B, Matejtschuk P (2015) The importance of formulation in the successful lyophilization of influenza reference materials. Biologicals 43 (2):110–116
9. Gaisford S, Kett V, Haines P (eds) (2016) Principles of thermal analysis and calorimetry, 2nd edn. Royal Society of Chemistry, Cambridge
10. Gatlin L, De Luca PP (1980) A study of the phase transitions in frozen antibiotic solutions by differential scanning calorimetry. J Parenter Drug Assoc 34(5):398–408
11. Gearing J, Malik KP, Matejtschuk P (2010) Use of dynamic mechanical analysis (DMA) to determine critical transition temperatures in frozen biomaterials intended for lyophilization. Cryobiology 61(1):27–32
12. Garcia-Fernandez CA, Artiaga R (2010) Comparative study of the dynamic glass transition temperature by DMA and TMDSC. Polym Test 29(8):1002–1006
13. Hatley RHM, Franks F (1991) Applications of DSC in the development of improved freeze-drying processes for labile biologicals. J Thermal Anal 37(8):1905–1914
14. Hawe A, Friess W (2006) Physicochemical characterisation of freezing behaviour of mannitol Human Serum Albumin formulations. AAPS PharmSciTech 7(4):E85–E94
15. Jones DS (1999) Dynamic mechanical analysis of polymeric systems of pharmaceutical and biomedical significance. Int J Pharm 179 (2):167–178
16. Kasraian K, DeLuca PP (1995) Thermal analysis of the tertiary butyl alcohol-water system and its implications on freeze-drying. Pharm Res 12(4):484–490
17. Kett V, McMahon D, Ward K (2004) Freeze-drying of protein pharmaceuticals-the application of thermal analysis. Cryo Letters 25 (6):389–404
18. Lachman L, DeLuca PP, Withnell R (1965) Lyophilization of pharmaceuticals. II. High-sensitivity resistance bridge for low-conductivity measurements at eutectic temperatures. J Pharm Sci 54(9):1342–1347
19. Liu W, Wang DQ, Nail SL (2005) Freeze-drying of proteins from a sucrose-glycine excipient system: effect of formulation composition on the initial recovery of protein activity. AAPS Pharm Sci Tech 6(2):E150–E157
20. MacKenzie AP (1964) Apparatus for microscopic observations during freeze-drying (AFBR freeze-drying microscope model 2). Biodynamica 9:213–222
21. MacKenzie AP (1975) Collapse during freeze-drying: qualitative and quantitative aspects. In: Goldblith SA, Rothmayr WW (eds) Freeze-drying and advanced food technology. Academic Press, New York, NY
22. Matejtschuk P, Harrison P, More JE (1995) Dry heat treatment of intravenous immunoglobulin—some practical considerations. Vox Sang 68(4):255–256
23. May JC, Brown F (eds) (1992) Biological product freeze-drying and formulation. Developments in biologicals, vol 74. Karger, Basel
24. Mehta M, Bhardwaj SP, Suryanarayanan R (2013) Controlling the physical form of mannitol in freeze-dried systems. Eur J Pharm Biopharm 85(2):207–213
25. Meister E, Gieseler H (2009) Freeze-dry microscopy of protein/sugar mixtures: drying behavior, interpretation of collapse temperatures and a comparison to corresponding glass transition data. J Pharm Sci 98(9):3072–3087
26. Meister E, Sasić S, Gieseler H (2009) Freeze-dry microscopy: impact of nucleation temperature and excipient concentration on collapse temperature data. AAPS PharmSciTech 10 (2):582–588
27. Mujat M, Greco K, Galbally-Kinney K, Hammer DX, Ferguson RD, Iftimia N, Mulhall P, Sharma P, Pikal MJ, Kessler WJ (2012) Optical coherence tomography-based freeze drying microscopy. Biomed Opt Express 3(1):55–63
28. Nail S, Tchessalov S, Shalaev E, Ganguly A, Renzi E, Dimarco F, Wegiel L, Ferris S, Kessler W, Pikal M, Sacha G, Alexeenko A, Thompson TN, Reiter C, Searles J, Coiteux P (2017) Recommended best practices for process monitoring instrumentation in

pharmaceutical freeze drying—2017. AAPS PharmSciTech 18(7):2379–2393
29. Price DM (1995) Temperature calibration of differential scanning calorimeters. J Thermal Anal 45:1285–1296
30. Rey LR (1960) Thermal analysis of eutectics in freezing solutions. Ann N Y Acad Sci 85:513–234
31. Rey LR (1961) Automatic regulation of the freeze-drying of complex systems. Biodynamica 8:241–260
32. Rey LR (2004) Glimpses into the realm of freeze drying: fundamental issues. In: Rey L, May JC (eds) Freeze-drying/lyophilization of pharmaceutical and biological products, 2nd edn. Marcel Dekker, New York, NY, pp 1–32
33. Rey LR (2010) Glimpses into the realm of freeze drying: classical issues and new ventures. In: Rey L, May JC (eds) Freeze-drying/lyophilization of pharmaceutical and biological products, 3rd edn. Informa, New York, NY, pp 1–28
34. Rieger J (2001) The glass transition temperature Tg of polymers – comparison of values from differential thermal analysis (DTA, DSC) and dynamic mechanical measurements (torsion pendulum). Polym Test 20(2):199–204
35. Royall PG, Huang CY, Tang SW, Duncan J, Van-de-Velde G, Brown MB (2005) The development of DMA for the detection of amorphous content in pharmaceutical powdered materials. Int J Pharm 301(1-2):181–191
36. Teagarden DL, Wang W, Baker DS (2010) Practical aspects of freeze-drying of pharmaceutical and biological systems using nonaqueous co-solvent systems. In: Rey L, May JC (eds) Freeze-drying/lyophilization of pharmaceutical and biological products, 3rd edn. Informa, New York, NY
37. Wang W (2000) Lyophilization and development of solid protein pharmaceuticals. Int J Pharm 203(1–2):1–60
38. Wang DQ (2004) Formulation characterization. In: Rey L, May J (eds) Freeze-drying/lyophilization of pharmaceutical and biological products. 2nd edition, revised and expanded. Marcel Dekker, New York, NY, pp 213–238
39. Ward K, Matejtschuk P (2010) The use of microscopy, thermal analysis and impedance measurements to establish critical formulation parameters for freeze-drying cycle development. In: Rey L, May J (eds) Freeze-drying/lyophilization of pharmaceuticals and biological products, 3rd edn. Informa Healthcare, New York, NY, pp 112–135
40. Ye P, Byron T (2008) Characterization of D-mannitol by thermal analysis, FTIR, and Raman spectroscopy. Am Lab 40(14):24–27
41. Zhai S, Taylor R, Sanches R, Slater NKH (2003) Measurement of Lyophilisation primary drying rates by freeze-drying microscopy. Chem Eng Sci 58:2313–2323

Chapter 2

Formulation and Process Development for Lyophilized Biological Reference Materials

Paul Matejtschuk, Kiran Malik, and Chinwe Duru

Abstract

Biologicals can often be inherently unstable in the liquid state and require lyophilization to ensure long-term stability. We describe our approach to the lyophilization of a wide range of biological reference materials, many prepared as part of our work on behalf of the WHO, to develop freeze-dried reference materials to assign biological activity. These can cover a wide range of materials, often purified proteins and sera but also including nucleic acids and viruses. Recent trends in optimizing our approach are presented; the importance of noninvasive monitoring is illustrated and the challenges of formulation design and cycle optimization are discussed.

Key words Biological reference materials, Formulation, Cycle optimization, Design of experiments, Nucleic acids, Viruses

1 Introduction

Biologicals cover the breadth of cell-produced, organism-derived, or synthetically-expressed macromolecules and as such, whether they are purified proteins, polysaccharide antigens, isolated nucleic acids, complexes of associated proteins, viral fragments, multi-component vaccines, or right through to whole cells, they are not entirely characterizable by physicochemical methods alone [1]. For this reason, there persists a need for physical reference materials with carefully assigned potency which can act as standards with which to compare such biologicals. As such, these reference materials may serve a role as primary standards such as those produced for the World Health Organization (WHO), and endorsed following international consultation under the auspices of the Expert Committee on Biological Standardization (ECBS) (http://www.who.int/biologicals/reference_preparations/en/),

Kevin R. Ward and Paul Matejtschuk (eds.), *Lyophilization of Pharmaceuticals and Biologicals: New Technologies and Approaches*, Methods in Pharmacology and Toxicology, https://doi.org/10.1007/978-1-4939-8928-7_2,

or may act as secondary reference preparations, such as those produced for use with Pharmacopeial methods, or indeed as assay run controls or working reagents for day-to-day assay assurance.

The National Institute for Biological Standards and Control (NIBSC) is a center of the Medicines and Healthcare Products Regulatory Agency in the United Kingdom, reporting to the UK Department of Health. Its mission is to safeguard and enhance public health through the standardization and control of biological medicines. At NIBSC we have for over 50 years been producing such reference materials on behalf of the WHO program. We have accumulated substantial experience in preparing and storing such materials, which because they require long shelf life stability, are typically lyophilized to minimize water-catalyzed degradation reactions. The manufacturing processes and technology to deliver these reference materials have been discussed previously [2, 3], but because the nature, formulation, and formats of such standards are constantly changing so our response to preparing them must also adapt. In this chapter, we present an overview of our approach to the development of such standards and then highlight some of the recent trends over the past 10 years. This would serve as a good illustration of the general strategies which can be adopted in the preparation of freeze-dried biological materials.

1.1 Candidate Biological Standards and Reference Materials Processed at NIBSC (Fig. 1)

Most of the materials we prepare are single batch products; indeed, the specific combination of biological material and formulants may not be encountered again until the reference material is replaced. Typically, a batch comprises a 0.5–1 g fill weight of material dispensed in some 100–20,000 containers, usually heat-sealed, type I neutral glass ampoules, although glass vials may alternatively be used for some reference materials. Although inherently more fragile than plastic, glass has superior properties that lend itself to long-term storage, for instance its impermeability to gases and resistance to water vapor ingress. In particular, a flame sealed homogeneous

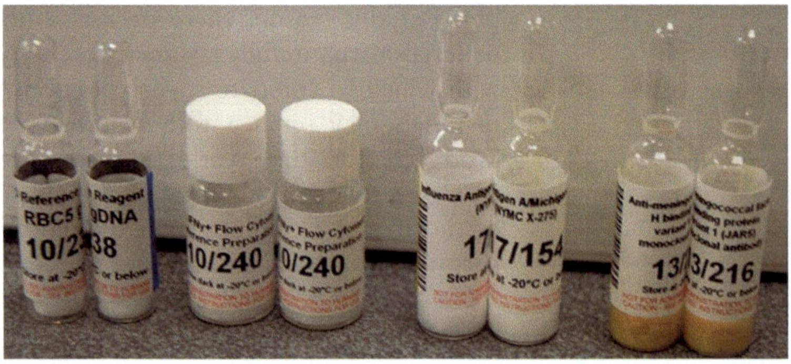

Fig. 1 Photograph of typical biological reference materials prepared by NIBSC showing different formats (ampoules and vials) and materials (DNA, cells, antibodies)

glass ampoule has the lowest risk from moisture ingress or change over storage time [4]. In general, freeze drying is tailored to yield a residual moisture of less than 1% weight of the non-volatiles' dry weight and dispensing is performed with a coefficient of variation of 1% or less for formulations with a plasma-like viscosity, or 0.25% or less for aqueous type materials. These parameters are in compliance with the general guidelines for the preparation of International Reference Preparations set out by the WHO [1].

NIBSC distributes biological standards and reference materials globally with a "handling" charge to account for the costs of storage and distribution by general mail or specialist carriage, such as those required for infectious materials, available from NIBSC's Internet web site http://www.nibsc.org

1.2 Quality Management System

NIBSC processing facilities operate under a quality management system independently certified to the international standard ISO 9001. This quality system is a visible sign of NIBSC's commitment to quality for the preparation of reference materials, as is the Institute's independent accreditation to ISO17025 for its regulatory batch release testing of biological medicines and other related testing activities. Other materials comply with the In Vitro Diagnostic (IVD) Directive ISO 13485 and are CE-marked. Compliance is facilitated by the use of an Institute-wide specific Reference Material Quality System and ISO9001 Quality Systems that control the reference material development from laboratory analytical work through to the process scale filling and distribution.

1.3 Approach to Reference Material Lyophilization

Due to the high throughput of different materials the lyophilization challenges we encounter are fundamentally different to those typical of a pharmaceutical manufacturer in that in the pharma process the same formulation and format is repeatedly processed, whereas at NIBSC we encounter many different formulations and rarely repeat exactly the same product/format combination within any given year. In order to address this over 10 years ago, NIBSC invested in a developmental freeze-drying approach, whereby small batches of the identical formulation and format are processed and the large-scale fill is then processed under the same conditions. This approach (as shown in Fig. 2) has been very successful in minimizing production scale failures and giving a high success rate for processing our standards "right first time".

Development scale freeze-drying processes are based upon previous experience of successful drying, combined with knowledge of the heat transfer properties of the container being used and the thermal analysis and freeze-drying microscopic data on the critical thermal properties of the formulation to be dried. This approach has been very successful but it is vital that on scale up there is no change in the formulation or the ratio of active material to excipients from those trialed at pilot scale and that no additional

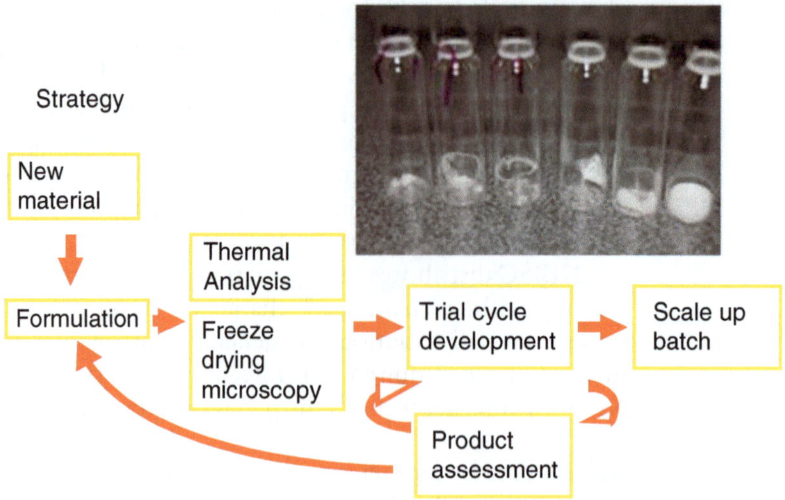

Fig. 2 Strategy for freeze-drying process development with inset example of various unsuccessful collapsed and successful well-formed freeze-dried cakes

processing has been introduced (e.g., sterile filtration that is well known can impact the ice nucleation properties of the material). The properties of the trial lyophilized material are studied for critical parameters (fill accuracy, residual moisture, and oxygen headspace content) as well as its biological potency post-lyophilization (compared to the material as dispensed, snap frozen in identical containers) and if necessary, the stability of the freeze-dried material is determined by accelerated thermal degradation stability studies. For this reason, trials are often performed several months before the definitive fill, to allow thermal stress stability testing if needed.

1.4 Characterization of Thermal Properties

The methods for determining critical physicochemical parameters have been widely described previously [5, 6] and are discussed in more detail in Chap. 1 of this volume. Practically, we have found that freeze-drying microscopy is the most versatile and widely applicable technology, although historically there was much focus on the thermal methods used in pharmaceutical characterization (differential thermal analysis, impedance, conductivity, and differential scanning calorimetry). While these approaches readily reveal eutectic temperatures, when crystallizable formulants solidify, these methods sometimes fail to reveal other critical thermal events (particularly the far weaker glass transitions, Tg′). Others have previously shown that with rising protein concentration a rise in the FDM (T collapse) temperature occurs whereas the Tg′ may remain largely unchanged [7]. The shelf temperature used in the freeze drying of these higher protein concentration products can be increased in line with the trend observed by the FDM and so cycles

Table 1
Influence of additional excipients on the critical thermal events of common formulants (as measured by impedance/differential thermal analysis using the Lyotherm 2) (Biopharma Process Systems Ltd, Winchester, UK)

Formulation	Impedance hysteresis (°C)	DTA event (°C)	Comments
0.9% NaCl	−21.2	−21.8 eutectic	Crystalline NaCl
1% trehalose 0.9% NaCl	−26.4	−24	Still some crystalline content
2% trehalose 0.9% NaCl	−35	No event	Amorphous
5% trehalose 0.9% NaCl	−30	No event	Amorphous

can be shortened and moisture contents reduced by using the more aggressive cycle conditions.

Tables of the Tg′ (and in fewer examples the Tc) of common formulants have been widely published, but in real-world formulations the impact of complex multi-excipient compositions means that the practical critical temperature may be different from that of the individual excipients used, as shown in Table 1.

1.5 Container Formats and Sublimation Impact

Selection of the appropriate format for the reference material to be freeze-dried is also important. A homogeneous and well-formed freeze-dried cake is the desired outcome; however, the container format can impact this. Too wide a diameter container and the freeze-dried cake formed may be too shallow and loose, resulting in an appearance that may deteriorate on manipulation, storage, and shipping, with breakup and shedding of fragments around the container. However, too narrow a diameter container may result in an excessive fill depth for that container (filling at one third to one half of the container volume is generally recommended) and this may impact the homogeneity of the cake appearance and also may result in increased frequency of container breakages in extreme cases. Deeper cakes are more likely to result in a cake with heterogeneities as the impact of any suboptimal cycle design will more likely be apparent in these cakes (often toward the base of the cake which represents the end of the primary drying process).

Telltale signs of inappropriate primary drying can be seen when cakes become pinched in the lower half of the cake, which has been dried during the later stages of the primary drying process (Fig. 3).

Sublimation rate is of course related to the diameter of the container and so a wider container will experience higher sublimation rates. This is illustrated in Fig. 4 where the sublimation rates of a given formulation in our common container formats are compared for the 20, 18, 15, and 13 mm diameter containers.

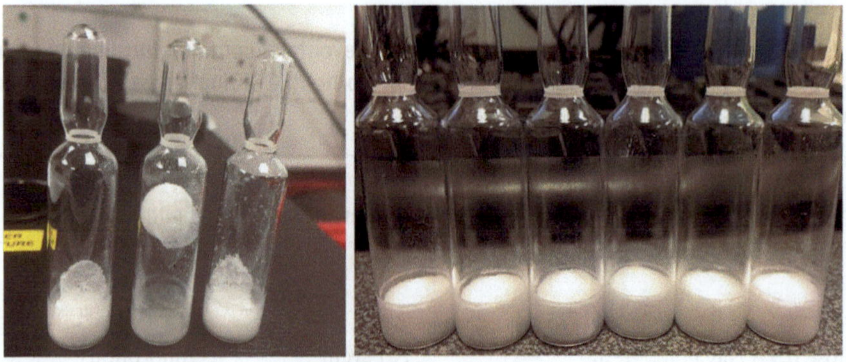

Fig. 3 Pinched and well-formed cakes of a formulated immunoglobulin. Initial study (left hand side) showed two defects, skin formation on top of cake and tapering cakes indicating collapse due to critical temperature being exceeded late in primary drying. A reduction in the inorganic salts content resulted in an acceptable appearance (right hand side image) though the primary drying shelf temperature used was 5 °C higher

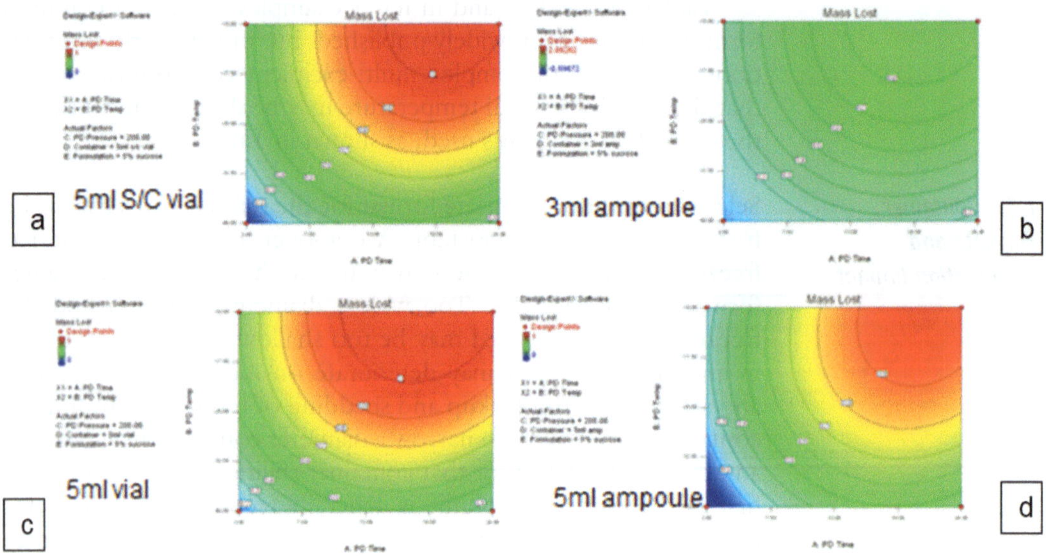

Fig. 4 The impact of container diameter on sublimation rate at a given shelf temperature—container diameters being (**a**): 20 mm, (**b**): 17 mm, (**c**) 14 mm and (**d**) 12 mm. Formulation (5% w/v sucrose in water) and fill volume being dried was the same in each case. Red indicates faster drying rates, through green to blue, indicative of slower rates. Y-axis shelf temperature and x-axis length of primary drying step

1.6 The Challenges of Infectious Materials

Freeze drying as a process can induce high rates of sublimation and this can potentially result in some loss of material from the vials into the drying chamber. This is less for well-formed freeze-dried cakes than for those with partial or total collapse but cannot be assumed not to occur even in well-formed freeze-dried cakes. Indeed, Adams [8] demonstrated this when considering the distribution of a bacterial suspension and we have similarly shown that plasmid nucleic acid can be similarly distributed during freeze drying (unpublished observation). So, freeze-drying infectious materials poses additional problems compared to non-infectious preparations.

- Consistent potency/viability
- Preventing exposure of environment/operators to pathogens
- Appropriate decontamination protocols
- Safe storage and shipping

In order to address these issues, we have at NIBSC introduced the use of a negative pressure isolator system interfaced to a steam sterilizable dryer and capable of decontamination with formaldehyde fumigation (Fig. 5).

Following the freeze-drying infectious materials also pose additional problems for quality control testing. Destructive testing of such materials would result in significant additional risk in conventional test procedures and so noninvasive test methods need to be introduced. Specifically, we have introduced noninvasive moisture and headspace gas analysis in our filling of infectious materials for reference materials.

Oxygen headspace analysis by noninvasive determination of the headspace gas contents has been available for a number of years now using frequency modulated infrared spectroscopy (typically at 760 nm), passing an infrared laser beam through the container and measuring the absorbed wavelengths on a system calibrated against known oxygen concentration standards in the identical format containers (Fig. 6).

These methods depend for their sensitivity on diameter of the container but in our hands can clearly demonstrate the headspace

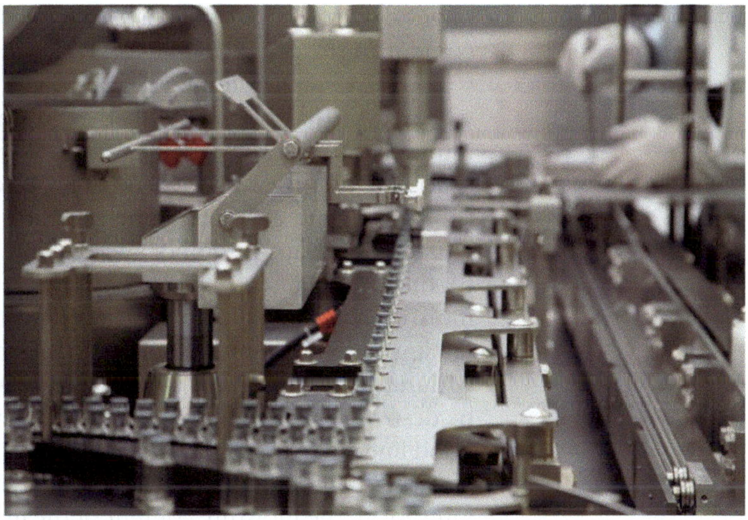

Fig. 5 Negative pressure isolator and freeze dryer assembly for freeze drying of infectious materials at NIBSC

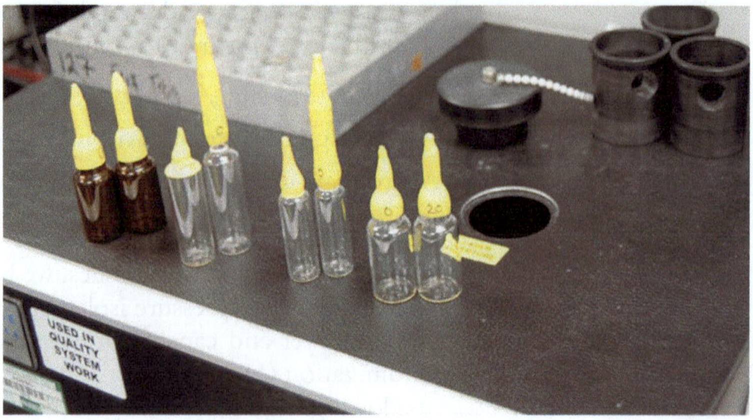

Fig. 6 Noninvasive oxygen headspace determination (FMS 760 Lighthouse Instruments, Charlottesville, VA, USA), calibrated using NIST-traceable oxygen standards in identical format containers

integrity (as our products are back-filled to atmospheric pressure with nitrogen) of the containers tested. Care must be taken when handling such containers of infectious materials that risk of breakage is minimized and this may require a temporary change in the containment status of the room in which the testing is located.

Noninvasive residual moisture FMS-based technologies can indeed measure water content when a wavelength suitable for the absorption spectrum of water is used and this can be a powerful means of demonstrating batch homogeneity and the impact of cycle development on product characteristics [9]. However, it has been shown [10] that such methods can give different moisture readings in the headspace fraction for different formulations with differing physical state and so the correlation of this value with the water content of the product needs careful validation.

An alternative noninvasive moisture-measuring technology which again has been published by numerous groups [11–13] is infrared absorption by the freeze-dried cake itself. Here, a suitable spectrum of infrared wavelengths is passed into the cake through the base of the container. The reflected against absorbed light is measured, the absorption of energies by the water being compared to those not absorbed in the IR spectrum. This is an indirect moisture determination and so we have calibrated containers containing identical freeze-dried formulation in the same format but without infectious agent and then have subjected these to testing by destructive coulometric Karl Fischer methods [14]. This gives a good linear correlation between the NIR readings and the absolute moisture content and this curve and equation can then be used to interpolate the moisture content of the infrared-analyzed infectious containers. As the relationship between the NIR signal and the moisture can be complicated by the overlapping NIR absorption spectra of excipients, especially sugars, it is necessary to create a freeze-dried calibration curve for each formulation, and to also calibrate this against Coulometric Karl Fischer titration. These can then be stored at sub-zero temperatures and the correlation re-checked on each occasion before a new infectious sample set is tested.

There are other limitations with this technology: the penetration of NIR into the cake is only into the nearest few mm of cake adjacent to the glass container and so the technique cannot reveal information on moisture in the deeper parts of the freeze-dried cake, and of course the technique requires an intact cake to be formed, as cracks or lateral shrinkage of the cake will interfere with the light absorption.

1.7 Use of Noninvasive Testing to Improve Quality Assurance

Noninvasive testing has been demonstrated to be very powerful for determining the moisture of infectious freeze-dried materials, but noninvasive testing can also be used to increase the quality assurance of non-infectious reference materials. In 2011, we were able to demonstrate this for a preparation of reference serum which was compromised in terms of the back-filling process such that there was a heterogeneity in the oxygen content of the headspace gas [15]. By using noninvasive testing, we were able to identify those ampoules that had compromised oxygen content and so were able to segregate and test the high oxygen against low-oxygen-containing ampoules, placing them both on elevated temperature thermal stressing to accentuate the rate of biological activity decay. As the biological assay could be done on ampoules where the oxygen content had previously been measured, we could correlate the activity to the oxygen content with complete confidence. For that material, the high oxygen content in the atmospheric headspace had no discernible impact on the biological activity and so the whole batch could be used.

Similar NIR technology has been used in line to test batch homogeneity and to assess the freeze-drying process as a Process Analytical Technology (PAT) tool [16, 17] and interest in NIR and Raman spectroscopy as PAT tools is ongoing.

The moisture uptake by different preparations when exposed to atmospheric (i.e., moist) air varies: Fig. 7 illustrates such uptake across a range of formulants used to generate freeze-dried cakes. The rate of uptake in a low-density material with a low freeze-dried residual cake weight is typically more rapid than a much denser material—e.g. human plasma—but the porosity of the cake is also important, as materials of similar dry weights can take up water at different rates.

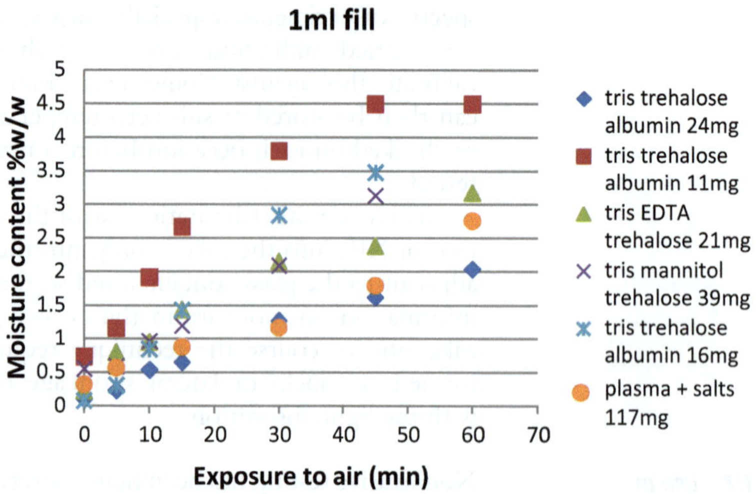

Fig. 7 Moisture uptake by hygroscopic freeze-dried cakes of different densities/formulation on exposure to atmospheric air

2 Novel Freeze-Dried Reference Materials

Although the majority of freeze-dried standards are purified proteins or animal/human sera, we have increasingly, in recent years, freeze dried more complex materials. Such complex materials pose additional challenges where intact viruses or even whole cells are to be freeze dried.

2.1 Viruses

Freeze drying of live virus preparations where infectivity must be obtained requires fast freezing rates to minimize the disruptive effect of ice crystal formation on the virus. As such, snap freezing of the product is performed (for instance on dry ice-acetone) and then loading is onto a shelf precooled to −50 °C so that the sample is held frozen before drying begins. For some materials, it may be possible to load as liquid but, to encourage freezing to occur as quickly as possible by loading onto a precooled shelf. Different stabilizers have been shown by others to be useful for different viruses (for example De Jonge et al. [18] recommended inulin for influenza vaccines, Pastorino et al. [19] advocated sorbitol as a specific stabilizer of viruses).

However, a good place to begin is with 1–5% nonreducing sugar (sucrose or trehalose), a pH modifier (buffer) at low mM concentration, and sufficient bulking material to allow the formation of a good cake (at least 5–10 mg mL^{-1}). Proteins such as albumin or gelatin and serum supplements (such as FCS) may be added to see if they improve stabilization. The Tg′ or Tc of the formulation (if necessary without virus) should be determined and used to guide the shelf temperature for primary drying and a modest secondary drying temperature (20–25 °C) of minimal duration (6–10 h) should be used to deliver a modest initial moisture content. From this starting point, other specific individual stabilizers can be tried and the cycle modified to produce lower or higher final moisture contents and the activity checked. Suitable containment and decontamination measures should be in place to prevent operator and environmental exposure to any material which may have ablated during drying [8] and suitable decontamination procedures used on condensate, before it is disposed of, and on the dryer before it is reused.

Recent NIBSC live virus reference materials for in-vitro detection have included those for Hepatitis B Virus [20], Cytomegalovirus [21], and Epstein Barr Virus [22]. The formulation of live viral vaccines for in-vivo use is outside of the scope of this chapter but has been reviewed recently by Hansen et al. [23].

2.2 Cellular Nucleic Acid

Freeze drying of mammalian cells usually results in the rupture of the cells and non-viability post-reconstitution. This has historically been attributed to reasons similar to those given above for viruses and focus around the disruptive effect of large ice crystals forming and then subliming from the cells. Some papers have reported the preservation of at least some bioactivity after drying [24, 25] by use of very small volumes and very rapid directional freezing. Others have optimized the formulation as well as freezing conditions to improve recovery of bioactivity [26, 27]. The scalability of some of these methods has yet to be demonstrated.

However, if the purpose of the cell preservation is not therapeutic or focused on recovery of bioactivity but rather the preservation of the nucleic acid, freeze-drying processes may be perfectly satisfactory. This has been demonstrated with the BCR-ABL RNA reference material established by WHO in 2010 [28] for quantification of the molecular defect resulting in a form of chronic myeloid leukemia and useful for early molecular-based diagnosis of relapse. Here, rather than isolate the nucleic acid, the un-fixed cells were freeze dried in different ratios of cells with the mutated and normal gene sequence. The nucleic acid is then extracted from the cells by the user, allowing better commutability to a patient sample, in that the extraction procedure used will be the same for sample and reference material.

For other genomic nucleic acid standards, the DNA has been first extracted and then lyophilized with excipients. Of course, if the nucleic acid is extracted and lyophilized in a stabilizing buffer, these preparations make reference material with excellent storage stability [29]. Originally, some difficulties were encountered with the physical appearance of such standards (Fig. 8), even though the materials themselves were perfectly stable to degradation. By careful modification of the drying conditions we have been able to

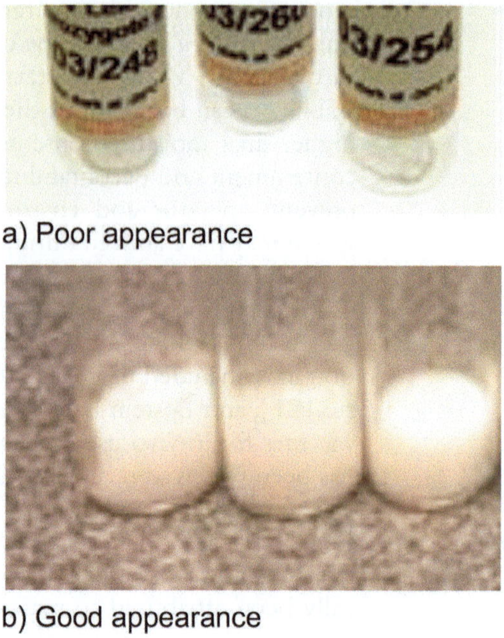

Fig. 8 Different appearance of freeze dried similarly extracted and formulated DNA preparations with low dry mass formulations (<10 mg per ampoule) reflecting appearance (**a**) before and (**b**) after cycle optimization

routinely deliver stable preparations with well-formed cakes (despite their low density) and modest moisture contents, even though the dry weights are little more than 10 mg per ampoule.

2.3 Lyophilization of Fixed Cells

Depending upon the application, pre-stabilization of cells using fixative solutions has rendered eukaryotic cells suitable for freeze drying. This has long been known for diagnostic applications such as immunoassay [30] where quite dilute solutions of fixative such as glutaraldehyde can render red blood cells capable of withstanding freeze drying without the clumping and aggregation caused by high levels of fixative. This allowed even antibodies attached to the surface of such cells to remain immunoreactive [31].

However, for some applications, the size and morphology of the cells is critical and NIBSC have recently prepared gently fixed peripheral blood monocytes as standards [32] for flow cytometry, where the gating window settings require the cells to retain both their immunological reactivity and their structure/size. There are applications for such reagents as controls in FACS-based diagnostic testing.

3 Formulation Strategy and Considerations

Excellent reviews of the role of various excipients in the stabilization of biologics in freeze drying exist [33, 34]. Each category of excipient type is listed and compared and so the reader is referred to these for advice on formulation. Figure 9 illustrates a generic approach to the formulation of biological materials in which the key components are identified. In general, ionic excipients such as sodium chloride or phosphate lower the Tg′ of the formulation and so should be avoided or kept to a minimum. Polymers, including proteins themselves, raise the Tg′ and so can result in more efficient cycles being possible. Disaccharides have intermediate Tg′ values in the region of −29 to −32 °C, but their inclusion is usually because of their benefit as lyoprotectants and so the lower Tg′ is tolerated or other excipients included which will allow for higher shelf temperatures in primary drying. For instance, the use of sucrose-mannitol mixtures has been illustrated as a generic formulation [35] because when crystallized by annealing, the mannitol results in a good product appearance even when using high primary drying temperatures, while the sucrose remains amorphous and so can stabilize the biological material.

3.1 One Factor at a Time (OFAT) Approach

This approach is very common in freeze-drying formulation development, where a known lyoprotectant is varied in concentration and its impact on preserving the biological activity and physical appearance of the freeze-dried cake is assessed. Other examples of where an OFAT development approach is appropriate are where a previous formulation is known to work effectively, but due to changes in either the format, fill depth or the product, the cycle is no longer suitable and an inferior or collapsed cake occurs. Modification to a single excipient component may suffice to restore a successful lyophilized appearance. Alternatively, in these cases,

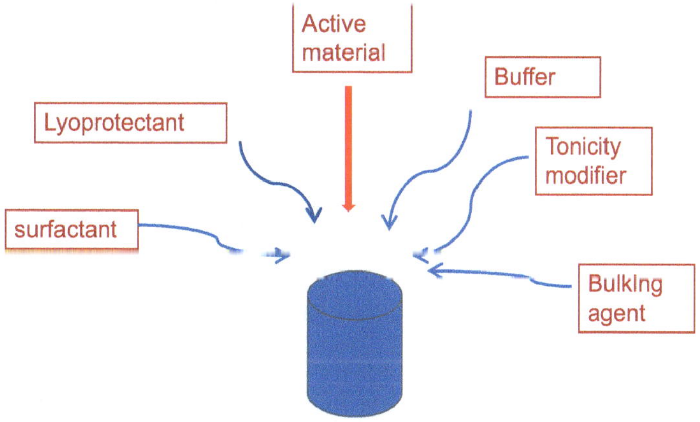

Fig. 9 Schematic of typical formulation components for lyophilization

simple modification in one of the cycle parameters in terms of the primary drying shelf temperature or vacuum setpoint may suffice to restore a successful lyophilization outcome. Careful thermal analysis is critical to identifying such shifts in the properties of the product and also the impact the OFAT changes introduced.

Influenza antigen preparations have long been produced by NIBSC to assist with the manufacture of influenza vaccines and also in serotyping of influenza viruses. In order to produce stable reagents, these materials are lyophilized with a commonly used formulation of 1% w/v sucrose in phosphate-buffered saline. On occasions, we have processed materials which instead of forming a well-supported, if not particularly dense, cake have resulted in a totally collapsed and sometimes even gelatinous appearance. This is unacceptable and will often result in an elevated residual moisture content. We have shown the utility of a modulated differential scanning calorimetry method (mDSC) to predict which formulations will be readily lyophilizable and which may result in a collapsed appearance on drying with our usual freeze-drying cycle [36]. We demonstrated a correlation of the freeze-dried appearance (see Fig. 10) to the presence and size of a eutectic event at −24 to −26 °C . This has been adopted at NIBSC for several years now and has prevented the preparation of collapsed freeze-dried batches, which can be both inconvenient and cause delays in the narrow time course available for the manufacturing and control process for seasonal influenza vaccines.

In other cases, there may initially be insufficient formulant present, for instance when we were developing drying protocols for polysaccharide antigens as serological markers for bacterial typing. Here, because the quantitation method was based on carbohydrate analysis, a simple formulation was chosen that would not interfere

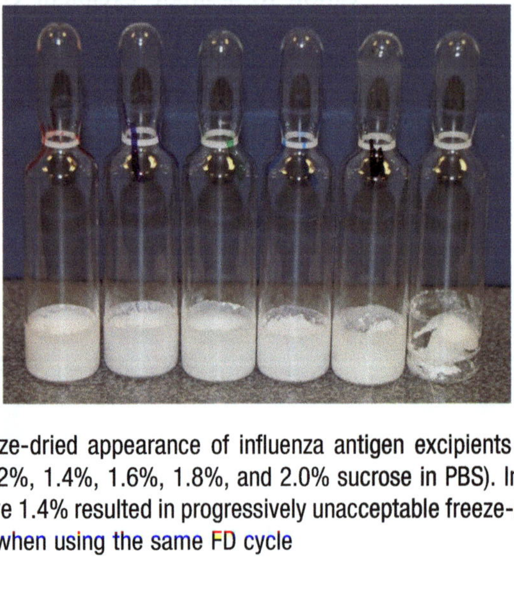

Fig. 10 Freeze-dried appearance of influenza antigen excipients (from left to right: 1%, 1.2%, 1.4%, 1.6%, 1.8%, and 2.0% sucrose in PBS). Increasing the sucrose above 1.4% resulted in progressively unacceptable freeze-dried product appearance when using the same FD cycle

Formulation	FDM °C	Dry weight	RMD (%w/w)	Appearance
6mM K_2HPO_4 4mM KH_2PO_4 0.1% trehalose, 0.5% HSA	-43	5mg	1.43	Good, well-formed, some cracking
60mM K_2HPO_4 40mM KH_2PO_4 0.2% trehalose, 0.5% HSA	-40	23mg	0.37	Good, some lateral shrinkage
6mM K_2HPO_4 4mMKH_2PO_4 0.2% trehalose, 0.5% HSA	-41	9mg	0.80	Good

Fig. 11 Formulation choice with resultant critical temperature (ascertained by FDM), trial freeze-dried appearance and moisture content for development of an interleukin-23 reference material (SS-068). HSA = human serum albumin

with the saccharide analytical methods being applied. However, there was initially insufficient dry mass and the resulting freeze dried cakes were poor in appearance at the upper surface and material ablated, such that the variation in the freeze-dried weight was unacceptably high. This was addressed by two alternative strategies—either raising the concentration of the active so that the dry weight was at least 5 mg mL^{-1} of the fill volume, or by the inclusion of neutral bulking agent which did not interfere with the polysaccharide quantitation method. The former was on this occasion deemed more acceptable and a successful reference material produced [37].

On other occasions, the evaluation of a number of formulation options can be undertaken and the outcome can be that all of the formulation options give reasonable freeze-dried cakes. However, other parameters need to be considered too and, in the example given in Fig. 11, the moisture content achieved was different, and so here a formulation was selected based on where the resultant moisture content was lowest.

It has been noted already that proteins will themselves raise the critical temperature required for freeze drying and so make more efficient cycles possible but also, we have shown that for some difficult materials, there may well be better stabilizers than sugars [38]. Although the inclusion of bulking or stabilizing proteins may not be possible for some applications, for others—especially diagnostic materials—they may prove a much more effective stabilizer and would also minimize nonspecific binding of low concentration active material proteins to surfaces during the filling process.

Adjuvanted materials and cellular materials may pose particular issues for freeze drying, not least because such materials may settle out during a prolonged freezing process. Although snap freezing with cryo-liquids may be useful at small scale, the use of precooled dryer shelves, down to −40 or −50 °C, may be needed to achieve successful scale-up.

3.2 Design of Experiment (DoE) Approaches to Formulation

In recent years we have, in conjunction with graduate students of Professor Paul Dalby at University College London, Department of Biochemical Engineering, investigated the use of rapid throughput formulation screening for freeze-drying optimization using a Design of Experiments (DoE) approach [39]. This has focused on the use of microtiter plates to allow for microscale freeze drying while evaluating numerous combinations and concentration options. Such cycles can be completed rapidly (typically overnight) and indeed the individual wells can be stoppered in situ with the use of 96-format lyocap cluster caps (Micronics, through Kinesis Ltd, St Neots, UK) to assist evaluation. A typical freeze-dried plate is shown in Fig. 12, and collapsed and well-formed cakes can be easily characterized. By application of Design of Experiment (DoE) approaches, a series of formulants can be rapidly evaluated and interactions between excipients can be readily identified. Such trends are easily investigated with proprietary software, such as Design Expert (Stat Ease Inc, Minneapolis, MN, USA). Such software can also be used to evaluate formulation interactions and optimization in traditional containers and so can be employed from early evaluation through development and scale-up. Grant et al. demonstrated this for the optimization of formulations for the freeze drying of low concentration granulocyte colony stimulating factor, a potent stimulator of blood cell proliferation [40]. Such fundamental formulation evaluation has proven less applicable to the scale up of many of our reference materials where the basic excipient choices and concentrations are already dictated often by the intended use of the materials. However, where freeze-drying formulation is required for a new biological material, especially one which is initially available in only very small amounts, this approach offers valuable time and active material savings, with the possibility of easily identifying potentially useful excipient interactions.

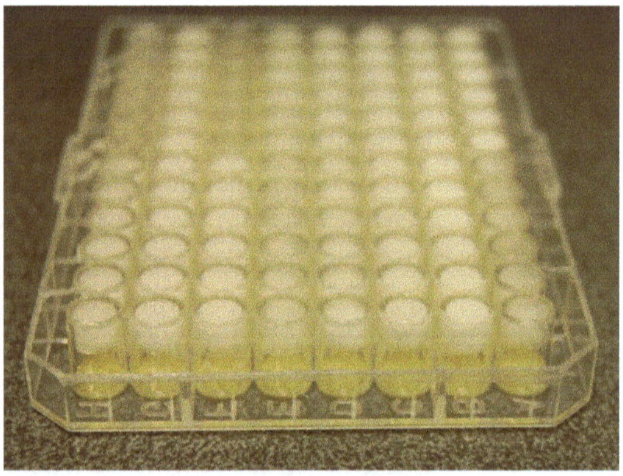

Fig. 12 Freeze drying in microplates for formulation screening/optimization of granulocyte colony stimulating factor

4 Cycle Optimization

4.1 Use of Critical Temperatures

The major transformation in freeze-drying cycle design in the past 20 years has been in the switch from a trial run empirical approach for cycle optimization to a more scientifically based process design based upon thermal analysis and freeze-drying microscopy data. This is addressed in greater detail in other chapters in this book, but here we will merely describe how we have addressed this process as it has developed for lyophilization of reference materials at NIBSC.

It is critical for successful drying to know in detail the formulation of the material to be dried and then to apply at least two of the many methods available to determine the critical temperature for this formulation. For instance, for a recent formulation of immunoglobulin, both the DMA and freeze-drying microscopy indicated that a critical temperature (in the range −14 to −18 °C) would be appropriate (see Fig. 13). After this temperature is determined, it can be built into a general cycle, allowing for some flexibility as the process of sublimation is endothermic and so heat will be drawn from the system—referred to as sublimative cooling—and this will allow a shelf temperature higher than the Tg′ or Tc to be used. The degree of difference will need to be based upon the sublimation rate, the performance of the freeze dryer being used and the dimensions of the container for any fill. This is still heavily based upon previous experience of what is likely to be successful, and a

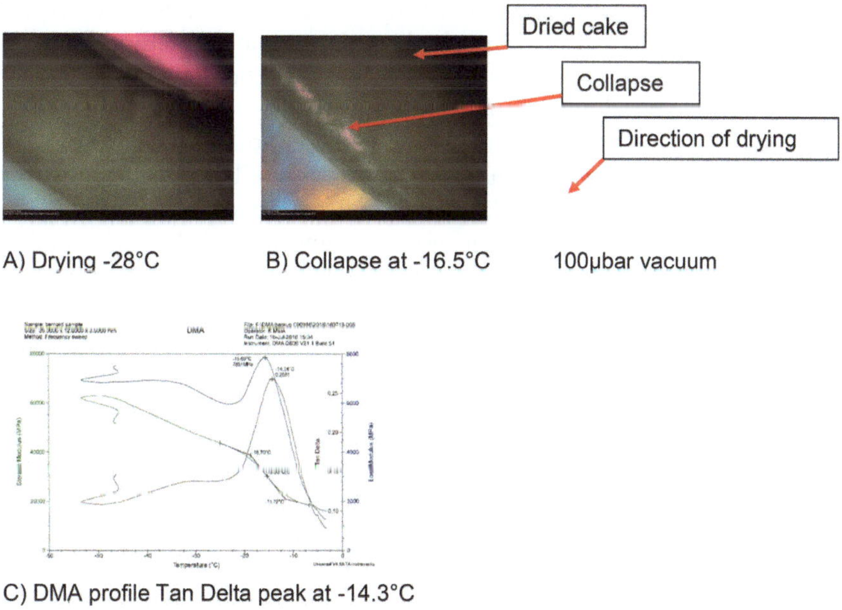

Fig. 13 (**A**, **B**) Freeze-drying microscopy and (**C**) sub-ambient dynamic mechanical analysis (DMA) of an immunoglobulin preparation both indicating a critical temperature in the region −14 to −18 °C

trial of 50–200 containers in a pilot dryer is applied ahead of scaling up the cycle to a batch size of between 3000 and 20,000 in a production dryer.

The stainless steel production dryer will differ in its performance due to factors such as the absence of a radiant heat, present for a pilot dryer due to its Perspex door, but also the capability of the vacuum pumps, heating rate, and temperature heterogeneity across a single shelf compared to a stack of much larger shelves, and indeed the mechanism of shelf cooling, which on a simple dryer may be electrothermal heating and on a larger dryer is almost always a coolant fluid. Once the Tg′/Tc is known from off-line analytical testing, then this data can be used to set the shelf temperature in the freeze-drying method, but the monitoring of the primary sublimation process is still an area of active development. Sublimation rates for frequently used containers can be measured by running gravimetric trials and measuring the weight of water loss after a given sublimation period, significantly less than that required for the full primary drying process step.

4.2 Monitoring of Freeze Drying

A number of technologies have been developed to monitor sublimation in real time within a freeze dryer and these are reviewed in other chapters. In our own experience, the inflection in a thermocouple or Pt 100 probe can provide useful data, if only indicative, as drying rate may be different in the majority of other non-probed vials. Other freeze dryer manufacturers supply an impedance or thermal analysis probe vial which can produce physicochemical data on a single vial in the batch. Most recently, we have been evaluating, as part of an Innovate-UK funded project, the applicability of a noninvasive impedance analysis method [41] which is also discussed in another chapter in this book by Prof. Geoff Smith, the developer of the technology.

As an alternative, there are a number of technologies that can measure the sublimation rate in the batch as a whole, for instance tunable diode laser absorbance spectroscopy (TDLAS)—as covered in Chap. 5 of this volume—and indeed the more straightforward pressure rise method and the comparative manometric method (comparing the pressure sensed by a Pirani vacuum gauge against that of a manometric gauge). These latter methods are illustrated in Fig. 14. In this illustration, the endpoint of comparative manometric method agrees well with the pressure rise test and indeed with that indicated by the thermocouples. This gives additional confidence in the suitability of these methods and in this cycle a marked reduction in the primary drying time would be possible, allowing substantial optimization of the process.

4.3 Ice Nucleation

One of the more recent process improvements in addressing heterogeneity in freeze-drying batch processes has been the introduction of induced ice nucleation methods. This minimizes the

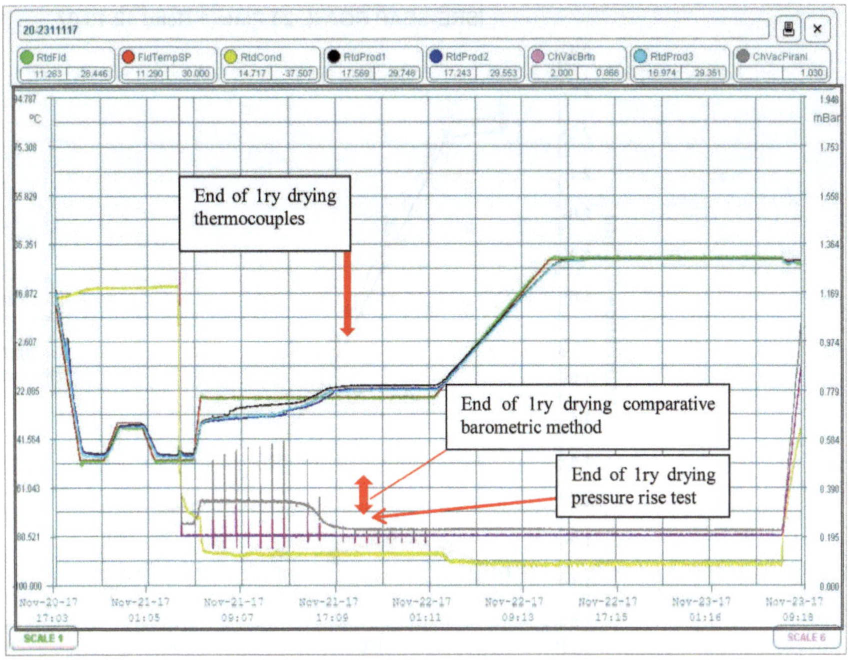

Fig. 14 Cycle optimization–endpoint determination methods on whole batch (pressure rise and comparative barometric readings) and individual probes (thermocouple) both indicating that the primary drying step in this cycle could be reduced in length significantly without impacting the end of this stage of drying (x axis time, y1 axis temperature(oC), y2 axis vacuum (mBar))

variability in the point of nucleation across a batch and this reduction in the heterogeneity in nucleation and hence the degree of supercooling across a batch may result in a cycle optimization time of the order of 10–30%. The methods for inducing controlled ice nucleation are the topic of other chapters in this volume (Chaps. 3 and 4) so will not be discussed further here.

4.4 Scale-Up

The process of scale-up for our cycles at NIBSC has been relatively straightforward as we tend to favor conservative shelf temperature and vacuum conditions for primary and secondary drying and so are likely to be operating well away from the limits of failure. This is illustrated by the scale-up presented in Fig. 15 where the performance of trial and production batch lyophilization for a cytokine reference material were shown to give good similarity between the resultant product in both physicochemical tests and biological activity.

This degree of caution may well not be possible for those developing more time-critical cycles but the underlying criteria we have discussed, of careful formulation development, including consideration of container selection, thorough pre-lyophilization stage analytical characterization of the critical thermal properties, and application of process analytical technologies where available, are sound principles to apply.

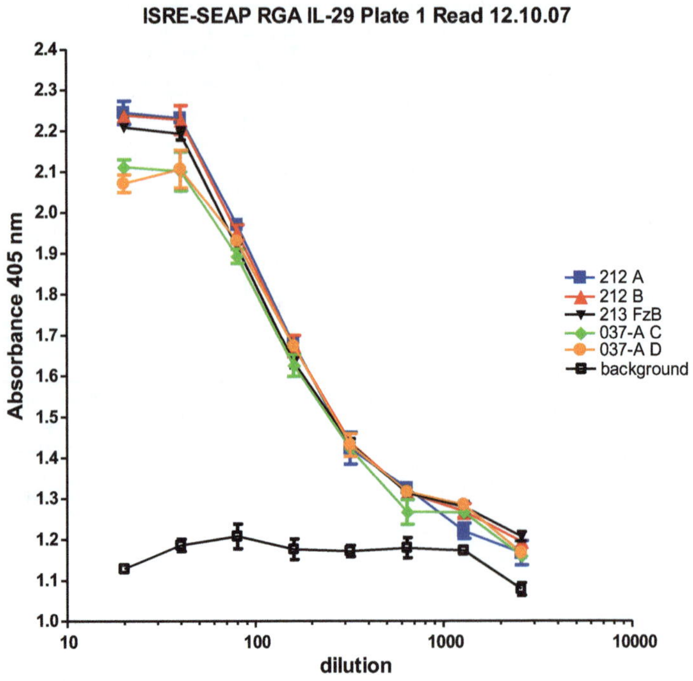

Fig. 15 Comparison of potency estimates for IL-29 trial (PM-037-A) and definitive fill (07/212) ampoules. IL-29 activity in reconstituted contents of ampoules of definitive fill 07/212 and trial fill PM-037-A was evaluated in two different reporter gene assays (RGA) calibrated with the frozen baseline 07/213 of the definitive fill. Typical dose-response data from the RGA are shown in the graphical plots. The geometric mean potency values for each of the two ampoules (A and B) of 07/212 (process batch) and each of the two ampoules (C and D) of PM-037-A (intermediate trial batch) do not differ significantly from one another or from 1.0, the value assigned to the FzB. Data courtesy of Dr A. Meager, NIBSC (retired)

4.5 Thermal Degradation Studies as a Predictor of Biological Stability

The assessment of real-time stability is a time-consuming and laborious process. The use of suitably studies can estimate the stability to a reasonable degree by use of temperatures significantly above the intended storage temperature and fitting the degradation rate using the Arrhenius relationship to predict the storage at the desired temperature [42]. This is approximation only, and has been shown on numerous occasions to over-estimate the real time degradation and may reveal degradation pathways which will not be operational at the lower intended storage temperature. However, where some indication of likely stability is required in the short term it is a useful comparator and has been used at NIBSC successfully to evaluate and compare lyo formulations in the short term (3–6 months) prior to selection for scale-up. The use of high-throughput screening methods based on molecular assessment of stability both in the freeze dried [43] and in reconstituted liquid states [44] may well find their place alongside such comparatively time-consuming studies in the future.

For some applications, standard processing in vials or ampoules may not be ideal as only very small quantities of liquid may need to be freeze dried per container due to the sensitivity of the assay method being applied to the biological. For such applications, we have been investigating alternative technologies, such as plastic microtubes. Whereas for some laboratory applications with proteins or polysaccharides that are highly stable these may be suitable, their general stability compared to classical containers remains to be demonstrated and the homogeneous flame-sealed glass ampoule remains a gold standard for the majority of our reference material applications at NIBSC [4].

5 Conclusions

Freeze drying remains the ideal format for biological reference materials where a long stable shelf life is required. In this overview, we have illustrated NIBSC's approach to the development of both formulation and cycle design for such freeze drying and its scale-up. Although applications in other areas—for instance, diagnostics or therapeutics development—may have different requirements, the principles outlined will hopefully have provided a starting point to those seeking advice in these activities.

Acknowledgments

We thank our many colleagues at NIBSC with whom development studies have been undertaken and those in the Standards Processing Division with whom we cooperate to deliver large-scale batches of lyophilized material. We also thank academic collaborators, especially Professor Paul Dalby, UCL and former students Drs. Mathew Robinson and Yitzchak Grant.

References

1. WHO (2006) Recommendations for the preparation, characterization and establishment of international and other biological reference standards (revised 2004), WHO technical report series, No. 932. WHO, Geneva, pp 75–131
2. Phillips P (1998) The preparation of International Biological Standards. Fresenius J Anal Chem 360:473–475. https://doi.org/10.1007/s002160050742
3. Matejtschuk P, Anderson M, Jefferson P (2010) Lyophilization of biological standards. In: Rey L, May JC (eds) Lyophilization/freeze drying of pharmaceutical & biological products, 3rd edn. Informa, New York, NY, pp 317–352
4. Matejtschuk P, Rafiq S, Johnes S, Gaines Das R (2005) A comparison of vials with ampoules for the storage of biological reference materials. Biologicals 33(2):63–70
5. Kett V (2009) Thermal Analysis - the use of DSC & MTDSC in analyzing freeze-dried formulations and products. Am Pharm Rev 12:24–29
6. Meister E, Gieseler H (2009) Freeze-dry microscopy of protein/sugar mixtures: drying behavior, interpretation of collapse

temperatures and a comparison to corresponding glass transition data. J Pharm Sci 98:3072–3087

7. Meister E, Sasi S, Gieseler H (2009) Freeze-dry microscopy: impact of nucleation temperature and excipient concentration on collapse temperature data. AAPS PharmSciTech 10 (2):582–588. https://doi.org/10.1208/s12249-009-9245-y
8. Adams GDJ (1991) The loss of substrate from a vial during freeze-drying using *Escherichia coli* as a trace organism. J Chem Technol Biotechnol 52(4):511–518
9. Cook IA, Ward KR (2011) Applications of headspace moisture analysis for investigating the water dynamics within a sealed vial containing freeze-dried material. PDA J Pharm Sci Technol 65:2–11
10. Cook IA, Ward KR (2011) Headspace moisture mapping and the information that can be gained about freeze-dried materials and processes. PDA J Pharm Sci Technol 65 (5):457–467. https://doi.org/10.5731/pdajpst.2011.00760
11. Jones JA, Last IR, MacDonald BF, Prebble KA (1993) Development and transferability of near-infrared methods for determination of moisture in a freeze-dried injection product. J Pharm Biomed Anal 11:1227–1231
12. Kamat MS, Lodder RA, DeLuca PP (1989) Near Infra red spectroscopic determination of residual moisture in lyophilized sucrose through intact glass vials. Pharm Res 6 (11):961–965
13. Lin TP, Hsu CC (2002) Determination of residual moisture in lyophilized protein pharmaceuticals using a rapid and noninvasive method: near infrared spectroscopy. PDA J Pharm Sci Technol 56(4):196–205
14. Malik KP, Duru C, Ahmed M, Matejtschuk P (2010) Analytical options for the measurement of residual moisture content in lyophilized biological materials. Am Pharm Rev 13 (5):42–47
15. Ferguson M, Wilkinson DE, Heath A, Matejtschuk P (2011) The first international standard for antibodies to HPV 16. Vaccine 29(38):6520–6526
16. De Beer TR, Vercruysse P, Burggraeve A, Quinten T, Ouyang J, Zhang X, Vervaet C, Remon JP, Baeyens WR (2009) In-line and real-time process monitoring of a freeze drying process using Raman and NIR spectroscopy as complementary process analytical technology (PAT) tools. J Pharm Sci 98(9):3430–3446. https://doi.org/10.1002/jps.21633
17. Kauppinen A, Toiviainen M, Korhonen O, Aaltonen J, Järvinen K, Paaso J, Juuti M, Ketolainen J (2013) In-line multipoint near-infrared spectroscopy for moisture content quantification during freeze-drying. Anal Chem 85(4):2377–2384
18. De Jonge J, Amorij JP, Hinrichs WL, Wilschut J, Huckriede A, Frijlink HW (2007) Inulin sugar glasses preserve the structural integrity and biological activity of influenza virosomes during freeze-drying and storage. Eur J Pharm Sci 32(1):33–44
19. Pastorino B, Baronti C, Gould EA, Charrel RN, de Lamballerie X (2015) Effect of chemical stabilizers on the thermostability and infectivity of a representative panel of freeze-dried viruses. PLoS One 10(4):e0118963. https://doi.org/10.1371/journal.pone.0118963
20. Fryer JF, Heath AB, Wilkinson DE, Minor PD (2017) A collaborative study to establish the 3rd WHO International Standard for hepatitis B virus for nucleic acid amplification techniques. Biologicals 46:57–63
21. Fryer JF, Heath AB, Minor PD, Collaborative Study Group (2016) A collaborative study to establish the 1st WHO International Standard for human cytomegalovirus for nucleic acid amplification technology. Biologicals 44 (4):242–251
22. Fryer JF, Heath AB, Wilkinson DE, Minor PD, Collaborative Study Group (2016) A collaborative study to establish the 1st WHO International Standard for Epstein-Barr virus for nucleic acid amplification techniques. Biologicals 44(5):423–433. https://doi.org/10.1016/j.biologicals.2016.04.010
23. Hansen LJ, Daoussi R, Vervaet C, Remon JP, De Beer TR (2015) Freeze-drying of live virus vaccines: a review. Vaccine 33(42):5507–5519. https://doi.org/10.1016/j.vaccine.2015.08.085
24. Natan D, Nagler A, Arav A (2009) Freeze-drying of mononuclear cells derived from umbilical cord blood followed by colony formation. PLoS One 4(4):e5240. https://doi.org/10.1371/journal.pone.0005240
25. Arav A, Natan D (2012) Freeze drying of red blood cells: the use of directional freezing and a new radio frequency lyophilization device. Biopreserv Biobank 10(4):386–394. https://doi.org/10.1089/bio.2012.0021
26. Ward K, Cowen A, Peacock T (2012) Freeze drying method. WO2012098358 A1
27. Loi P, Iuso D, Czernik M, Zacchini F, Ptak G (2013) Towards storage of cells and gametes in dry form. Trends Biotechnol 31(12):688–695.

https://doi.org/10.1016/j.tibtech.2013.09.004
28. White HE, Matejtschuk P, Rigsby P, Gabert J, Lin F, Wang YL, Branford S, Müller MC, Beaufils N, Beillard E, Colomer D, Dvorakova D, Ehrencrona H, Goh HG, El Housni H, Jones D, Kairisto V, Kamel-Reid S, Kim DW, Langabeer S, Ma ES, Press RD, Romeo G, Wang L, Zoi K, Hughes T, Saglio G, Hochhaus A, Goldman JM, Metcalfe P, Cross NC (2010) Establishment of the 1st World Health Organization International Genetic Reference Panel for quantitation of BCR-ABL mRNA. Blood 116(22): e111–e117. https://doi.org/10.1182/blood-2010-06-291641 PMID: 20720184
29. Gray E, Hawkins JR, Morrison M, Hawkins M, Byrne E, Kitchen S, Jennings I, Makris M, Preston FE, Metcalfe P (2006) Establishment of the 1st International Genetic Reference Panel for factor V Leiden (G1691A), human gDNA. Thromb Haemost 96:215–219
30. Cranage MP, Gurner BW, Coombs RR (1983) Glutaraldehyde stabilisation of antibody-linked erythrocytes for use in reverse passive and related haemagglutination assays. J Immunol Methods 64(1-2):7–16
31. Matejtschuk P, Easter G, Thorpe R, Coombs RR (1988) Experimental studies on red cell-based assays for total IgE and allergen-specific IgE. Int Arch Appl Immunol 86(1):106–111
32. Stebbings R, Wang L, Sutherland J, Kammel M, Gaigalas AK, John M, Roemer B, Kuhne M, Schneider RJ, Braun M, Engel A, Dikshit DK, Abbasi F, Marti GE, Sassi MP, Revel L, Kim SK, Baradez MO, Lekishvili T, Marshall D, Whitby L, Jing W, Ost V, Vonsky M, Neukammer J (2015) Quantification of cells with specific phenotypes I: determination of CD4+ cell count per microliter in reconstituted lyophilized human PBMC prelabeled with anti-CD4 FITC antibody. Cytometry A 87(3):244–253. https://doi.org/10.1002/cyto.a.22614
33. Wang W (2000) Lyophilization and development of solid protein pharmaceuticals. Int J Pharm 203:1–60
34. Costantino HR (2004) Excipients for use in lyophilized pharmaceutical peptide, protein and other bioproducts. In: Costantino HR, Pikal MJ (eds) Lyophilization of biopharmaceuticals. AAPS Press, Arlington, VA, pp 139–228
35. Johnson RE, Kirchhoff CF (2002) Gaud HT (2002) Mannitol–sucrose mixtures—versatile formulations for protein lyophilization. J Pharm Sci 91:914–922
36. Duru C, Swann C, Dunleavy U, Mulloy B, Matejtschuk P (2015) The importance of formulation in the successful lyophilization of influenza reference materials. Biologicals 43(2):110–116. https://doi.org/10.1016/j.biologicals.2014.12.001
37. Mawas F, Bolgiano B, Rigsby P, Crane D, Belgrave D, Corbel MJ (2007) Evaluation of the saccharide content and stability of the first WHO International Standard for *Haemophilus influenzae* b capsular polysaccharide. Biologicals 35(4):235–245
38. Stickings P, Rigsby P, Coombes L, Malik K, Matejtschuk P, Sesardic D (2010) Collaborative study for the calibration of a replacement international standard for diphtheria toxoid adsorbed. Biologicals 38(5):529–538
39. Grant Y, Matejtschuk P, Dalby PA (2009) Rapid optimization of protein freeze-drying formulations using ultra scale-down and factorial design of experiment in microplates. Biotechnol Bioeng 104:957–964
40. Grant Y, Matejtschuk P, Bird C, Wadhwa M, Dalby PA (2012) Freeze drying formulation using microscale and of experiment approaches: a case study using granulocyte colony-stimulating factor. Biotechnol Lett 34(4):641–648. https://doi.org/10.1007/s10529-011-0822-2
41. Smith G, Arshad MS, Polygalov E, Ermolina I, McCoy TR, Matejtschuk P (2017) Process understanding in freeze-drying cycle development: applications for through-vial impedance spectroscopy (TVIS) in mini-pilot studies. J Pharm Innov 12:26. https://doi.org/10.1007/s12247-016-9266-5
42. Matejtschuk P, Phillips PK (2008) Product stability and accelerated degradation studies. In: Stacey G, Davis JM (eds) Medicines from animal cell culture. Wiley, Chichester, UK pp 503–522
43. Robinson MJ, Matejtschuk P, Bristow AF, Dalby PA (2018) Tm-values and unfolded fraction can predict aggregation rates for granulocyte colony stimulating factor variant formulations but not under predominantly native conditions. Mol Pharm 15:256. https://doi.org/10.1021/acs.molpharmaceut.7b00876
44. Malik K, Matejtschuk P, Thelwell C, Burns C (2013) Differential scanning fluorimetry: rapid screening of formulations that promote the stability of reference preparations. J Pharm Biomed Anal 77:163–166

Chapter 3

Controlled Ice Nucleation Using ControLyo® Pressurization-Depressurization Method

Jacob Luoma, Graham Magill, Lokesh Kumar, and Zakaria Yusoff

Abstract

Controlling the ice nucleation temperature during the freeze phase of lyophilization is an area that has grown significantly in importance in the recent past. Different Controlled Ice Nucleation (CIN) techniques investigated in the pharmaceutical industry are discussed in this chapter, along with their limitations for commercial implementation. Recent work using the ControLyo® pressurization and depressurization technology is further discussed, along with a discussion of CIN cycle design. This book chapter also explores how ControLyo® CIN technology could be used to enable a Quality by Design (QbD) approach for the freeze phase of lyophilization cycles.

Key words Freeze drying, Lyophilization, Ice nucleation, Controlled ice nucleation, ControLyo® Technology, Quality by design, QbD, Mechanistic understanding

1 Introduction

Lyophilization (or freeze drying) is an established technique to stabilize unstable active pharmaceutical ingredients (API), including biologics [1]. It is a batch process that, in most instances, is long and consumes a lot of energy, time, and resources. Pharmaceutical manufacturers of parenteral drugs must often freeze dry their products in order to extend their shelf life, which enables them to be safely transported all over the world under various climate conditions and to assure preservation of product quality. In less developed regions of the world where the supply chain and transportation systems may be less robust, having a product that can tolerate these types of logistic challenges can be very important from a business and patient care perspective.

A typical lyophilization cycle consists of a freezing phase, primary drying, and secondary drying. A more elaborate explanation of a lyophilization process is discussed in other chapters of this book.

Kevin R. Ward and Paul Matejtschuk (eds.), *Lyophilization of Pharmaceuticals and Biologicals: New Technologies and Approaches*, Methods in Pharmacology and Toxicology, https://doi.org/10.1007/978-1-4939-8928-7_3,

During the freezing phase, it is well documented that the vials in a batch nucleate randomly, with each vial nucleating at a different degree of supercooling. When the product is in the liquid state, but still colder than its thermodynamic freezing point, the difference between the product temperature and thermodynamic freezing point of the formulation is often referred to as its degree of supercooling [2]. The further the product temperature is below the thermodynamic freezing point, the greater is the degree of supercooling. When vials nucleate at greater degrees of supercooling, smaller ice crystals are generated. Further, when the upper layer of ice is sublimed from the frozen formulation, it leads to a narrow and tortuous path for the water vapor from the bottom part to escape, thus yielding higher dry layer resistance to vapor flow.

The temperature at which a vial nucleates depends on many factors including the formulation composition and the vial geometry. Additionally, vial imperfections and particulate load in the vial can both provide ice nucleation sites from which ice crystals can grow further. In a laboratory environment where the particulate level in the air is not well controlled, ice nucleation may occur at temperatures as low as 20 °C below the thermodynamic freezing point. In environments where particulate level is strictly controlled, such as in a Class 100 or Grade A zone, ice nucleation may occur at temperatures as low as 30 °C or more below the thermodynamic freezing point [3]. Therefore, the dry layer resistance (and therefore primary drying time) of a formulation during lyophilization may be higher when lyophilized in controlled areas. It has been demonstrated that for each 1 °C increase in ice nucleation temperature, the primary drying time can be reduced by about 3% [4, 5].

For formulations with proteins and/or amorphous excipients, the freezing phase typically involves a single ramp to the final freezing temperature. For formulations with crystalline excipients, an additional annealing step is generally required to fully crystallize the excipients. It is important to ensure complete crystallization of crystalline bulking components, such as mannitol or glycine, during the freezing phase to avoid vial breakage during primary drying as well as potential storage stability issues resulting from crystallization during storage [6].

Freezing heterogeneity, or uncontrolled vial nucleation, during the freezing phase could result in variable dry layer resistance in a batch. Lyophilization cycles must be conservative to ensure that the drying conditions do not lead to collapse in the vials with higher dry layer resistance. However, this leads to extra primary drying time to ensure that sublimation is complete in all vials prior to proceeding to secondary drying, while at the same time avoiding collapse in all vials. This may result in higher manufacturing costs, in an attempt to accommodate the heterogeneity associated with intra and inter-batch variations.

Reproducibility, repeatability, consistency, and process control are key objectives of the manufacturing process for parenteral drugs to ensure that each batch meets final product specifications [5]. Controlled Ice Nucleation (CIN) presents such an opportunity for users, by allowing for reduced variability in drug product resistance as well as reduced intra and inter- batch variability of product quality attributes. Further, with CIN, a more aggressive cycle can be achieved, without collapse.

This chapter will first address the various methods for inducing CIN along with some of their limitations. Then, the discussion will shift to the focus of this chapter: the ControLyo® Technology. Information about the technology will be presented, along with a discussion of the proposed mechanism for induction of ice nucleation. This will be followed by a discussion of the impact of process parameters on CIN process behavior along with a potential approach for developing a commercial CIN process in accordance with Quality by Design (QbD) principles.

2 Approaches to Control Ice Nucleation

There are many approaches with diverse mechanisms for inducing CIN. For instance, similar to ControLyo® Technology, the chamber pressure may be modulated by the SynchroFreeze™ Technology from HOF. While the ControLyo® Technology involves pressurization and then rapid depressurization of the chamber, the SynchroFreeze™ Technology involves decreasing the chamber pressure to approximately the vapor pressure of the solution to induce ice nucleation [7].

Alternatively, ice crystals may be seeded into the vials through the introduction of an ice fog into the chamber. This approach has been extensively studied for induction of ice nucleation [8, 9]. The VERISEQ™ Technology from IMA life is an example of a commercially available technology that uses ice fog to induce nucleation in the vials.

More exotic approaches may involve the addition of chemical nucleants or additives such as silver iodide, *Pseudomonas syringae* bacteria, or crystalline cholesterol [10]. Other approaches involve the use of electrofreezing [11] or mechanically induced nucleation through the use of ultrasonic vibration, shaking, tapping, or physical agitation [12]. Finally, vials may be pretreated by intentionally roughing, scratching, or otherwise creating imperfections on the finished surfaces to facilitate ice nucleation [13].

2.1 Commercial and Safety Considerations for Manufacturing Implementation

While the techniques described above have been proven to induce CIN in lab scale freeze dryers, there are fundamental concerns in implementing some of these techniques in commercial freeze dryers. In manufacturing sterile parenteral drugs, the use of chemical nucleants or additives may not be acceptable as these agents could be harmful to patients. Similarly, care must be taken to ensure that ice fog techniques do not impact patient safety by introducing chemical or biological contaminants into the product.

CIN can also be induced by mechanical shaking of the lyophilizer. The challenge of CIN via mechanical induction within larger commercial manufacturing freeze dryers, however, lies in providing consistent practical force needed to induce ice nucleation in all the vials. In addition, scalability issues and concerns of particle generation as a result of the mechanical disturbances within the chamber would require extensive assessment.

Methods involving pressure modulation are unlikely to present patient safety concerns. However, the pressure-rating of the lyophilizer should not be exceeded if the lyophilizer is pressurized to induce ice nucleation.

2.2 The ControLyo® Technology

The use of pressurization and depressurization as a potentially viable CIN technology for controlling ice nucleation was inspired by the observation of ice formation when opening a supercooled carbonated soda drink. When the pressurized container was opened, the contents immediately froze. This simple observation led to research evaluating the applicability of this observation to induce ice nucleation in vials in the freeze dryer. In collaboration with a contract manufacturing organization, researchers at Praxair, Inc. conducted several studies in larger commercial lyophilizers to demonstrate that the technology was viable for CIN during lyophilization process [5].

Praxair investigated CIN technology in 2005 in collaboration with the Center for Pharmaceutical and Processing Research (CPPR) research team. To better control and address the random ice nucleation observed in laboratory and manufacturing environments, Praxair piloted the CIN technology originally known as ControLyo® Nucleation On-Demand Technology, to provide a more consistent and reproducible method of controlling the ice nucleation during the freezing phase of lyophilization. Commercial introduction of this technology to the industry inspired many researchers to undertake additional CIN studies aimed at gathering a more coherent understanding of its benefits to product quality attributes and its overall application to commercial lyophilization manufacturing [3, 5].

In 2015, SP Industries, Inc. acquired ControLyo® Technology and all related patents from Praxair, Inc. Acquisition of the ControLyo® Technology by a full-scale equipment manufacturer were a major milestone in bringing this technology from the laboratory research and development environment to commercial manufacturing settings including retrofitting onto existing units regardless of lyophilizer manufacturer.

2.3 Overview of the ControLyo® Technology

ControLyo® Technology involves pressurization of the lyophilizer chamber with an inert gas followed by rapid depressurization to induce simultaneous ice nucleation in all the vials in the lyophilizer chamber, regardless of their location. A series of manifolds are installed to assist with the rapid depressurization of the inert gas. The manifold assembly is external to the lyophilizer chamber and, therefore, does not interfere with internal vapor flow, nor does it require supplementary piping internal to the chamber, which may otherwise necessitate further consideration during clean in place (CIP) process for effective cleaning coverage by spray nozzles or spray balls. Inert gas such as nitrogen, which is already an integral part of a lyophilization process at-scale, or argon can be easily and efficiently utilized in the CIN technique for pressurization and depressurization. It is important to note that sterile inert gas usage does not alter the formulation and does not require an abundance of development work to demonstrate its impact or lack thereof, to the stability of the formulation. In a typical process, sterile filter(s) are used at the inert gas inlet to the lyophilizer chamber. Filter integrity testing is conducted before and after use to demonstrate that the integrity of the filter remained intact for sterility assurance of the process. It may also be noted that use of the ControLyo® Technology is optional and controllable within the software, allowing the same dryer to easily accommodate products not requiring CIN. The ability to run any type of cycle without any changes to the internal and external equipment makes this technique a practical solution to maximizing usage and improving production output.

2.4 ControLyo® Technology: Case Studies

Examples mentioned in this section are intended to highlight how the CIN technology has evolved and to demonstrate the benefits of CIN in general. Early investigation of this technology explored the use of argon as inert gas for the experiments and demonstrated it to be more effective at inducing CIN than nitrogen. Additionally, CIN was demonstrated to result in cakes with significantly larger effective pore size and lower dry layer resistance than cakes produced with stochastic nucleation [3].

In a separate work, researchers from University of Connecticut examined the correlation between freezing heterogeneity and protein degradation [14]. The research work compared CIN and annealing process, for their impact on sodium phosphate buffer crystallization and degradation of β-galactosidase. Formulations were lyophilized using an annealing process during the freezing phase or ControLyo® Technology, without an additional annealing step. The lyophilized cakes were analyzed and the stability of the enzyme determined by enzyme activity assay, high performance liquid chromatography (HPLC), fluorescence spectroscopy, and dynamic light scattering (DLS). Annealed lyophilized formulations showed 12–40% loss of activity. In contrast, CIN formulations showed 9–14% loss of activity. Similar trends were observed for formulations without sodium phosphate buffer.

In another research work, Wang et al. investigated CIN for high and low concentration protein formulations and its application in vials and dual cartridge syringes [15]. Product temperature profiles for the CIN cycle demonstrated more uniform product temperatures. Improved cake appearance as compared to similar products run without CIN was observed during product visual inspection. Further, cycle time reduction for the products lyophilized with CIN was dramatically reduced by approximately 20%. It was also found that the reconstitution time for all formulations was shorter for products lyophilized with CIN. Shorter reconstitution time was attributed to the large pores that are the result of higher ice nucleation temperature during the freezing phase. For the highly concentrated product, CIN did not impact protein aggregation in high concentration protein formulations.

Awotwe-Otoo et al. used model monoclonal antibody (mAb) to determine the impact of ice nucleation temperature on lyophilization performance and quality attributes [16]. The nucleation temperatures as observed via product thermocouples (TC) installed in the vials ranged from −10 to −16.4 °C for the stochastic cycle. On the other hand, the nucleation temperatures for the CIN cycle occurred within a narrow temperature range of −2.3 °C to −3.2 °C. Warmer ice nucleation temperatures in the CIN cycle benefited the primary drying process by creating larger ice crystals and pores for removal of water vapor during the sublimation process. Product temperatures were observed to be lower than those of the stochastic cycle during primary drying. A higher sublimation rate was reported because of the lowered dry layer resistance for the CIN lyophilization cycle. Improvements in product quality attributes such as cake appearance, cake morphology, and vial to vial homogeneity were observed in products lyophilized with the CIN cycle.

3 Mechanism of Ice Nucleation Using the ControLyo® Technology

This section presents the authors' viewpoint on the mechanism behind ice nucleation during the pressurization-depressurization events of the ControLyo® Technology. A mechanistic understanding of the mechanism can help inform the selection of CIN parameter setpoints. The information presented here was derived from experiments conducted at Genentech [17].

Studies evaluating gas temperature changes during depressurization: The Joule-Thompson effect, a non-ideal temperature change in gases upon adiabatic expansion, has previously been proposed as the mechanism behind the induction of ice nucleation (unpublished data). For nitrogen gas with a pressure drop of 18 psi the expected magnitude of the Joule-Thompson effect is −0.33 °C.

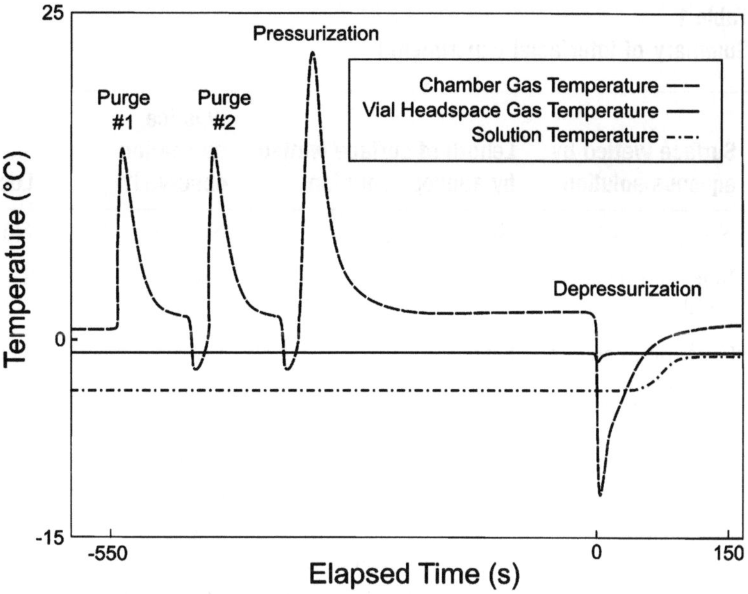

Fig. 1 Schematic of temperature changes upon purging and depressurization with nitrogen gas for a model aqueous formulation in glass vial

This theory is inconsistent with experimental data in which temperature changes of about −15 °C and about −1 °C were observed in the lyophilizer chamber gas and headspace of the vial respectively (Fig. 1). The observed temperature changes are more consistent with the gas doing work as it escapes the lyophilizer chamber through the restriction of the exhaust valve and competing mechanisms of heat transfer (radiation and gas conduction) contributing to the smaller change in the vial headspace.

Visual observation of ice nucleation events: The following observations were made using an aqueous drug solution contained in a glass vial. Shortly following depressurization, the first visual signs of ice nucleation can be seen at the liquid surface. These ice nuclei are only observed at the liquid surface and are notably absent from the liquid bulk. Within the next minute the ice nuclei grow to form dendritic ice crystals that grow as a front from the liquid surface and propagate toward the bottom of the vial. During this initial phase of ice growth, a small fraction of the water in the solution crystallizes. This initial fraction of crystallized water was estimated to be about 19% by Overcashier et al. when the nucleation temperature is −15 °C [18]. The remaining liquid solution after ice nucleation warms to the thermodynamic freezing point. The heat from the liquid solution is removed by the cold shelf surface and the remaining liquid solution freezes from the bottom of the vial upward.

Studies to understand the role of the liquid-gas interface: The highly localized origination of ice nuclei at the liquid surface suggests that a surface process could be a major contributing factor to the

Table 1
Summary of interfacial experiments

Surface wetted by aqueous solution	Length of surface wetted by aqueous solution	Was ice nucleation observed?	Location of ice nucleation
None	None	No	None
Inner perimeter of vial	Large	Yes	Thin aqueous film wetting inner perimeter of vial
Outer perimeter of glass tube	Small	Yes	Thin aqueous film wetting outer perimeter of glass tube

induction of ice nucleation. In order to probe the importance of the gas-liquid interface, several experiments were conducted in which the surface was modified by addition of silicone oil to the surface of the aqueous solution (Table 1). If vials are prepared such that a thin layer of silicone oil covers the entire surface and wets the vial walls, ice nucleation by depressurization is completely inhibited. If instead vials are prepared in such a way that the aqueous solution wets the walls of the vial (with silicone oil covering the remainder of the surface), ice nuclei are observed to originate in the thin film of aqueous solution exposed to the gas around the periphery of the vial. Such an experiment was further varied to introduce other small, hydrophilic glass objects penetrating the surface that can be wetted by the aqueous solution. In those cases, nuclei origination was only observed at the small liquid-gas interface. These observations suggest that the mechanical impulse of the depressurization alone is not responsible for CIN induction; rather a surface process involving direct contact of the aqueous drug solution with the gas plays a critical role in induction of ice nucleation. The fact that the surface process can operate effectively on the thin film of wetted surface also suggests that it acts over an extremely short length scale.

Possible ice nucleation mechanism: Based on these observations, the following mechanism is hypothesized (Fig. 2). Prior to the depressurization of the chamber, the concentration of water vapor in the vapor phase boundary layer above the aqueous solution is in equilibrium with the solution. Upon depressurization, the concentration of water in the vapor phase boundary layer decreases as the chamber pressure decreases, pulling the system away from equilibrium. To reestablish equilibrium, as part of an evaporative process, water is evolved from the liquid surface into the gas phase of the boundary layer. The water molecules most likely to move from the liquid phase to the gas phase are those with the highest energy, taking their kinetic energy with them as they leave the liquid phase. When viewed in the context of the thermodynamics, what results is a decrease in the average kinetic energy, and therefore temperature,

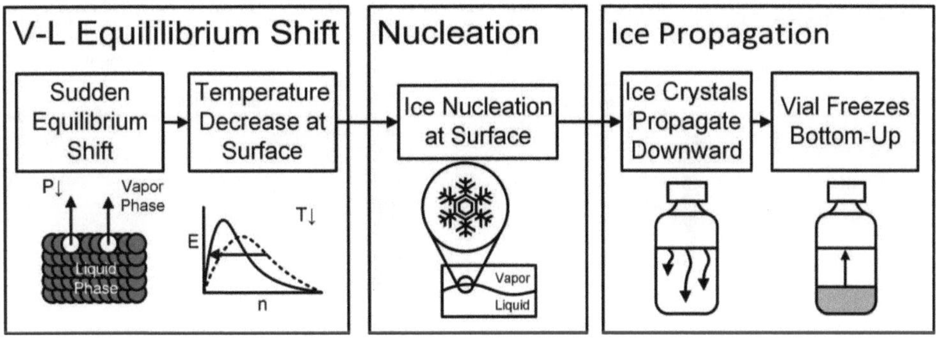

Fig. 2 Theory of operation hypothesis

of the surface of the liquid phase. It is hypothesized that this sudden, localized decrease in temperature is responsible for the induction of ice nucleation. In other words, the hypothesized mechanism of ice nucleation induction is evaporation driven by the depressurization of the chamber.

4 Important CIN Process Parameters

The CIN process can be conceptually divided into three phases, as illustrated in Fig. 3. These phases are Pre-Ice Nucleation Equilibration, Ice Nucleation, and Post-Ice Nucleation Freezing. The process parameters associated with each phase impact the ice nucleation and cake attributes. Therefore, an understanding of the effect of each process parameter is essential.

In a typical lyophilization cycle with CIN, vials are loaded onto the shelf at 5 °C and allowed to equilibrate. The chamber is purged with nitrogen (or argon) gas and then pressurized to the target CIN pressure. The shelf temperature setpoint is ramped to a temperature which will adequately supercool the vials and the vials are allowed to equilibrate. The chamber is then rapidly depressurized to induce ice nucleation in all the vials. The shelf temperature setpoint may then be maintained for a set amount of time to allow for ice crystal growth or may immediately be ramped to the final freeze temperature. After equilibration at the final freezing temperature, the lyophilization cycle then proceeds to the drying phase.

4.1 Pre-Ice Nucleation Equilibration

The purpose of the pre-ice nucleation equilibration phase is to ensure that the temperature at the liquid surface in each vial is cold enough to achieve reliable ice nucleation. Theoretically, the temperature at the liquid surface needs only to be colder than the thermodynamic freezing point of the formulation. This temperature is around −1 to −2 °C in many aqueous sucrose-based pharmaceutical formulations [19]. In practice, the liquid surface

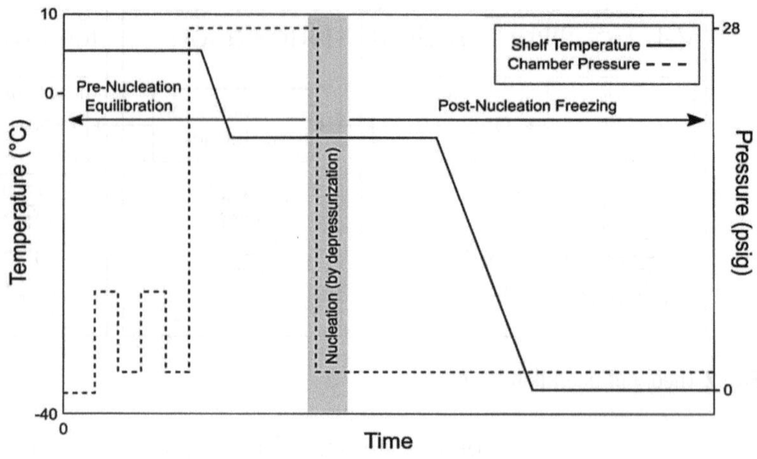

Fig. 3 Outline of CIN phases and parameters

temperature may be required to be 3–10 °C colder than the thermodynamic freezing point to ensure robust ice nucleation (ice nucleation in all vials).

The parameters most important in controlling the liquid surface temperature are the shelf temperature setpoint and the hold time prior to depressurization. These two parameters should be set to ensure that the liquid surface temperature has equilibrated prior to proceeding to the ice nucleation phase to ensure consistent behavior between different lyophilization runs. Equilibration behavior can be impacted by a number of factors including shelf temperature variability, shelf wetness (wet shelves facilitate faster cooling), and vial fill height. Importantly, the temperature at the bottom of the vial will be different from the temperature at the liquid surface. Therefore, when determining the necessary equilibration time, it is helpful to have thermocouples placed at the top of the liquid.

Note that a shelf temperature setpoint that is too cold may result in some vials stochastically nucleating before the ice nucleation step which can alter the ice crystal size and impact cake attributes (further discussed in Sect. 4.3). This is a bigger concern in the lab environment where the ambient particle load is higher, but is also a concern in a production environment. We have found that a shelf temperature setpoint between −5 and −10 °C strikes a good compromise between ice nucleation robustness and ice crystal size for most vial sizes. The impact of process parameters on ice crystal size is discussed in Sect. 4.3.

4.2 Ice Nucleation

Once all vials have equilibrated at the shelf temperature set point for CIN, the chamber is rapidly depressurized to induce ice nucleation. As described in Sect. 3, it is theorized that depressurization causes extremely localized surface cooling, resulting in ice nucleation. The extent of cooling at the liquid surface is controlled by the depressurization rate and the depressurization time. The depressurization rate may be inferred from the depressurization time and the total pressure drop. This has important implications for Quality by Design (QbD) strategy, as only depressurization time and total pressure drop are easy to quantify.

Of the depressurization rate, depressurization time, and total pressure drop, none are directly controllable process parameters. These variables are instead controlled by the initial chamber pressure setpoint, final chamber pressure setpoint, the depressurization offset, and the exhaust system of the lyophilizer. Controlling these parameters to maximize the depressurization rate and pressure drop will result in greater ice nucleation robustness. For instance, on the LyoStar 3 freeze dryer equipped with ControLyo® Technology, the initial chamber pressure setpoint can be set to a maximum of 28.5 psig and the final chamber pressure setpoint is frequently set to 2 psig. Without any restriction of the exhaust vent and a depressurization offset of 2 psig, the depressurization time is approximately 2 s. These nucleation parameter settings, combined with a proper shelf temperature, result in robust ice nucleation for most vial sizes, fill volumes, and formulations. Anecdotal experience within the industry is that use of argon may result in slightly more robust ice nucleation than nitrogen [3]. However, due to ready availability of nitrogen in the manufacturing environment, use of nitrogen is recommended.

It is important to define what is meant by the terms "depressurization time," "final chamber pressure," and "depressurization offset." As can be seen in Fig. 4, during depressurization, the pressure reaches a minimum and then recovers to some final value. It is believed that the surface cooling process happens quickly relative to the depressurization rate, meaning that evaporation (and therefore cooling) only occurs during the initial phase of

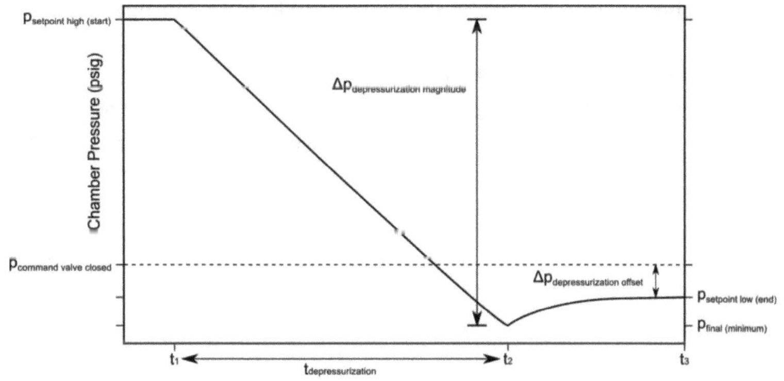

Fig. 4 Diagram of CIN depressurization process with labeled values

depressurization. On that basis, we have defined depressurization time to be the time from the moment the pressure begins to drop to the minimum of the pressure trace. Additionally, we have defined the final chamber pressure to be the pressure value at the minimum of the pressure trace. This is not the only way to define these variables, but these definitions facilitate the development of a QbD methodology and are believed to reflect the physical processes at work during depressurization. Finally, the depressurization offset defines the pressure value at which the chamber exhaust valve will start to close. To appreciate the impact of the depressurization offset, consider the sequence of events for the depressurization illustrated in Fig. 4. The chamber exhaust valve opens and the chamber depressurizes. The final chamber pressure is set to 2 psig and the depressurization offset is also set to 2 psig—their sum is 4 psig. Once the pressure reaches 4 psig, the chamber exhaust valve begins to close. The valve does not close instantaneously, so the chamber pressure continues to drop until it reaches 2 psig and the chamber valve is completely closed. The pressure then increases as the formerly moving gas becomes static.

Setting the depressurization parameters is somewhat of a trial and error exercise. Control of the depressurization time and pressure drop requires simultaneously setting the initial chamber pressure setpoint, final chamber pressure setpoint, the depressurization offset, and the level of exhaust path restriction. Table 2 has been included to provide the reader with an intuitive sense of how these parameters interact. This data set was generated on a Lyostar 3 equipped with ControLyo® Technology. A DiaFlo rotary valve was used to restrict the exhaust flow path. The number of valve turns refer to the number of turns from fully open (zero valve turns means the valve is fully open and the exhaust flow path is unrestricted; four turns mean that the valve is fully closed).

Table 2
Example parameters to control depressurization time and final chamber pressure in Lyostar 3

Initial chamber pressure setpoint (psig)	Final chamber pressure setpoint (psig)	Pressure offset (psig)	Number of valve turns	Depressurization time (s)	Final chamber pressure (psig)
27	2	4	0	2.1	2.2
22	2	3.5	1.25	2.2	2.3
17	2	3.1	1.5	1.9	2.2
12	2	2	2.25	2.3	2.1

There are three important considerations for commercial scale lyophilizers. First, the maximum pressure rating of the lyophilizer limits the achievable initial chamber pressure. While most commercial lyophilizers are rated for steam-in-place pressures, the actual pressure rating can vary from lyophilizer to lyophilizer. A safety margin is also applied based on that rating. For instance, a lyophilizer rated for 25 psig may only be pressurized to 20 psig during routine operation. It is important that the limits of the lyophilizers in the network be considered when developing CIN conditions in the lab.

Second, the depressurization rate of a commercial lyophilizer depends on the number and size of available ports on the machine. A fast depressurization time (e.g., 2 s) may require the use of multiple ports connected to an exhaust manifold or may otherwise be unfeasible. This in itself brings up two important points:

One: Different lyophilizers may depressurize at different rates. It is easiest to transfer CIN parameters from one lyophilizer to another in the network if they can achieve similar depressurization times, so an effort should be made to achieve comparable performance. Vendors are able to provide estimates of depressurization time at-scale based on an understanding of the at-scale chamber volume, exhaust dimensions, and desired pressurization and depressurization values. Depending on isolation valve rating, condenser chamber volume may also need to be considered. These estimates may be used as part of an assessment of CIN retrofit options and its overall feasibility for a given lyophilizer.

Two: When developing a CIN protocol in the lab, worst-case depressurization times should be evaluated (i.e., they should exceed the expected depressurization times of the commercial lyophilizers). This facilitates transfer of CIN protocols to lyophilizers with longer depressurization times in the future as well as helps to establish the design space which can be leveraged to cover manufacturing deviations. More details of developing a CIN protocol following QbD methodology are discussed in Sect. 5.

Third, it is important to note that, regardless of whether the lyophilizer is vented into the unclassified maintenance space or into an exhaust manifold, the sterility of the lyophilizer must be maintained through all operations (including multiple pressurization and depressurization cycles, if allowed by the CIN strategy). This can be accomplished with an appropriately designed valve and automation strategy. This approach requires that positive pressure be maintained within the lyophilizer any time the valve(s) is/are open and that valve sequencing facilitate multiple pressurizations and depressurizations.

4.3 Post-ice Nucleation Freezing

The lyophilized cake structure is strongly influenced by the thermal treatment protocol post-ice nucleation [20]. During CIN, only a small fraction of the water in each vial is frozen, and further crystal growth ensues during the post-ice nucleation freezing phase. Therefore, subsequent thermal treatment strongly influences the ice crystal growth rate and thus the ice crystal size and structure. This, in turn, impacts lyophilized cake attributes including residual moisture, cake-specific surface area (SSA), and potentially the stress degradation profile and reconstitution time.

The relevant thermal treatment parameters for controlling ice crystal size are the shelf temperature, post-ice nucleation hold time, and freeze ramp rate. Ice crystal size increases with warmer shelf temperatures, longer post-ice nucleation hold times, and slower freeze ramp rates. As an example, holding nucleated vials at the ice nucleation temperature prior to initiating the freeze ramp will result in larger ice crystals than immediately beginning the freeze ramp. Similarly, holding the vials at a warmer temperature (but still colder than the thermodynamic freezing point) will result in larger crystals. It should be expected that smaller vials with lower fill volumes will take less time to freeze than larger vials with higher fill volumes due to their lower thermal mass. This means that a shorter post-nucleation hold is required to completely freeze smaller vials.

The freeze ramp rate can also be modified to control the cake structure. Slower ramp rates will result in larger ice crystals. To maximize ice crystal size, we have found that it is generally quicker to do a post-ice nucleation hold rather than a very slow ramp to the final freeze temperature. Note that larger ice crystals decrease cake SSA and cake resistance [18], and the residual moisture may increase if the secondary drying time or temperature is not increased to compensate [16].

In addition to maximizing ice crystal size (and therefore, minimizing the cake resistance and primary drying time), CIN results in less inter-vial variability in certain critical quality attributes including SSA and residual moisture content, as compared to lyophilized drug product with conventional stochastic ice nucleation. Due to the stochastic nature of conventional ice nucleation, all vials freeze at different temperatures and therefore also experience different post-ice nucleation thermal treatment during the freeze ramp. By ensuring that all vials freeze at similar temperature and experience the same thermal treatment post-ice nucleation, CIN results in lower inter-vial variability.

Table 3
Parameters impacting CIN

Parameters impacting success of CIN	Typical range	Criteria for more robust nucleation
Shelf temperature setpoint (before ice nucleation)	−5 to −15 °C	Colder shelf temperature
Hold time (before ice nucleation)	2–4 h	Longer hold time
Initial chamber pressure	15–30 psig	Higher initial chamber pressure
Final chamber pressure	1–4 psig	Lower final chamber pressure
Depressurization time	1–3 s	Shorter depressurization time
Parameters impacting cake attributes	**Typical range**	**Criteria for larger ice crystals**
Shelf temperature setpoint (after ice nucleation)	−5 to −15 °C	Warmer shelf temperature
Hold time (after ice nucleation)	0–5 h	Longer hold time
Ramp rate (after ice nucleation)	0.1–1 °C min^{-1}	Slower ramp rate

4.4 Summary and Practical Considerations

The Pre-Ice Nucleation Equilibration and Ice Nucleation steps impact the robustness of ice nucleation during CIN, whereas the Post-Ice Nucleation Freezing step impacts the resultant cake structure. Table 3 summarizes the important parameters, common ranges, and their general effect on ice nucleation robustness.

When designing a CIN process, it is important to bear in mind that smaller vials have been observed to be more difficult to nucleate, compared to larger vials. This may necessitate the use of colder shelf temperatures or altering other parameters. If the shelf temperature is decreased to improve nucleation robustness, be aware that some vials may nucleate early if the shelf temperature is set too cold.

5 Quality by Design for Controlled Ice Nucleation Component of a Lyophilization Cycle

Quality by design (QbD) refers to the philosophy of building, rather than testing, quality into the product. For the CIN component of the lyophilization cycle, a QbD approach would ensure that the employed CIN parameters are robust and lead to successful, reproducible CIN performance, from one batch to another, and for all the vials within a batch.

CIN parameters and their overall impact on CIN performance are defined in Sect. 4. Table 3 divides CIN parameters into the parameters impacting ice nucleation initiation (i.e., success of CIN) and those impacting cake attributes (including SSA, residual moisture, and stress degradation). Each parameter type is discussed in subsequent subsections.

To develop the CIN component of a lyophilization cycle, a risk ranking and filtering (RRF) approach should be first performed, to identify the CIN parameters of importance for the product under consideration. Further, using the QbD approach, the multivariate acceptable ranges (MAR) for each of the identified CIN parameters can be defined using small-scale experiments. Small-scale CIN studies could be performed to define and demonstrate robustness of the CIN MARs and then the CIN MARs can be verified at-scale during technical and product performance qualification (PPQ) CIN lyophilization runs.

5.1 Studies to Assess Parameters Impacting Success of Controlled Ice Nucleation

Figure 5 visually depicts the impact of CIN parameters on success of CIN. Figure 5 has been simplified to two dimensions for visualization purposes. The red zone represents a combination of CIN parameters that could lead to failed CIN (i.e., successful CIN in only some or no vials in the batch). The light green zone depicts a multivariate zone that represents a successful CIN outcome (i.e., successful CIN in all the vials). Pursuant to the QbD approach, CIN experiments could be performed to define conditions near the green-red interface in Fig. 5. This approach therefore avoids testing for conditions that are theoretically known to lead to unsuccessful CIN (i.e., the red zone), and thus saves both time and resources. The green-red interface represents the minimum successful conditions for CIN. Once the interface parameter settings are delineated, target CIN parameter settings could be finalized for at-scale CIN operation. Target CIN conditions should be based on both small-scale CIN MAR ranges as well as at-scale manufacturing limitations (e.g., achievable pressure drop for CIN at-scale). To ensure successful and reproducible CIN at-scale, a conservative approach should be pursued, wherein target CIN parameters are further restricted

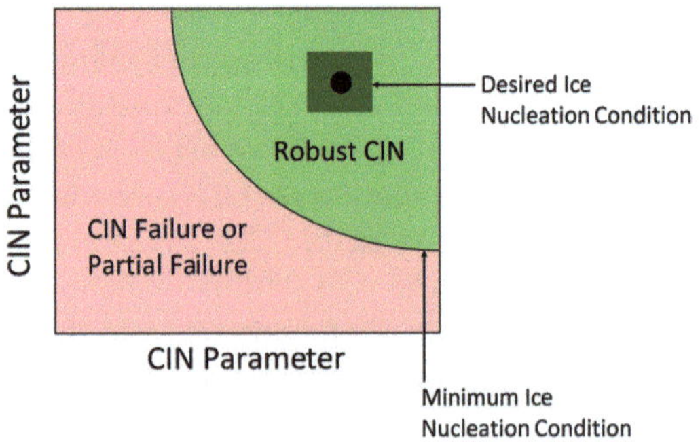

Fig. 5 Strategy to evaluate CIN parameters for impact on ice nucleation initiation. The red and green zones represent unsuccessful and successful CIN conditions, respectively. CIN parameters include shelf temperature, hold time before ice nucleation, initial chamber pressure, final chamber pressure, and depressurization time

within the MAR space, as illustrated by the dark green square box within the green zone, in Fig. 5.

In one development approach, the shelf temperature for CIN can be selected first, followed by determination of minimum ice nucleation conditions at the selected target shelf temperature for CIN. The shelf temperature setpoint for CIN is generally selected by the process development team, based on factors delineated in Sect. 4.1. Additionally, shelf temperature variability at-scale may be available based on existing shelf mapping studies at-scale. Once the shelf temperature set point for CIN and shelf temperature variability are known, a small-scale study could be performed at the worst-case CIN shelf temperature set point (based on at-scale shelf temperature variability), to determine the minimum hold time needed to reach solution equilibration at the CIN shelf set point. For example, if the desired shelf temperature set point for CIN is −10 °C, and the at-scale shelf temperature variability is ±2 °C, the small-scale study should be performed at −8 °C. Multiple thermocouples in representative vials (edge and center) could be used to determine the minimum hold time for CIN. Since ice nucleation happens at the solution surface, the liquid surface temperature could be used as a marker to determine vial equilibration, and thus the hold time. It may, however, be noted that the hold time determined at small-scale needs to be verified at-scale due to scale-up differences, including differences in shelf cooling, shelf wetness, and vial quantity between small-scale and at-scale. Confirmation of the hold time can be performed during CIN technical runs at-scale.

Depending on the lyophilizer exhaust manifold and depressurization valve design, theoretical depressurization time could further be predicted, as mentioned in Sect. 4.2. Once CIN shelf temperature, hold time, and the worst-case depressurization time are defined, additional small-scale CIN studies could be performed to determine the minimum pressure needed for successful CIN, which can be assessed visually.

In an orthogonal approach to determine CIN MARs, especially for small vial sizes or for cases where pressurization to a higher value is limited, the maximum possible pressure drop at-scale could first be determined theoretically and then the target worst-case shelf temperature needed to achieve CIN could be determined. In both cases, a very low temperature for CIN should not be selected as it may lead to stochastic ice nucleation, before inducing CIN, as well as lead to smaller ice crystals, and thus higher dry layer resistance to sublimation.

To determine CIN MARs, small-scale CIN experiments should be performed using the same CIN technology (i.e., pressurization/depressurization) as intended for the at-scale use. Further, use of statistics could be employed to ensure predictability of at-scale CIN behavior for a large set of vials, based on small-scale CIN studies utilizing fewer vials. Multiple small-scale CIN studies may be performed at the worst-case CIN conditions, to determine the reproducibility of CIN at small-scale, and to help select robust CIN parameters for at-scale CIN operation. Also, since pressure drop and depressurization time are the main determinants for success of CIN by pressurization/depressurization technique, data generated with small-scale experiments (to determine the minimum ice nucleation conditions for CIN) can be considered representative of at-scale CIN performance, as long as similar pressure drop and depressurization time are achieved at-scale.

5.2 Studies to Assess the Parameters Impacting Cake Attributes

This section discusses studies to evaluate CIN parameters impacting cake attributes (e.g., SSA and residual moisture), including the CIN shelf temperature setpoint and post-ice nucleation hold time.

In certain unforeseen instances, there may be a delay in ramping down to the final freeze temperature after successful CIN and/or hold time at CIN shelf set point. To cover for such deviations, a range of hold times post CIN (e.g., 0–12 h) could be evaluated in a small-scale CIN study. This study should be performed at both edges of shelf temperature set point for CIN, based on shelf temperature variability (generally ±2–3 °C) at-scale. For example, if the target shelf temperature set point for CIN is −10 °C, and the at-scale shelf temperature variability is ±2 °C, the small-scale study should be performed at −8 °C and −12 °C. Impact on product quality attributes (such as SSA, residual moisture, and stress degradation) could be evaluated, based on the RRF for the lyophilized product under consideration. This study would define the minimum/maximum allowable hold time post-ice nucleation at-scale, before ramp down to the final freezing temperature.

Generally, target post-ice nucleation hold time is defined by the lyophilization cycle. However, this study may also include evaluation of a minimum post-ice nucleation hold time, thus covering a broader range of post-ice nucleation hold time. Any manufacturing deviation longer than the validated post-ice nucleation hold time may need to be supported with additional studies, including assessment of impact to product quality.

Scale-up differences due to factors including differences in vial heat transfer coefficient (K_v), differences in ice nucleation temperature, as well as lyophilizer design impart differences in lyophilization performance between small-scale and at-scale. Since CIN eliminates scale-up variability due to differences in ice nucleation temperature (because the product is nucleated at the same CIN shelf temperature at both small-scale and at-scale), the CIN data developed at small-scale can be considered to better represent the at-scale CIN performance.

5.3 Strategy to Assess Impact of Deviations in Controlled Ice Nucleation

In certain unforeseen situations, the process may perform outside the MARs (as confirmed by temperature and/or pressure-time traces during depressurization step) and thus the CIN run may be unsuccessful. In this case, the strategy for the batch should be clearly outlined. One possible option is to repeat the CIN operation (i.e., perform a second pressurization and depressurization) of the whole batch, at the same shelf temperature setpoint for CIN, as used for the first depressurization. The assumption here is that during the repeat CIN operation, vials that did not nucleate in the first failed (or partially failed) CIN operation, would nucleate during the second CIN, as the conditions may be more optimal during second CIN (i.e., within the CIN MARs). To achieve this, vials may be maintained at the same shelf temperature setpoint for CIN after the first failed CIN, pressurized to the set value, held for a certain duration, and then depressurized again to induce CIN in the non-nucleated vials. However, if there were a repeat failure to achieve the acceptable CIN parameters (i.e., during CIN reprocessing), it could be up to the process development team to decide if a third CIN operation (i.e., third CIN pressurization and depressurization) should be performed.

One of the underlying questions regarding the second CIN operation could be its impact on product quality. In case of a partially successful CIN operation, some of the vials may nucleate while the others may fail to nucleate. In such cases, a second CIN operation would subject the already nucleated vials (hereinafter referred to as the first nucleators; nucleated during the first pressurization-depressurization) to a second pressurization-depressurization. The impact of second CIN operation on product quality attributes (including residual moisture, SSA and stress degradation) should be assessed.

Another possible manufacturing variable for the second CIN operation is the maximum allowable hold time after the first failed CIN operation, before performing the second CIN operation. For the "first nucleators" resulting from the first (fully or partially failed) CIN operation, the hold time before the second CIN operation would be akin to a post-ice nucleation hold time, which may reduce the SSA of the resulting lyophilized cake, as well as progressively increase the residual moisture of resultant lyophilized drug product. It is to be noted that this would only happen in the "first nucleators," and not in the rest of non-nucleated vials from the first CIN operation. Small-scale CIN study comparing a "re-nucleation" batch to a "single CIN" batch could be performed to define the impact of renucleation on drug product attributes as well as to determine the maximum allowable hold time before which renucleation needs to be performed. Data from the small-scale CIN study to evaluate impact of post-ice nucleation hold time on product attributes (e.g., SSA, residual moisture and stress degradation) could also be leveraged.

5.4 Design of a Robust Controlled Ice Nucleation Cycle

Based on CIN ranges determined at small-scale, MARs for at-scale CIN operation can be defined. Furthermore, scale-up of CIN conditions may be evaluated during at-scale technical CIN runs, and could be performed with target or worst-case CIN parameters determined at small scale.

Successful at-scale CIN performance can be evaluated by CIN depressurization traces, visual assessment of the resultant lyophilized cake for the presence of characteristic long ice crystals, as well as assessment of resultant cake attributes (i.e., SSA, residual moisture, and stress degradation). Since CIN may lead to perceptible differences in cake structure, visual evaluation of cake structure could be a useful additional indicator of successful CIN. Furthermore, CIN generally leads to a significantly lower SSA and higher residual moisture (compared to cakes prepared with uncontrolled ice nucleation), which could be used as an indicator of successful CIN.

Based on successful CIN performance at-scale, final validation batches with target CIN parameters may be performed.

6 Summary

CIN is a recent breakthrough technology aimed at optimizing the freezing phase of the lyophilization cycle. CIN technology reduces intra and inter-vial variability, and has the potential to improve lyophilized cake attributes, including residual moisture, reconstitution time and cake appearance as well as reduce the primary drying time.

Numerous CIN technologies, varying in their mechanical design, are available. The ControLyo® technology involves pressurization and depressurization of the chamber and has been extensively studied. Experiments to identify the mechanism by which ControLyo® induces CIN suggest surface evaporation as the contributing factor.

Design of a robust CIN lyophilization cycle requires an understanding of the impact of process parameters (including shelf temperature, hold times, and chamber pressure) on ice nucleation robustness as well as the resulting cake structure and primary drying behavior. A QbD approach is proposed to develop the at-scale CIN lyophilization cycle by performing multivariate small-scale CIN experiments to determine the minimum ice nucleation conditions, to understand the impact of CIN variables on cake attributes, and to cover deviations, followed by at-scale experiments to verify performance. Such an approach would ensure reproducible CIN performance at-scale from one batch to another, and between different vials in a lyophilization cycle.

References

1. Schneid SC, Gieseler H (2012) Rational approaches and transfer strategies for the scale-up of freeze-drying cycles. Chemistry Today 30(2):9–12
2. Tang X, Pikal MJ (2004) Design of freeze-drying process for pharmaceuticals: practical advice. Pharm Res 21(2):191–200
3. Konstantinidis AK, Kuu W, Otten L, Nail SL, Sever RR (2011) Controlled nucleation in freeze-drying: effects on pore size in the dried product later, mass transfer resistance, and primary drying rate. J Pharm Sci 100(8):3458–3470
4. Searles JA, Carpenter T, Randolph TW (2001) The ice nucleation temperature determines the primary drying rate of lyophilization for samples frozen on a temperature controlled shelf. J Pharm Sci 90(7):860–871
5. Bursac R, Sever R, Hunek B (2009) A practical method for resolving the nucleation problem in lyophilization. BioProcess Int 7(9):66–72
6. Williams NA, Lee Y, Polli GP, Jennings TA (1986) The effects of cooling rate on solid phase transitions and associated vial breakage occurring in frozen mannitol solution. J Parenter Sci Technol 40(4):135–141
7. Allmendinger A et al (2016) Controlled nucleation during freeze drying using vacuum-induced surface freezing. Database no. 633018. http://www.researchdisclosure.com
8. Rambhatla S, Ramot R, Bhugra C, Pikal MJ (2004) Heat and mass transfer scale-up issues during freeze drying: II. Control and characterization of the degree of supercooling. AAPS PharmSciTech 5(4):54–62
9. Winter G (2015) Current trends and challenge in freeze drying of biologics. ISLFD 7th International Conference, Barcelona
10. Morris GJ, Acton E (2013) Controlled ice nucleation in cryopreservation – a review. Cryobiology 66(2):85–92
11. Petersen A, Schneider H, Rau G, Glasmacher B (2006) New approach for freezing aqueous solutions under active control of the nucleation temperature. Cryobiology 53(2):248–257
12. Hobbs PV (1974) Ice physics. Oxford University Press, New York, NY
13. Tsotsas E, Mujumdar AS (2011) Modern drying technology, volume 3: product quality and formulation. Wiley-VCH, Weinheim
14. Mudhivarthi VK (2015) Controlled ice nucleation in freeze drying: freezing heterogeneity and protein stability. SP Scientific Lyolearn Webinar. http://www.spscientific.com/LyoTech-Center/LyoLearn-Webinars-Archive.aspx
15. Wang B (2016) Application of controlled nucleation during lyophilization to improve cake appearance and product quality. SP Scientific Lyolearn Webinar. http://www.spscientific.com/LyoTech-Center/LyoLearn-Webinars-Archive.aspx
16. Awotwe-Otoo D, Agarabi C, Read EK, Lute S, Brorson KA, Khan MA, Shah RB (2013) Impact of controlled ice nucleation on process performance and quality attributes of a lyophilized monoclonal antibody. Int J Pharm 450 (1-2):70–78
17. Magill G (2015) Application of controlled ice nucleation for lyophilization of a low glass transition temperature solution. PepTalk Conference Podium Presentation–Cambridge Healthtech Institute's 14th Annual Conference
18. Patapoff T, Overcashier D (2002) The importance of freezing on lyophilization cycle development. BioPharm 15(3):16–21 72
19. Pongsawatmanit R, Miyawaki O (1993) Measurement of temperature-dependent ice fraction in frozen foods. Biosci Biotechnol Biochem 57(10):1650–1654
20. Bhatnagar BS, Bogner RH, Pikal MJ (2007) Protein stability during freezing: separation of stresses and mechanisms of protein stabilization. Pharm Dev Technol 12(5):505–523

Chapter 4

Alternative Methods of Controlling Nucleation in Freeze Drying

Roberto Pisano

Abstract

The control of freezing, and particularly of the nucleation temperature, is one of the most challenging aspects of the development of a lyophilization cycle. Technological advances of recent years have increased the efficiency with which nucleation temperature can be adjusted. This chapter discusses these technologies, as well as some emerging technologies that might play an important role in near future. In particular each technology is presented in terms of easy to be implemented, scalability on industrial units, influence on product morphology, protein preservation, intra-vial and vial-to-vial heterogeneity, and process performance.

Key words Control, Freezing, Nucleation

Abbreviations

HES Hydroxyethyl starch
SSA Specific surface area
VISF Vacuum-induced surface freezing

Symbols

D_p Pore size, m
J_w Vapour flux, kg m^{-2} s^{-1}
M_w Molecular weight of water, kg mol^{-1}
P_{ice} Vapour pressure of ice, Pa
P_w Partial pressure of water inside the drying chamber, Pa
R_p Resistance to mass transfer, m s^{-1}
R Ideal gas constant, J mol^{-1} K^{-1}
T_g' Glass transition temperature, K
T_{eu} Eutectic temperature, K
T_n Nucleation temperature, K

Kevin R. Ward and Paul Matejtschuk (eds.), *Lyophilization of Pharmaceuticals and Biologicals: New Technologies and Approaches*, Methods in Pharmacology and Toxicology, https://doi.org/10.1007/978-1-4939-8928-7_4,

Greek Letters

ε Porosity of the lyophilized product, –
τ Tortuosity of the lyophilized product, –

1 Introduction

Freezing is a process in which water is separated, as ice crystals, from a supercooled solution. The typical temperature trend that can be observed during freezing of a pharmaceutical solution is shown in Fig. 1. The solution is first cooled until nucleation of ice occurs. This event results in a rapid increase in product temperature and corresponds to step $\overline{AB}$ in Fig. 1. The second step ($\overline{BC}$) is the growth of these new crystals, which promote the cryo-concentration of the solution. During this step, product temperature remains constant until the completion of the solidification process. Then, the frozen solution is further cooled down ($\overline{DE}$) and equilibrated at a specified temperature. It must be noted that, in lyophilization science, there exists a clear distinction between the rate of cooling and that of freezing. The former refers to the rate at which a solution is cooled, while the latter measures the rate of

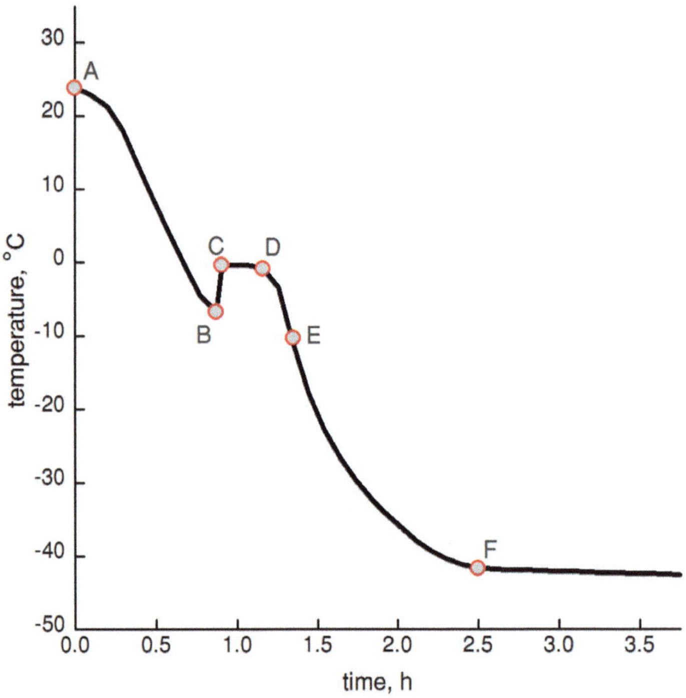

Fig. 1 The temperature profile of a pharmaceutical solution during freezing

decrease in temperature, as observed in a specified position within the sample, once nucleation occurred. It follows that the freezing rate also depends on the extent of supercooling and can thus differ from the cooling rate. It is well established that ice crystal size and, hence, other product and process parameters correlate to the nucleation temperature, which thus plays a key role in the development of a successful lyophilization cycle. To make sense of this, and to understand how the various methodologies impacts on product quality and overall process performance require some knowledge of crystallization and freezing. In this chapter, the basics of freezing and the most recent controlled nucleation technologies are discussed, with emphasis on the benefits that these technologies can offer in terms of product quality, vial-to vial and batch-to-batch uniformity, and scalability of a lyophilization cycle.

2 Fundamentals of Freezing

A pharmaceutical solution does not spontaneously freeze at its thermodynamic freezing point when it is cooled down but remains liquid far below this temperature. The difference between the thermodynamic freezing point and the temperature at which the first ice crystals are formed, also known as the nucleation temperature, is termed supercooling. Supercooling strongly depends on the composition of the solution, as well as on the freezing methodology. As aforementioned, crystallization of ice from a solution can be described as a two-step process, nucleation, and crystal growth or solidification. Nucleation corresponds to the phase separation of new crystals, which become larger and larger during crystal growth.

Nucleation can be divided into two further steps, primary and secondary nucleation [1]. Primary nucleation corresponds to the formation of the first stable nuclei and is followed by secondary nucleation, also referred to as crystallization, which proceeds with a velocity of mm s^{-1} and involves a larger portion of the liquid volume [2]. Secondary nucleation terminates as the nucleated liquid approaches its equilibrium freezing point. Primary nucleation occurs independently of the presence of crystalline surfaces which, by contrast, are actively involved in secondary nucleation. Primary nucleation can then occur through two mechanisms, homogeneous and heterogeneous nucleation. Because of suspended impurities and physical features, primary nucleation is mostly heterogeneous. This is true for all pharmaceutical solutions, which are sterile-filtered and use water for injection; water clusters are thus formed via adsorption of water molecules on a foreign substance such as the vial wall, particulate, or some proteins [3]. Nonetheless, although homogeneous nucleation is rarely observed in practice, it has been largely investigated because it constitutes the basis for several nucleation theories.

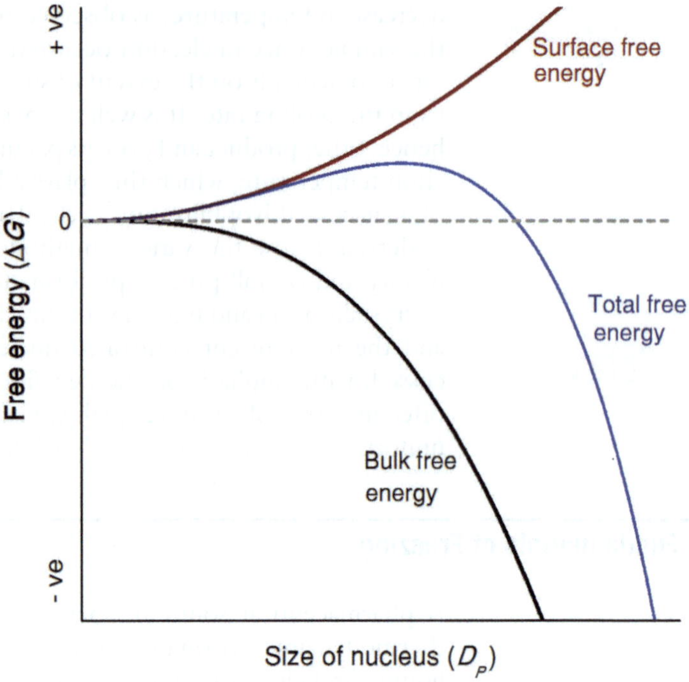

Fig. 2 Free energy diagram for the nucleation of spherical nuclei

The supercooled solution is not in equilibrium. Although the mean density of the solution is constant, local fluctuations in concentration give rise to ordered structures or clusters, with persistent hydrogen bonds [4], and structurally similar to ice crystals. The Gibbs free energy for the formation of these clusters is the sum of the change in free energy resulting from the formation of the nucleus surface (a positive quantity) and that for the phase transformation (a negative quantity). As can be seen in Fig. 2, the nucleation is a spontaneous process (decrease in free energy) only if clusters are greater than a critical size. It follows that smaller clusters tend to dissolve, whereas larger clusters grow until they reach a critical size beyond which a new phase is formed.

It is well known that the presence of a foreign substance reduces the free energy barrier to be overcome for nucleation. Consequently, nucleation in a heterogeneous system occurs at a higher temperature than a homogeneous system, i.e., −40 °C for pure water [5]. Besides, Volmer [6] observed that the decrease in free energy correlates with the contact, or wetting, angle of the solid phase.

Once stable nuclei have been formed, they grow larger by the addition of further water molecules from the progressively cryo-concentrated solution. This process is referred to as crystal growth and, along with nucleation, determines the final distribution of ice crystal size. It must be noted that this process is not instantaneous since only a part of the supercooled water can immediately freeze. In fact, the supercooled solution can absorb 15 cal g^{-1}, whereas the heat released by the solidification process is 79 cal g^{-1} [7]. Consequently, once crystallization takes place, the product temperature suddenly increases up to the thermodynamic freezing point. Then, heat is continuously removed by further cooling and allows the product temperature to remain constant as the crystallization of the remaining water occurs. Once all water has been frozen, the product temperature starts to decrease as shown in Fig. 1 (EF).

The number of stable nuclei formed during nucleation, the rate of ice crystal growth, and the mean size of ice crystals strongly depend on the extent of supercooling. An understanding of this relationship is important and very useful in the selection of the most appropriate freezing methodology and process conditions. Generally, a very low nucleation temperature promotes the formation of many stable nuclei and hence very small ice crystals. By contrast, the higher the nucleation temperature, the smaller the number of stable nuclei, and the larger the final ice crystals formed. The rate of freezing depends on both the degree of supercooling and the cooling rate. As concerns this last dependence, the rate of freezing is inversely correlated with the cooling rate only in the case of global supercooling, whereas it is directly correlated for the directional freezing. The global supercooling is typical, e.g., of shelf-ramped freezing, which is characterized by almost uniform supercooling and solidification occurs within the entire already-nucleated volume of solution. By contrast, directional freezing is common in quench freezing when only a small portion of the solution volume is supercooled and, thus, the fronts of nucleation and solidification are in close proximity in space and time [8]. In conclusion, the extent of supercooling, or nucleation temperature, and rate of freezing play a key role in the definition of the average size of ice crystals and their distribution. Uncontrolled nucleation greatly affects the desired size distribution and is responsible for vial-to-vial heterogeneity in terms of product morphology and drying behavior. A substantial improvement in this area might be achieved by the most recent controlled nucleation technology.

3 Conventional Freezing Methods for Lyophilization

3.1 Conventional Freezing

In a conventional lyophilization cycle, vials are filled in with a given volume of solution, partially stoppered, and loaded on the temperature-controlled shelves of the freeze-dryer. This operation is usually carried out at room temperature, but in some cases, at 5–10 °C. This is particularly true for those formulations containing organic solvents, e.g., *t*-butyl alcohol, that are very volatile or when the active pharmaceutical ingredients are very unstable at room temperature [9]. After loading, shelf temperature is decreased over 2–5 h and held at low temperature until all the vials freeze completely. The final shelf temperature and its holding time have to carefully be selected so as to ensure the complete solidification of the material being freeze-dried. In particular, the final shelf temperature has to be below T_g' for non-crystallizing excipients or below T_{eu} of crystalline materials. While the final shelf temperature is product-specific, the holding time essentially depends on the filling volume. As general guidelines, Tang and Pikal [10] found that 1 h is long enough for samples having a filling depth of 1 cm or smaller, while at least 2 h are necessary for those samples with a filling depth of greater than 1 cm.

The rate of cooling is another parameter that can be adjusted during freezing so as to control ice morphology and hence drying performance. However, this effect is strongly limited by the narrow range of cooling rates that can effectively be employed in a conventional freeze-dryer, i.e., less than 2 °C min^{-1}. For example, Searles et al. [8] observed a weak correlation between the cooling rate, ranged from 0.05 to 1 °C min^{-1}, and the nucleation temperature. However, this correlation might be stronger if much higher cooling rates were employed [11]. High cooling rates, such as those obtained by quench freezing, can effectively increase the supercooling extent, promote the formation of small pores and, hence, slower primary drying. If it is true that fast freezing is not beneficial to process performance, slow freezing should be avoided for all those formulations prone to phase separation, e.g., those containing polymers as stabilizers [12]. In fact, if the cooling rate is too slow, below 0.5 °C min^{-1}, protein and stabilizer have enough time to separate and any stabilization effect will be lost [13]. Besides, such conditions provide enough time for biomolecular degradation reactions to occur, because they prolong the time the protein exists in a concentrated fluid state. Because of all these considerations, Tang and Pikal [10] suggest the use of moderate cooling rates, about 1 °C min^{-1}, because it does not dramatically impact the supercooling extent and, at the same time, is suitable for all those formulations prone to phase separation.

One of the major drawbacks of this method is the lack of control of the degree of supercooling, which is responsible for a great variability in both process performance and product quality. A first attempt to reduce this variability was given by Liu et al. [14] by the two-step freezing: shelf temperature is first decreased to −5 °C and held for 0.5–1 h and, then, to the final shelf temperature till the completion of solidification. This last method was found to be particularly beneficial to product quality by reducing the vertical heterogeneity within the porous cake, but ineffective in reducing vial-to-vial variability.

3.2 Quench Freezing

In quench freezing, vials are immersed into cryogenic fluids (liquid nitrogen, dry ice/acetone, or dry ice/ethanol) for a specified time that allows its complete solidification [15–17]. Then, the frozen vials are loaded on precooled shelves [18] and freeze-dried. The rapid cooling results in very low randomly distributed nucleation temperatures and high freezing rates, which produce very small ice crystals. The method, as originally conceived, does not give any control to the extent of supercooling. Zhou et al. [21] designed a special freezing system that, to some extent, allows a more precise control of nucleation temperature and freezing rate. The vials are loaded onto porous metal plates within a confined cooling chamber. Then, they are rapidly cooled down via forced convection by a laminar and unidirectional flow of cryogen. Another porous metal surface, placed above the container, promptly removes the cryogen gas, after its contact with the vials, and prevents any recirculation of the cryogen within the cooling chamber. The exhausted gas is recycled, as warm nitrogen gas, to cryogen intake circuit. Through this configuration, heat is uniformly removed from the various vials that, thus, undergo the same freezing conditions. The precise control of the cooling rate is achieved by adjusting the temperature of the cryogen. More specifically, cryogen temperature is adjusted by mixing a specified volume of cold liquid nitrogen with that of nitrogen gas at room temperature. If it is true that this apparatus can precisely control the cooling rate, the nucleation temperature still remains stochastically distributed. Zhou et al. [21] partially solved this problem by adjusting both the temperature and pressure of cryogen. In detail, vials are first equilibrated at a specified temperature, below the thermodynamic freezing temperature of water, and held for a few minutes. Then, a decrease in pressure is performed so as to initiate nucleation and, after that, atmospheric pressure is re-established and, simultaneously, the cryogen temperature is decreased to −80 °C. This last method, as will be described later, is similar to the vacuum-induced surface freezing.

To date, there is not any evidence of application of this method to lyophilization; this is likely due to the fact that it is hardly scalable on a production unit. This problem might be solved by freezing vials using the apparatus proposed in [21] and then loading the frozen vials into the freeze-dryer.

3.3 Precooled Shelf Method

In the precooled shelf freezing, the vials are loaded on the freeze-dryer once its shelves have been cooled at very low temperature, i.e., −40 °C or −45 °C. During this operation, the freezing chamber is slightly pressurized with anhydrous nitrogen in order to prevent the condensation of humid air on the shelf surface. The influence of this freezing method on the average nucleation temperature is controversial. Searles et al. [8] found that nucleation occurred at a higher average temperature (−9.5 °C) with respect to the conventional shelf-ramped freezing protocol (−13.4 °C) while

Hottot et al. [19] did not observe any statistically significant variation in nucleation temperature between precooled and conventional freezing. Besides, it has been observed that the vial geometry and filling volume dramatically impact the freezing dynamics and particularly the freezing rate [19, 20]. All the authors agree that the loading at very low temperature does not provide any improvement in the nucleation temperature distribution and hence on the freezing-induced heterogeneity.

3.4 Annealing

Annealing is a post-freezing treatment during which the frozen solution is held at a specified temperature, 10–20 °C above the glass transition temperature of the formulation [10], for a period of time. Above the glass transition temperature, ice partially melts and its rate of melting is inversely correlated with the size of its crystals [22]; the smaller the ice crystals, the faster the rate of freezing. The increase in water content and temperature then promotes the mobility of the glassy phase and of all the components included in it, resulting in the relaxation into physical states characterized by lower free energy [22]. Besides, Ostwald ripening facilitates dissolution of ice crystals smaller than a critical size and their deposition onto larger crystals, contributing to their growth. Lifshitz and Slyozov [23] demonstrated that the increase in the cube of the average pore size directly correlates with the annealing time. Consequently, those samples containing smaller ice crystals will grow up faster than those characterized by larger crystals, reducing vial-to-vial heterogeneity in pores structure and drying behavior [22]. Upon refreezing of the annealed sample, these large crystals serve as nucleation sites for recrystallization inhibiting the formation of new smaller crystals, resulting in a frozen structure characterized by much larger ice crystals.

The annealing treatment is commonly used to promote the crystallization of pharmaceutical active ingredients [24] and some bulking agents such as glycine and mannitol [25], as well as the completion of freeze concentration by crystallization of amorphous water [26–28]. Besides, it has been observed that annealing promotes the formation of much larger ice crystals, eliminating the dependence of their size and morphology on the nucleation temperature. Because of that, various authors [9, 29, 30] hypothesized that annealing accelerates the sublimation process. Contrary to these results, Esfandiary et al. [31] observed that annealing makes primary drying 20% longer than that without annealing. This last result was likely the consequence of lack of control on drying conditions, resulting in poor cake appearance with shrinkage. Searles et al. [32] also observed that annealing enlarges the pores on the top surface of the cake, decreasing the dry layer resistance to vapor flow. This post-freezing treatment has been successfully combined with various protocols from the conventional shelf-ramped freezing method to controlled nucleation technologies.

4 Methods of Controlling Nucleation Temperature

In lyophilization, controlled nucleation technology is generally used to eliminate any freezing-induced heterogeneity and, more recently, to control the product morphology. This technology should respond to the following requirements,

1. The nucleation event is initiated within the solution being frozen irrespective of the scale of the freeze-dryer, geometry of the vial, type of stopper, formulation, and filling volume.
2. Nucleation is effectively initiated in all the vials of the batch within a narrow range of temperature (<1 °C) and time (<30 s). This factor is essential to reduce vial-to-vial variability.
3. It can easily be replicated, minimizing batch-to-batch variability.
4. The equipment can effectively perform the freezing conditions employed by the controlled nucleation method (temperature, pressure, rate of cooling, rate of depressurization, etc.).
5. The methodology is easily scalable from the laboratory to production units.
6. It does not alter the aseptic conditions of the process.
7. Its application does not adversely impact the critical quality attributes of the product.

4.1 Nucleating Agents

The addition of insoluble impurities to the solution to be frozen can serve as ice nucleating agents, promoting the formation of stable nuclei at higher temperatures compared to those at which nucleation spontaneously occurs. A common nucleating agent is silver iodide, which has been widely investigated for cloud seeding. Its capability to initiate nucleation was ascribed to its similarity in structure with ice, as well as to electric field mechanisms [33]. In food science, various bacteria were found to have the potential to serve as nucleating agents [34], but *Pseudomonas syringae* was the most investigated [35]. Again, its capability to promote the formation of ice nucleation was due to structural similarity with ice, but also because of its high hydrophobicity [36]. However, it must be noted that these agents initiate nucleation event at higher temperatures than those at which nucleation spontaneously occurs but cannot be used to regulate the nucleation temperature. In addition, various authors claimed it did not improve intra batch uniformity and the addition of such materials is likely to be incompatible with parenteral pharma processes [8].

4.2 Electro-Freezing

In 1951, Rau [37] demonstrated that a high voltage, applied to metal electrodes, can initiate nucleation in supercooled water. Various scientists tried to explain the basic mechanisms of electro-freezing, which include the formation of bubbles and their breakdown [38], influence on structural and dynamical properties of water [39], and formation of hydrated metal-ion complexes [40]. Although the underlying mechanisms of this methodology have not been clearly understood yet, it is widely recognized that the application of an electric field is beneficial to the formation of stable nuclei.

The use of high voltage to initiate nucleation within a sample at controlled temperature, which is then lyophilized, was first reported by Petersen et al. [41]. According to their procedure, samples are first equilibrated at the desired temperature, at which nucleation is promoted by the application of an electric pulse of 4.5 kV, and then the nucleated samples are cooled down to −45 °C. Petersen et al. [41] proposed two possible configurations for the electro-freezer. In the first configuration, named direct electro-freezing, the electrode probe was directly inserted into the liquid being frozen. However, the authors observed that the presence of excipients, and particularly of ionic salts, makes this method less reproducible and, in some cases, inhibited the nucleation event at temperatures higher than that observed for spontaneous nucleation. For these reasons, they proposed a second configuration of the device where the electrodes are immersed into a cap containing 100 μL of pure water. In this way, nucleation can be initiated into pure water and then ice crystals are forced to grow through a narrow tube into the liquid sample, starting its crystallization [41, 42].

4.3 Gap Freezing

Kuu et al. [43, 44] employed a special spacer, having low thermal conductivity, which allows heat to be removed essentially by radiation. This configuration allows the freezing front to move from the bottom and the top simultaneously, inhibiting the formation of a compact layer on the top surface of the cake and hence resulting in a dramatic increase in rate of drying. The authors claimed that the average nucleation temperature can effectively be initiated at a higher temperature than that observed for conventional freezing, and nucleation temperature can, to some extent, be regulated by employing different spacers. However, this system can hardly be coupled with the automatic loading and unloading system of the lyophilizer. Capozzi and Pisano [45] proposed as an alternative to suspend the vials over a track, while cooling essentially occurs via natural or forced convection. This configuration resulted in a significant increase in the average nucleation temperature that, however, could not be directly controlled.

4.4 Ice Fog Technique

In 1990, Rowe [46] demonstrated that ice nucleation of a solution to be freeze-dried can be forced to occur at a specified temperature by introducing cryogenic gas into the drying chamber. More specifically, this method includes the following steps:

1. The solution is equilibrated at the desired temperature, below its thermodynamic freezing point.
2. A specified flow rate of cold nitrogen gas (from −40 to −50 °C) is introduced into the drying chamber, thereby promoting the spontaneous nucleation in water vapor. The presence and growth of these nuclei allow cloud or fog formation [47] that, in contact with the top surface of the supercooled solution to be freeze-dried, initiates its nucleation.
3. The nucleated vials are then cooled down to −45 °C.

Rambhatla et al. [48] applied this protocol to the lyophilization of a 5% (w/w) sucrose solution and could successfully initiate ice nucleation in a wide range of temperatures, from −1 to −12 °C. However, they observed that complete nucleation of all the vials of the batch only occurred after 30 min. This wide distribution in nucleation time resulted in vial-to-vial heterogeneity in terms of morphology of the lyophilized samples and drying behavior. In fact, because of this time span, the earlier nucleated vials undergo different freezing conditions during or after the completion of the solidification process. Rambhatla et al. [48] proposed an alternative plant configuration which employs a circular tube with regularly, spaced-distributed holes to bleed the cold gas within the freeze-drying chamber. This configuration allows a more uniform distribution of the cold gas and reduces the nucleation time span to 5 min. However, some vials still remained excluded from the forced nucleation process, because the suspended ice crystals could not reach all the vials of the batch. This problem was partially solved by Patel et al. [49] who proposed to depressurize the drying chamber to 66 mbar prior to the introduction of the cold gas. By this modification, ice nucleation was achieved in all the vials of the batch within 1 min, but only if the freeze-dryer is partially loaded. In the case of a full load freeze-dryer, this procedure had to be repeated several times to complete ice nucleation within the entire batch of vials. It follows that, for full load runs, the problem of large nucleation time span persists although it is less evident compared to that observed in the absence of depressurization. This problem is more and more evident with larger freezing chambers, representing the major obstacle to the scale-up of this technology to commercial lyophilizers. Demarco et al. [50] used an ejector to generate the ice fog, which is then uniformly and rapidly distributed throughout the freezing chamber. The ice fog is produced by mixing liquid nitrogen, water, and the ice fog exiting the freezing chamber itself. The authors showed that their technology can induce ice nucleation in all the vials of the batch within 30–50 s on both the laboratory and pilot scale unit. In addition, process sterility is preserved since the cold gas is sterile filtered and, of course, the freezing chamber is sterilized by steam before vials are loaded onto the shelves.

Since the use of cryogenic gas might be technically demanding, attention was recently placed on the development of technologies that can generate the ice fog without using liquid nitrogen. For example, Weija [51] used an external condenser to generate the ice fog. More specifically, once the vials have been loaded and equilibrated at the desired temperature, the freezing chamber is isolated from condenser, closing the valve separating the two environments, and its pressure is decreased to 67 mbar. The condenser surfaces are cooled down to very low temperature and placed in contact with the humidified gas, thereby generating the ice fog. Then, the isolation valve is open, and the ice fog enters the freezing chamber thanks to its low pressure. The final pressure for the depressurization step has to be low enough to promote the inlet of the ice fog, but high enough to prevent any boiling of the solution to be lyophilized. Since this pressure may vary with the formulation being frozen, it needs to be determined experimentally prior to its application. As an alternative, Geidobler et al. [52] proposed to reduce the pressure of the entire lyophilizer, freezing chamber, and condenser, to 3.7 mbar. Then, atmospheric pressure is re-established by opening the venting valve on the condenser. The venting gas, in contact with the cold surfaces of the condenser, reduces its temperature and then flows into the freezing chamber. Here, the cold gas enters in contact with the water vapor, produced by the vacuum evaporation of the solution into the vials, and forms the ice fog. However, there might be a risk of contamination, as a result of this process back flushing particles from the condenser.

4.5 Ultrasound-Induced Ice Nucleation (UIIN)

It is well known that ultrasonic vibrations trigger ice nucleation in supercooled water [53]. This result was widely used in food industry to control the freezing process during ice cream manufacturing [54, 55]. Later, Inada et al. [56] showed that the ultrasonic vibrations can effectively be used to initiate ice nucleation at the desired temperature. In a follow-up study, Zhang et al. [57] demonstrated that the probability of phase change is directly correlated with the number of bubbles formed by acoustic cavitation, but the mechanism that triggers nucleation in a supercooled solution exposed to ultrasonic waves is still controversial. Two models have been proposed in the literature. Hickling [53] hypothesized nucleation is initiated by the decrease in the equilibrium freezing temperature of water caused by the dramatic increase in local pressure (1 GPa) produced by the collapse of a cavitation bubble, while Hunt and Jackson [58] stated that nucleation is promoted by the negative pressures following the collapse of a bubble. Both hypothesis, however, correlated the initiation of nucleation with the collapse of a cavitation bubble. Recently, Zhang et al. [59] observed that this phenomenon alone is not sufficient to describe the initiation of ice nucleation, but other secondary factors, e.g., the motion of cavitation bubbles, can play a critical role.

The application of ultrasonic vibrations to control the nucleation temperature in a lyophilization cycle was first reported by Nakagawa et al. [60]. They showed that the ultrasound technology can effectively be used to trigger ice nucleation at the desired temperature for both amorphous and crystallizing formulations. Subsequently, it has been found that, besides the extent of supercooling, the acoustic power also plays a critical role in the freezing process. For example, Hottot et al. [61] found that the acoustic power influenced the type of mannitol polymorphs obtained after lyophilization, while Saclier et al. [62] correlated the average size and structure of ice crystals with both the extent of supercooling and the acoustic power. In all these studies, the generator of ultrasonic waves was positioned externally, and vibrations are transferred to the vials through an aluminum plate, which was in tight contact with the temperature-controlled shelf of the freeze-dryer. The authors also claimed that silicone oil had to be used to ensure good contact between the vials and the vibrating surface. Furthermore, Acton [63] demonstrated that ice nucleation can be facilitated if pressure is reduced or a volatile fluid is dissolved in the solution prior to the application of ultrasonic vibrations. It can easily be understood that the complexity of this configuration makes the upscaling of this technology very difficult. In Passot et al. [64], a prototype freeze-dryer is described, containing one temperature-controlled shelf directly equipped with the ultrasound technology and, thus, eliminating some of the heat transfer problems observed in the previous configuration. However, this controlled nucleation technology was only partially successful because only 80% of the vials nucleated at the desired temperature. Additionally, the scalability of this technology to the manufacturing equipment is still limited by the fact that ice nucleation fails if vials are placed on the so-called nodal points, which are characterized by the lowest ultrasonic intensity [60]. This problem can be mitigated if the ultrasonic probe is positioned below the temperature-controlled shelf. However, this plant configuration requires the frequent degassing of the silicone oil and interfered with the vial stoppering operation. As an alternative, the ultrasound probe could be positioned on the shelves, and transducers could be activated in sequence and scanned over a wide range of wavelengths to avoid the presence of nodes in specified positions (Miguel Galan, Azbil Telstar, personal communication). However, the implementation of this solution would be technically complex and may require adaptations to be compatible with GMP sterility requirements.

4.6 High-Pressure Shift or Depressurization Freezing

The use of compression and/or expansion cycles to control the nucleation temperature was first reported by Kanda et al. [65]. They used this technology to increase the degree of supercooling during freezing of tofu, promoting the formation of smaller ice crystals, similar to those obtained by quench freezing in liquid nitrogen [66] and thus limiting damage to food structure [54]. Sanz et al. [67] also observed that high-pressure treatments in agar gel promoted uniform subcooling within the whole sample and, hence, fast and uniform nucleation and ice crystal growth. Knorr et al. [68] identified three different high-pressure freezing methods: high-pressure-assisted freezing, high-pressure-shift freezing, and high-pressure-induced freezing. The phase transition occurs under constant pressure conditions in the high-pressure-assisted freezing, while it is initiated by a pressure release in the high-pressure-shift freezing [69, 70] and by a pressure increase followed by an isobaric phase for the high-pressure-induced freezing. It must be evidenced that all these methodologies have been proposed for food science applications and only the high-pressure-shift method effectively found application in pharmaceutical lyophilization [71, 72]. This last application is often referred to as depressurization method and involves the following operations,

1. Once the vials have been loaded, the drying chamber is pressurized with argon to 1.5–4.5 bar. Various types of gas can be used as pressurizing gas, e.g., air, carbon dioxide, helium, nitrogen, xenon, etc. Konstantinidis et al. [73] observed that the efficacy of the method is strongly connected with the type of gas used during the pressurization phase, and argon was found to be the most efficient.
2. Samples are equilibrated at a temperature below the equilibrium freezing point of the solution and then the drying chamber is rapidly depressurized. This method can effectively initiate the nucleation event in all the vials of the batch, provided that the rate of depressurization is higher than 0.8 bar min^{-1}.
3. The nucleated vials are then cooled down to the final shelf temperature, i.e., −40 °C or lower.

The underlying mechanism by which depressurization freezing induces nucleation is not yet clear. Several potential mechanisms have been hypothesized by Gasteyer et al. [71] which, although speculative, deserve attention and need to be experimentally confirmed. One possible mechanism is that depressurization promotes the release of the gas dissolved in the solution, forming bubbles over which nucleation initiates. In fact, the initial high pressure increases the concentration of gas dissolved into the liquid to be frozen, which is rapidly released as soon as pressure is reduced during the depressurization phase, triggering ice nucleation. Another possibility is that depressurization promotes local evaporation of the solution, resulting in a dramatic decrease in its temperature at the top surface which can trigger the nucleation event. As an alternative, it has been hypothesized that the cold gas, resulting from evaporation, freezes some water vapor close to the top surface, and these crystals, entering in contact with the solution, act as nucleating sites. A fourth hypothesis [73] is that the rapid depressurization generates pressure waves which facilitate the initiation of nucleation by mechanical vibrations.

This procedure is easy to realize in both laboratory and production units, and is fully compatible with aseptic manufacturing and does not require any changes in the drug formulation. However, it can be implemented only if the freeze-dryers can withstand 0.5–3 bar overpressure during freezing. Most of the production freeze-dryers have been designed to resist such conditions, e.g., during steam sterilization; otherwise, the application of the depressurization method requires the modification of the equipment which might be quite expensive [74].

4.7 Vacuum-Induced Surface Freezing

The application of vacuum to promote the rapid decrease in temperature, via evaporation of surface water, of some vegetables was largely investigated in food industry as an innovative cooling method, called evaporative or vacuum cooling. This method is widely used as a precooling treatment of some horticultural products such as lettuce and mushrooms [75]. It must, however, be pointed out that in this application, much attention was given to the selection of the processing conditions, temperature and pressure, so as to avoid any freezing of the product, because crystallization of ice was correlated with cellular and structural damage of food.

The basic principle of evaporative or vacuum cooling was later used by Kramer et al. [76] to develop the vacuum-induced surface freezing method (VISF). VISF is a general method for controlling nucleation temperature and is based on the perturbation of chamber pressure. As originally proposed by Kramer et al. [76], this method encompasses the following steps,

1. The vial is loaded on the freeze-dryer at room temperature and atmospheric pressure,
2. The liquid being frozen is cooled down to +10 °C and maintained at that temperature for 1 h,
3. Pressure inside the drying chamber is reduced to a given value, that is product specific, as fast as possible and maintained at that value for 5 min,
4. Atmospheric pressure is re-established and the nucleated vials are cooled down to 3–4 °C below the eutectic temperature,
5. The frozen product is cooled down to −40 °C, at 1 °C min^{-1}, and maintained for at least 1 h.

As discussed above, the application of vacuum promotes the partial evaporation of water and thus a sudden decrease in the liquid temperature which triggers the nucleation event. This method is gaining increasing interest within the lyophilization community because it is easy to realize, does not require any additional device, and allows the precise control of nucleation temperature. However, the protocol described in Kramer et al. [76] promoted the formation of a thin frozen layer at the top of the sample, having a thickness of 1–3 mm, while the part underneath remained unfrozen and crystallized only once shelf temperature was reduced toward −40 °C. This process resulted in a two-layer solidification because the heat removed by evaporation was not enough high to supercool the entire volume of solution. Liu et al. [14] showed that if the vacuum step is performed after the solution has been equilibrated at −10 °C, the formation of ice occurs rapidly throughout the whole sample. Recently, Zhou et al. [21] claimed that the depressurization can be used to induce nucleation of ice into samples cooled by quench freezing. More particularly, the cooling system proposed by the authors makes it possible to adjust the nucleation temperature, while samples undergo high cooling rates, 4.5–5 °C min^{-1}. Unfortunately, some aesthetic defects remained unresolved, e.g., the formation of flakes on the top surface of the product and blow-up of the frozen plug, which are detrimental to the elegance of the final product and can cause its rejection during quality control testing. In addition, some vials could spontaneously nucleate during the quench freezing, before the desired vacuum is achieved.

A substantial improvement in the VISF performances was achieved by Oddone et al. [77], who essentially modified the step 3 of the above procedure. As soon as the desired vacuum has been reached, the drying chamber is isolated from condenser for approximately 1 min and, then, atmospheric pressure is re-established. The isolation of the drying chamber has been found to be effective in blow-up suppression because it slows down the rate of water evaporation and hence makes blow-up less probable. Furthermore, vacuum time as short as 1 min was found to be sufficient to initiate nucleation within all the vials of the batch, and short enough to avoid boiling and blow-up. Overall, this simple change was found to eliminate both blow-up and flakes formation, making VISF much more competitive with other controlled nucleation technologies. All the validation tests were carried out in a pilot-scale freeze-dryer working under full load conditions, i.e., approximately 800 vials (10R type).

5 Influence of Controlled Nucleation Technology on Product Quality and Process Performance

5.1 Morphology of the Lyophilized Product and Intra-Vial Heterogeneity

It is well known that ice crystal size and the extent of supercooling are strongly correlated. In 1989, Roy and Pikal [78] observed that vials with internally placed thermocouples nucleated at higher temperatures compared to those without thermocouples, and completed ice sublimation much sooner. Similarly, Searles et al. [8] manipulated the average nucleation temperature, using ice nucleators, and observed that primary drying rate inversely correlates to the extent of supercooling. As the rate of sublimation is directly correlated to the average size of ice crystals [79], we deduce that a higher degree of supercooling produces small ice crystals which, upon sublimation during primary drying, leave smaller pores and hence higher resistance to mass transfer, and result in a dramatic increase in the primary drying time. It follows that if the average nucleation temperature can be controlled, to some extent, product morphology can also be controlled.

Depending on freezing conditions, we can observe two basic mechanisms of freezing: directional solidification and global supercooling. In the case of directional solidification, only a portion of the liquid volume is sufficiently supercooled to promote primary and secondary nucleation. Consequently, once nucleation occurred, the nucleation front moves into the non-nucleated liquid and, in close proximity, is followed by the solidification front. Generally, freezing by directional solidification occurs if the extent of supercooling is small, less 5 °C, resulting in large chimney-like pores. For example, if VISF is carried out at +5 °C as proposed by Kramer et al. [76], nucleation will occur at a temperature close to the equilibrium freezing point, producing chimney-like and extremely large pores having a diameter of approximately 200 μm or larger. To provide an example, Fig. 3 shows the internal porous structure of 5% mannitol after lyophilization and using VISF to control nucleation [77]. The vacuum was applied after product equilibration at +5 °C, thus we can presume that nucleation occurred at a temperature very close to the equilibrium freezing point and, hence, freezing preferentially proceeded by directional solidification. Because of vacuum, the liquid solution is cooled down more efficiently close to its upper surface, promoting the formation of temperature gradients within its volume. The extent of temperature gradient substantially depends on the temperature at which vacuum is applied. The higher that temperature is, the larger the extent of the temperature gradient is. Consequently, if the vacuum is performed at +5 °C, large temperature gradients are expected and, hence, small pores are produced close to the top surface, that exhibits the lowest temperature, and much larger pores at the bottom [80].

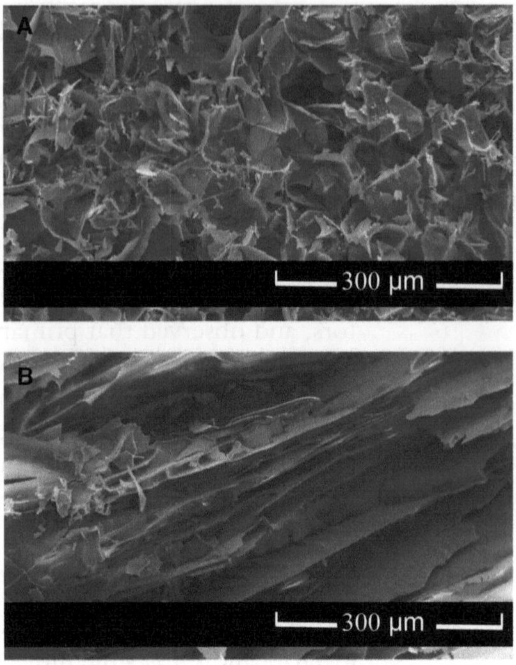

Fig. 3 SEM micrographs of lyophilized samples of 5% mannitol in the case of (**A**) uncontrolled freezing and (**B**) VISF at +5 °C. Cake cross-sections at 90° to the vial axis

If nucleation is induced at or below −5 °C, the extent of supercooling is quite uniform within the entire liquid volume, and the secondary nucleation zone spreads (from top to bottom) within the whole sample volume in few seconds [81]. Oddone et al. [81] also observed that the solidification/freezing front moves from the bottom of the vial toward the top surface of the product being frozen independently of the freezing technology used. They also observed that samples produced by VISF have much larger pores compared to those obtained by uncontrolled freezing. The average pore size ranges from 80 to 140 μm for VISF, and 15–20 μm for uncontrolled freezing. Furthermore, if VISF is employed and we exclude peripheral zones (0.5 mm from the top and bottom surfaces), the average size of pores is very uniform within the remaining sample volume.

Besides the average pore size, freezing can also influence the morphology of the crystalline excipients; for example, lyophilized mannitol can contain three polymorphs (α, β, δ), which have different thermodynamic stability and can thus influence the stability of the active molecules differently during storage. β-mannitol is strongly desirable because it is the thermodynamically stable form, while both α and δ are metastable [82].

High freezing rates, typical of quench freezing, promote the formation of amorphous mannitol, which tends to be transformed into a metastable form over time. On the contrary, all the other methods, which involve freezing rates below 2 °C min^{-1}, promote the formation of crystalline mannitol [83]. The physical state seems to be strongly related to mannitol concentration and the freezing rate. Generally, fast freezing promotes the formation of the δ-polymorph for 10% mannitol, and prevalently the β-polymorph (with traces of α and δ) for 5% mannitol [82–84]. Slow freezing was found to promote the formation of the β-form for both 5% mannitol and 10%, while the precooled shelf freezing promotes the formation of the α-polymorph with traces of the β-form. It might, however, be considered that the presence of proteins or other co-solutes may strongly influence the physical state of mannitol [85, 86].

As concerns VISF, Oddone et al. [80] observed that uncontrolled freezing promoted the formation of all the three mannitol polymorphs and their composition dramatically differed from vial to vial. On the contrary, the control of the nucleation temperature by VISF promoted the formation of only one of these forms, while the others were present only in traces. More specifically, XRD analyses revealed that if nucleation is induced at −5 °C or at a higher temperature, the lyophilized mannitol is prevalently made of δ with traces of α. In addition, Raman spectroscopy showed that in all the samples α-mannitol was concentrated within a thin layer close to the top surface of the cake, while the remaining part was made of δ-mannitol. On the contrary, if nucleation is induced at a lower temperature, e.g., −10 °C, the mannitol samples were essentially pure and contained only the β-form. In the VISF runs, mannitol hydrate was absent. These results are very interesting because they show that the control of nucleation temperature is important not only because it can alter the ice morphology, but also the crystalline state of crystallizing excipients.

Limited literature is available about the relationship between freezing conditions and reconstitution time because this quality attribute depends on numerous factors: aesthetic defects such as collapse, shrinkage and melting back, product morphology including pore size and interconnectivity, specific surface area, and physical state of the various excipients. To provide an example, Searles et al. [32] observed that annealing promotes fast reconstitution of HES samples, while 2 years later Webb et al. [87] found that, for the same formulation, annealing was not beneficial but slows down its reconstitution. However, these results cannot be compared, because there is another parameter to be accounted for, i.e., the samples lyophilized by Searles et al. [32] had holes that promote pore interconnectivity and thus liquid permeation during reconstitution. It is agreed that annealing and all those techniques that promote the formation of larger pores, including the most recent controlled nucleation temperature technologies, tend to prolong the reconstitution time. However, it is difficult to give a general guideline, because as aforementioned the reconstitution time is the results of the combination of various factors besides pore size and specific surface area [88].

5.2 Process Performance

5.2.1 Primary Drying

As aforementioned, freezing dramatically impacts both size and conformation of ice crystals and the nucleation temperature plays a key role in this process. Size and distribution of ice crystals were found to influence both the quality attributes of the lyophilized samples and drying performance.

As concerns primary drying, rate of sublimation J_w inversely correlates with the resistance to mass transfer R_p,

$$J_w = \frac{(P_{ice} - P_w)}{R_p} \tag{1}$$

where P_{ice} is the vapor pressure of ice and depends on the product temperature at the interface of sublimation, and P_w is the partial pressure of water inside the drying chamber. The resistance to mass transfer is determined by both the average size (D_p) and interconnectivity of pores left after sublimation of ice crystals [89]. Rambhatla et al. [48] found that the resistance to mass transfer is inversely correlated to the pore size,

$$R_p = \sqrt{\frac{\pi R T}{8 M_w}} \frac{3\tau^2}{\varepsilon} \frac{1}{D_p} \tag{2}$$

where M_w is the molecular weight of water, R the ideal gas constant, T the vapor temperature in Kelvin, ε the cake porosity, while τ is linked to pores' interconnectivity and is often set to 1.5 [96]. It follows that if freezing can alter product morphology, it also influences the resistance to mass transfer and hence the primary drying rate. Pisano et al. [90] showed that the primary drying time indirectly correlates with the average size of pores. To provide an example, Fig. 4 shows that the primary drying time of 5% mannitol nonlinearly decreases with the average pore size of the lyophilized samples but, beyond a threshold value, it levels off and the influence of pore size is negated. It is well known that sublimation is not rate-controlled by mass transfer if the product resistance to mass transfer is too low. In this case, the rate of sublimation is determined by heat transfer, and product temperature reaches a plateau level at which vapor pressure of ice equals the partial pressure of water inside the drying chamber [92, 93]. If follows that all those freezing methodologies, which indirectly manipulate the product morphology, can effectively impact primary drying performance until the primary drying rate becomes under control of the pore size.

Most of the controlled freezing technologies initiate nucleation at higher temperatures compared to uncontrolled freezing, increasing the primary drying rate. Searles et al. [8] observed that the primary drying time of a 10% (w/v) hydroxyethyl starch (HES) solution was approximately 4% shorter for each degree of additional supercooling. For the same formulation, a similar result was

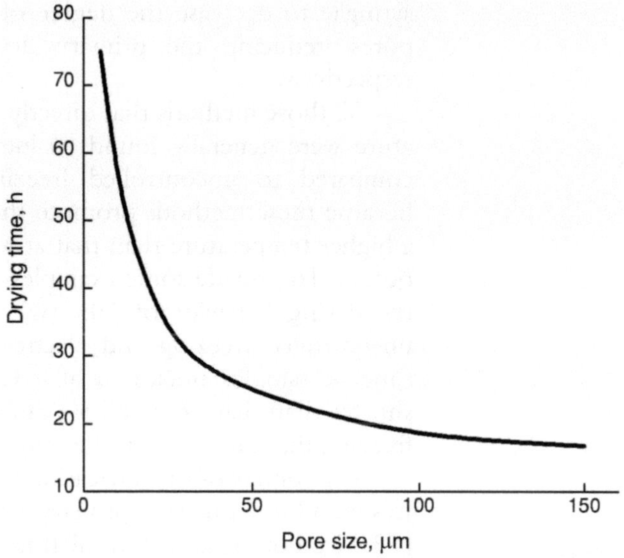

Fig. 4 The relationship between the primary drying time and the average pore size for lyophilized mannitol samples. Data were obtained using the bi-dimensional mathematical model described by Velardi and Barresi [91], while drying was carried out at −10 °C and 10 Pa

observed by Petersen et al. [42] using electro-freezing to regulate the nucleation temperature.

If the nucleation temperature cannot be controlled, the rate of sublimation can still be increased, e.g., using the precooled shelf method or adding an annealing treatment to the conventional freezing step. The precooled shelf method reduces the primary drying time by 14–18% [8, 64], while the annealing technologies up to 50% or larger [9, 18, 32]. However, it must be remarked that the effect of annealing on the dry layer resistance and drying time varies with the formulation being freeze-dried. In some cases, annealing can contribute to the increase of the resistance to mass transfer, because it changes the physical state of the lyophilized sample. For example, Lu and Pikal [28] observed that annealing influences the crystallization process of mannitol–trehalose–sodium chloride-based formulations, decreasing its amorphous content. Consequently, the resistance to mass transfer increases, making the primary drying time longer.

Quench freezing and all those technologies that increase the extent of supercooling promote the formation of small pores, thereby extending primary drying [74, 94]. Besides the formation of small pores, the horizontal direction of the pores, from the vial wall toward the middle of the cake, further obstructs the pathways for vapor escape [18]. Searles et al. [8] and Passot et al. [64] observed that addition of a nucleation agent like Pseudomonas syringae to decrease the degree of supercooling produces larger pores, reducing the primary drying time by 60% and 30% respectively.

All those methods that directly control the nucleation temperature were generally found to increase the rate of sublimation, compared to uncontrolled freezing; this result was expected because these methods promote the formation of stable nuclei at a higher temperature than that at which nucleation spontaneously occurs. To provide some examples, Petersen et al. [42] compared the drying behavior of 10% (w/v) HES samples produced via uncontrolled freezing and electro-freezing. The primary drying time of samples nucleated at −1.5 °C was approximately 70% shorter than that observed for samples produced by uncontrolled freezing that nucleated in the range of −11.5 to −17.1 °C.

The control of the nucleation temperature via depressurization was found to reduce the primary drying time of 5% sucrose by 27% [73, 95]. For the same formulation, Rambhatla et al. [48] observed that the primary drying time can be reduced by 30% by initiating nucleation at −1 °C via the ice fog technique. A similar result was found for 10% mannitol, 10% sucrose, and BSA 5% formulations by using ultrasounds to initiate nucleation at a temperature close to the equilibrium freezing point [60, 61]. For example, Nakagawa et al. [60] observed that if a solution of mannitol (10% by weight) is nucleated at −2 °C, the primary drying rate will be 60% shorter compared to an uncontrolled nucleation cycle.

Generally, the VISF method was found to be beneficial to primary drying performance. However, in order to obtain maximum benefit, attention has to be paid to the selection of an appropriate temperature at which the vacuum application is performed. For example, if the vacuum is performed at +5 °C, the primary drying time was 15% and 25% shorter for mannitol 2% and sucrose 2% respectively [76]. Similarly, Oddone et al. [77] observed that drying time saving for mannitol and lactose-based formulations varied in the range of 20–70%, depending on the nucleation temperature. However, it must be noted that if nucleation was induced at a temperature too close to the equilibrium freezing point, the porous structure was not uniform within the cake [80].

5.2.2 Secondary Drying

The specific surface area (SSA) is inversely correlated to the pore size. If we assume a capillary tube model, SSA in $m^2\ g^{-1}$ can be expressed as [48],

$$\mathrm{SSA} = \frac{4\varepsilon}{\rho_s(1-\varepsilon)}\frac{1}{D_p} \tag{3}$$

where ρ_s is the mass density of the dry solid. For a given solid content ε, SSA is determined only by pore size and, since pore size is substantially determined by the extent of supercooling, we can deduct that SSA and nucleation temperature are well correlated. More specifically, high supercooling promotes the formation of large pores and hence small SSA. To provide an example, Konstantinidis et al. [73] observed that SSA, as determined by a Krypton adsorption analysis, of lyophilized mannitol (5% by weight) was 2.78 $m^2\ g^{-1}$ for samples nucleated at approx. −3 °C and 5.54 $m^2\ g^{-1}$ in the case of uncontrolled nucleation.

Although this was proven to be beneficial to primary drying performance, an opposite effect was observed for the secondary drying rate. For example, various authors observed that, on constant secondary drying temperature and time, all those freezing methodologies that produce larger pores result in an increased residual moisture content [8, 14–76, 87].

A first order mechanism has been hypothesized for the desorption process [97],

$$\begin{cases} \frac{\mathrm{d}C_{\mathrm{w}}}{\mathrm{d}t} = -k\left(C_{\mathrm{w}} - C^0\right) \\ C_{\mathrm{w}}(t=0) = C_{\mathrm{wo}} \end{cases} \tag{4}$$

where C_{wo} is the residual moisture of the lyophilized product at the end of primary drying, C^0 is the equilibrium water content as determined from the moisture sorption isotherm, and k is the rate constant for the desorption process. Such a mechanism was initially proposed for glassy materials [97, 98] but was then found to be adequate also for crystallizing materials [99]. The rate constant for the desorption process is directly correlated to SSA and, hence, to the nucleation temperature.

Although it has been hypothesized that controlled nucleation technologies have a negative effect on the secondary drying rate, this aspect has been poorly investigated. An early investigation on the impact of controlled nucleation on both primary and secondary drying performance was given by Oddone et al. [100]. They found that VISF reduces the extent of supercooling for mannitol-based formulations, promoting the formation of larger ice crystals which resulted in 55% decrease in the primary drying time. However, they also observed that, if this result was beneficial to primary drying performance, it dramatically slowed down the desorption process and, thus, increased the time necessary to achieve a target moisture specification. It is, however, true that any increase in the secondary drying time is expected to be only a minor contribution to the overall lyophilization cycle time. For example, Oddone et al. [100] observed that the application of VISF to control the nucleation temperature resulted in 10–20% decrease in the overall cycle time.

5.3 Vial-to-Vial Heterogeneity

Controlled nucleation is beneficial to drying performance, but also to vial-to-vial uniformity. Recent studies showed that the precise control of the nucleation temperature reduces the variation within a batch of vials for the specific surface area [49], residual moisture

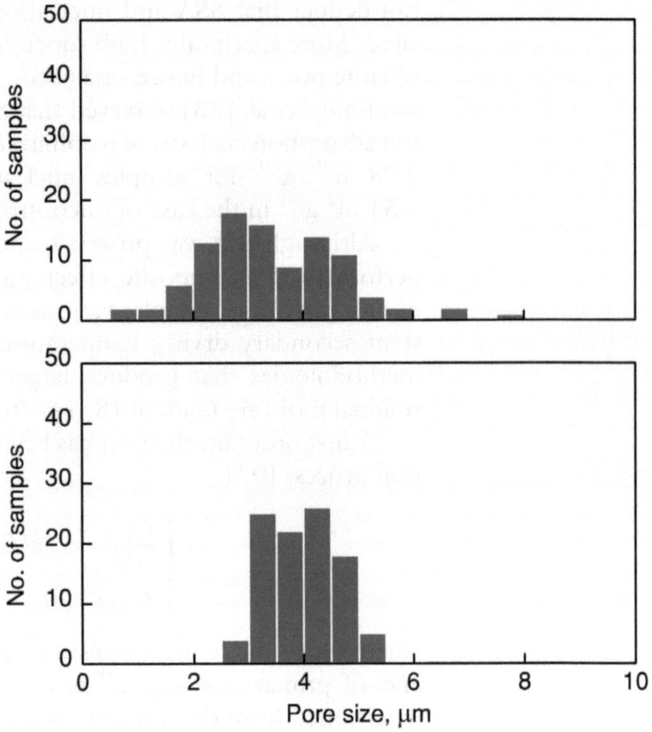

Fig. 5 Statistical distribution of the residual moisture content as observed at the end of primary drying for 5% mannitol samples produced by (upper graph) uncontrolled nucleation and (lower graph) VISF

content [100], and primary drying time [64, 77, 80]. For example, Oddone et al. [80] evaluated the dispersion of the primary drying time distribution from the difference between the onset and the offset time of the pressure ratio curve [64, 77] for three formulations containing lactose, mannitol, and sucrose. They observed that the primary drying time distribution of uncontrolled samples was 30–60% larger than that observed for samples produced by VISF. In addition, VISF showed a more uniform distribution of the residual moisture throughout the batch of vials. Figure 5 shows the statistical distribution of the residual moisture at the end of primary drying for uncontrolled freezing and VISF. It can be observed that the two distributions had similar mean values, 3.8% vs. 4.0%, but samples produced by VISF had the lowest standard deviation, 0.6% vs. 1.3%. These values agree with those reported in the literature for crystalline materials, which usually ranges from 1% for glycine [101] to 10% for mannitol [97, 102]. Furthermore, the residual moisture was lower than 5% for 98% of VISF samples but for only 85% of uncontrolled nucleation samples. These results confirmed that the control of nucleation temperature plays a crucial role in the production of homogeneous batches, provided that the controlled nucleation technology can promote the nucleation event in all the vials of the batch within a narrow range of time and temperature. It must, however, be remarked that these benefits can be achieved only if nucleation is initiated at high temperatures, much higher than that at which samples spontaneously nucleate. If nucleation is induced at lower temperatures, below −10 °C, controlled nucleation competes with the spontaneous process and part of its benefit, mainly in terms of batch uniformity, will be lost [74].

5.4 Activity and Stability of Lyophilized Proteins

Freezing, and more specifically controlled nucleation, acts on various factors that affect the stability of protein-based drugs. The main factors that could destabilize or unfold proteins include crystallization of buffer components and/or co-solutes, and the extent of ice-water interface. As concerns this last parameter, it is well known that some proteins tend to be adsorbed onto the interface separating ice and the cryo-concentrated solution, and hence change their secondary and tertiary structures [103]. For these proteins, stability is directly correlated with the extent of the ice-water interface which is essentially determined by freezing rate and nucleation temperature [104].

All those methods that entail high freezing rates and nucleation at low temperatures, e.g., quench freezing, promote the formation of large ice-water interface and, thus, protein aggregation or changes in its structure [105–107]. Other authors could not find a clear correlation between protein activity/stability and freezing rate. For example, Jiang and Nail [20] found that the activity of LDH was best preserved by precooled freezing at −40 °C, while the conventional shelf-ramped freezing (and 0.5 °C min^{-1} as cooling rate) gave intermediate recovery. Quench freezing in liquid nitrogen instead resulted in the lowest LDH activity. If this comparison is based on cooling rate, these results seem to be in contrast with other observations reported in the literature. Nonetheless, the area of the ice-water interface is not determined by the cooling rate, but by the actual freezing rate. Consequently, if it is true that the cooling rate of precooled shelf freezing was higher than that of the conventional method, this was not true for the freezing rate. In fact, the freezing rate was higher for the conventional freezing because of its higher degree of supercooling and more uniform thermal equilibrium within the sample volume [88]. Similarly, annealing produces smaller ice-water interface and, hence, better preserves the protein stability [107]. This result can effectively be achieved if we assume that protein denaturation induced by adsorption on the ice-water interface is reversible in the liquid state and becomes irreversible only after lyophilization. Of course, these results are valid only if the protein denaturation is predominantly due to its adsorption onto the ice-water interface, while other factors, e.g., phase separation, play a minor role.

If the adsorption onto the ice-water interface is the predominant mechanism of denaturation/destabilization of the proteins, we can deduce that the controlled nucleation technologies are beneficial to the recovery of their activity. In fact, these technologies were found to dramatically decrease SSA of lyophilized samples and, thus, the area of the ice-water interface formed during freezing [117]. Consequently, they should decrease the probability of protein adsorption on the ice crystals surface and its denaturation. However, this hypothesis has not been experimentally confirmed in the literature to date.

5.5 Scalability to Manufacturing Units

Despite their advantages, not all the controlled nucleation technologies can effectively be applied in large-scale units. For example, electro-freezing can hardly be implemented in industrial equipment because of the limitations in the salt content of the solutions and the high voltage required to promote the formation of the ice crystals. By contrast, the addition of nucleating agents is potentially applicable in large-scale units but is hardly compatible with the regulatory requirements of the pharmaceutical products. Ultimately, the application of ultrasound to initiate nucleation is not applicable for all the freeze-dryers and process conditions need to be adjusted for partially and full-loaded freeze-dryers. At the present time, commercially available equipment can control nucleation by either the ice-fog method, pressurization-depressurization freezing, or vacuum-induced surface freezing [108]. Their application to industrial scale freeze-dryers is discussed below.

Martin Christ developed the LyoCoN technology [109]. The ice fog is produced in a dedicated condenser, which operates at atmospheric pressure, and is then naturally transferred to the freezing chamber, which works at 10 mbar, as soon as the isolation valve that separates the two units is open. A similar apparatus is commercially distributed by Millrock Technology, named FreezeBooster, which uses an external ice seed generator to instantly distribute the ice fog. This unit has been designed for a pilot-scale freeze-dryer, with shelf areas from 0.5 to 9 m^2, and is currently being tested in large-scale equipment, with a shelf area of 20 m^2. This last technology includes some technical improvements to the conventional ice fog method [110]. For example, a predetermined volume of condensed frost is created on the inner surface of the condenser, which is maintained at high pressure to promote the transition to turbulence as soon as the product chamber and condenser are connected. The turbulence breaks the frost formed on the condenser surface into large ice crystals, which last longer in the product chamber and therefore increase the probability to trigger nucleation of all the product vials.

The ice fog method as modified by Geidobler [52] has been implemented by GEA for both a laboratory freeze-dryer, with a shelf area of 5 m^2, and an industrial one, with a shelf area of

$42\ m^2$ [111]. Preliminary tests of this technology, named LYOSPARK, demonstrated that some vials spontaneously nucleated before venting and others did not nucleate at all. Therefore, careful control of the venting pressure is required and may need to be adjusted depending on the apparatus design and size.

Linde and IMA further optimized the ice fog method, in terms of sterility, density, and uniformity of the ice fog [112], to make it suitable for industrial applications. In this technology, named VERISEQ, the cryogenic gas is filtered and then mixed with sterile steam [113] or a humid gas [114] through an injector, producing the ice fog under controlled sterile conditions. This technology has been tested in an industrial apparatus, with a shelf area of $56\ m^2$, and allowed the instantaneous nucleation of 195,000 vials [115].

The pressurization-depressurization method has been patented by Praxair [71, 72, 116], initially licensed to SP Scientific and GEA, and then exclusively to SP Scientific. This technology, named ConTroLyo, can easily be installed onto manufacturing units with steam-in-place capability, while it is generally not compatible with a laboratory unit because of the high operating pressure required by this method. In addition, the high rate of depressurization, $0.014\ bar\ s^{-1}$, may represent a limiting factor to their application in large equipment. This method has been tested, showing good performance, in pilot-scale freeze-dryers, with shelf areas from 1 to $5\ m^2$, and more recently in a large-scale unit, with a shelf area of $28\ m^2$ [108]. This technique is more fully described in Chap. 3 by Luoma et al.

The VISF method was originally patented by Bayer [118], but then abandoned because of aesthetic defects of the lyophilized products. However, Oddone et al. [77] have demonstrated that these product defects can be avoided, e.g., if the solution is degassed prior to freezing and if the product chamber is isolated as soon as the desired vacuum is achieved. They also noted that the optimal pressure at which the solution nucleates varies with its formulation and proposed a simple procedure to determine it [119]. The application of this method to industrial scale freeze-dryers is currently being investigated by Azbil-Telstar (VIN) and by HOF (SynchroFreeze). HOF further improved the SynchroFreeze technology by including, in addition to the automatic degasification of the solution to be lyophilized, a further step that allows a rapid pressurization of the product chamber as soon as nucleation occurs [120]. Azbil-Telstar has implemented the VISF technology in some manufacturing units, with shelf areas from 12 to $30\ m^2$, and the results were satisfactory (Miquel Galan, personal communication). However, the precise control of the rate of depressurization/pressurization is still problematic and needs to be further investigated.

6 Future Prospects

The most recent controlled ice nucleation technologies have dramatically increased the efficiency with which the mean nucleation temperature and its distribution can be adjusted. Their ability to initiate the ice nucleation at higher temperatures, compared to that at which spontaneously occurs, results in larger pores and shorter primary drying, whereas the secondary drying rate was reduced. Despite this negative effect, the overall drying time is dramatically shorter and has also been hypothesized that the larger pores are beneficial to the preservation of the protein activity. All these advantages did not generally require any change in the composition of the drug formulation. Some of these technologies (such as the depressurization method, VISF, etc.) also allow a dramatic reduction in vial-to-vial variability and some authors claimed that might make the scale up of a cycle from the laboratory to the industrial units easier. Despite these advances, most of these technologies are still in their early development and are far from being employed on industrial scale units. By contrast, other technologies have already been implemented; the preliminary tests seem to be promising, but some technical problems still remain unresolved. The limiting factors vary with the type of technology considered and finding practical solutions to these problems might be a promising area for future technology development.

References

1. Myerson AS (ed) (2002) Handbook of industrial crystallization. Butterworth Heinemann, Boston, MA
2. Blond G (1988) Velocity of linear crystallization of ice in macromolecular systems. Cryobiology 25(1):61–66
3. Wilson PW, Heneghan AF, Haymet ADJ (2003) Ice nucleation in nature: supercooling point (SCP) measurements and the role of heterogeneous nucleation. Cryobiology 46 (1):88–98
4. Matsumoto M, Saito S, Ohmine I (2002) Molecular dynamics simulation of the ice nucleation and growth process leading to water freezing. Nature 416(6879):409–413
5. Mason BJ (1958) The supercooling and nucleation of water. Adv Phys 7(26):221–234
6. Volmer M (1939) Kinetic der Phasenbildung. Steinkoff, Dresden
7. Lide DR (2008) CRC handbook of chemistry and physics, 88th edn. CRC Press Taylor & Francis, New York, NY, pp 6–8
8. Searles JA, Carpenter JF, Randolph TW (2001) The ice nucleation temperature determines the primary drying rate of lyophilization for samples frozen on a temperature-controlled shelf. J Pharm Sci 90(7):860–871
9. Pisano R, Fissore D, Barresi AA, Brayard P, Chouvenc P, Woinet B (2013) Quality by design: optimization of a freeze-drying cycle via design space in case of heterogeneous drying behavior and influence of the freezing protocol. Pharm Dev Technol 18:1–16
10. Tang XC, Pikal MJ (2004) Design of freeze-drying processes for pharmaceuticals: practical advice. Pharm Res 21:191–200
11. Hsu CC, Nguyen HM, Yeung DA, Brooks DA, Koe GS, Bewley TA, Pearlman R (1995) Surface denaturation at solid-void interface--a possible pathway by which opalescent particulates form during the storage of lyophilized tissue-type plasminogen activator at high temperatures. Pharm Res 12(1):69–77

12. Heller MC, Carpenter JF, Randolph TW (1999) Application of a thermodynamic model to the prediction of phase separations in freeze-concentrated formulations for protein lyophilization. Arch Biochem Biophys 363(2):191–201
13. Heller MC, Carpenter JF, Randolph T (1999) Protein formulation and lyophilization cycle design: prevention of damage due to freeze-concentration induced phase separation. Biotechnol Bioeng 63(2):166–174
14. Liu J, Viverette T, Virgin M, Anderson M, Dalal P (2005) A study of the impact of freezing on the lyophilization of a concentrated formulation with a high fill depth. Pharm Dev Technol 10(2):261–272
15. Snell GD, Cloudman AM (1943) The effect of rate of freezing on the survival of fourteen transplantable tumors of mice. Cancer Res 3 (6):396–400
16. Talstad I, Dalen H, Scheie P, Røli J (1981) Patterns in quench frozen, freeze-dried, blood proteins. Scan Electron Microsc (Pt 2):319–326
17. Scheie P, Dalen H, Saetersdal T, Myklebust R (1982) Freezing patterns in quench frozen, freeze-dried polyvinylpyrrolidone (PVP). J Microsc 126(3):237–242
18. Patapoff TW, Overcashier DE (2002) The importance of freezing on lyophilization cycle development. Biopharm 15(1):16–21
19. Hottot A, Vessot S, Andrieu J (2007) Freeze drying of pharmaceuticals in vials: influence of freezing protocol and sample configuration on ice morphology and freeze-dried cake texture. Chem Eng Process 46(7):666–674
20. Jiang S, Nail SL (1998) Effect of process conditions on recovery of protein activity after freezing and freeze-drying. Eu J Pharm Biopharm 45(3):249–257
21. Zhou Y, Gasteyer TH, Grinter NJ, Cheng AT, Ho S Y-C, Sever RR (2014) Method and system for nucleation control in a controlled rate freezer (CRF). Patent US 8,794,013 B2, 5 Aug 2014
22. Searles JA (2004) Freezing and annealing phenomena in lyophilization. In: Rey L, May JC (eds) Freeze-drying/lyophilization of pharmaceutical and biological products, 2nd edn. Marcel Dekker, New York, NY, pp 109–145
23. Lifshitz IM, Slyozov VV (1961) The kinetics of precipitation from supersaturated solid solutions. J Phys Chem Solid 19(1-2):35–50
24. Gatlin L, Deluca PP (1980) A study of the phase transitions in frozen antibiotic solutions by differential scanning calorimetry. J Parenter Drug Assoc 34(5):398–408
25. Carpenter JF, Pikal MJ, Chang BS, Randolph TW (1997) Rational design of stable lyophilized protein formulations: some practical advice. Pharm Res 14(8):969–975
26. Simatos D, Faure M, Bonjour E, Couach M (1975) The physical state of water at low temperatures in plasma with different water contents as studied by differential thermal analysis and differential scanning calorimetry. Cryobiology 12(3):202–208
27. Sahagian ME, Goff HD (1994) Effect of freezing rate on the thermal, mechanical and physical aging properties of the glassy state in frozen sucrose solutions. Thermochim Acta 246(2):271–283
28. Lu X, Pikal MJ (2004) Freeze-drying of mannitol–trehalose–sodium chloride-based formulations: the impact of annealing on dry layer resistance to mass transfer and cake structure. Pharm Dev Technol 9 (1):85–95
29. Gatlin LA, Nail SL (1994) Freeze drying: a practical overview. In: Harrison R (ed) Protein purification process engineering, 1st edn. Marcel Dekker, New York, NY, pp 317–367
30. Franks F (1998) Freeze-drying of bioproducts: putting principles into practice. Eu J Pharm Biopharm 45(3):221–229
31. Esfandiary R, Gattu SK, Stewart JM, Patel SM (2016) Effect of freezing on lyophilization process performance and drug product cake appearance. J Pharm Sci 105 (4):1427–1433
32. Searles JA, Carpenter JF, Randolph TW (2001) Annealing to optimize the primary drying rate, reduce freezing-induced drying rate heterogeneity, and determine Tg' in pharmaceutical lyophilization. J Pharm Sci 90 (7):872–887
33. Layton RC (1973) Ice nucleation by silver iodide: influence of an electric field. J Colloid Interface Sci 42(1):214–217
34. Margaritis A, Bassi AS (1991) Principles and biotechnological applications of bacterial ice nucleation. Crit Rev Biotechnol 11 (3):277–295
35. Lindong W, Shannon NT, Anisa S, Shannon LS, Mehmet T (2017) Controlled ice nucleation using freeze-dried *Pseudomonas syringae* encapsulated in alginate beads. Cryobiology 75(4):1–6
36. Cochet N, Widehem P (2000) Ice crystallization by Pseudomonas syringae. Appl Microbiol Biotechnol 54(2):153–161
37. Rau W (1951) Eiskeimbildung durch dielektrische Polarisation. Zeitschrift für Naturforschung A 6(11):649–657

38. Shichiri T, Araki Y (1986) Nucleation mechanism of ice crystals under electrical effect. J Cryst Growth 78(3):502–508
39. Wei S, Zhong C, Su-Yi H (2005) Molecular dynamics simulation of liquid water under the influence of an external electric field. Mol Simulat 31(8):555–559
40. Hozumi T, Saito A, Okawa S, Eshita Y (2003) Effects of shapes of electrodes on freezing of supercooled water in electric freeze control. Int J Refrig 26(5):537–542
41. Petersen A, Schneider H, Rau G, Glasmacher B (2006) A new approach for freezing of aqueous solutions under active control of the nucleation temperature. Cryobiology 53 (2):248–257
42. Petersen A, Rau G, Glasmacher B (2006) Reduction of primary freeze-drying time by electric field induced ice nucleus formation. Heat Mass Transfer 42(10):929–938
43. Kuu W-Y, Doty MJ, Rebbeck CL, Hurst WS, Cho YK (2013) Gap-freezing approach for shortening the lyophilization cycle time of pharmaceutical formulations-demonstration of the concept. J Pharm Sci 102 (8):2572–2588
44. Kuu W-Y, Doty MJ, Hurst WS, Rebbeck CL (2017) Optimization of nucleation and crystallization for lyophilization using gap freezing. Patent US 9,625,210 B2, 18 Apr 2017
45. Capozzi LC, Pisano R (2016) Freeze-drying of suspended vials: the first step toward continuous manufacturing. In: Proceedings of the 2nd international symposium on continuous manufacturing of pharmaceuticals, Cambridge, 26–27 September 2016
46. Rowe TD (1992) A technique for the nucleation of ice. In: Brown F, May JC (eds) Proceedings of international symposium on biological product freeze-drying and formulation, Bethesda, 24-26 October 1990. Developments in biological standardization, vol 74. Karger, New York, NY, p 377
47. Mason BJ, Ludlam FH (1951) The microphysics of clouds. Rep Prog Phys 14 (1):147–195
48. Rambhatla S, Ramot R, Bhugra C, Pikal MJ (2004) Heat and mass transfer scale-up issues during freeze drying: II. Control and characterization of the degree of supercooling. AAPS PharmSciTech 5(4):54–62
49. Patel SM, Bhugra C, Pikal MJ (2009) Reduced pressure ice fog technique for controlled ice nucleation during freeze-drying. AAPS PharmSciTech 10(4):1406–1411
50. Demarco F, Renzi E, Lee R, Chakravarty P (2012) Ice fog as a means to induce uniform ice nucleation during lyophilization. Biopharm Int 25(1):33–38
51. Weija L (2012) Controlled nucleation during freezing step of freeze drying cycle using pressure differential ice fog distribution. Patent US 8,839,528 B2, 23 Sept 2014
52. Geidobler R, Mannschedel S, Winter G (2012) A new approach to achieve controlled ice nucleation of supercooled solutions during the freezing step in freeze-drying. J Pharm Sci 101(12):4409–4413
53. Hickling R (1965) Nucleation of freezing by cavity collapse and its relation to cavitation damage. Nature 206(4987):915–917
54. Li B, Sun D-W (2002) Novel methods for rapid freezing and thawing of foods – a review. J Food Eng 54(3):175–182
55. Petzold G, Aguilera JM (2009) Ice morphology: fundamentals and technological applications in foods. Food Biophys 4(4):378–396
56. Inada T, Zhang X, Yabe A, Kozawa Y (2001) Active control of phase change from supercooled water to ice by ultrasonic vibration 1. Control of freezing temperature. J Heat Mass Transfer 44(23):4523–4531
57. Zhang X, Inada T, Yabe A, Lu S, Kozawa Y (2001) Active control of phase change from supercooled water to ice by ultrasonic vibration 2. Generation of ice slurries and effect of bubble nuclei. J Heat Mass Transfer 44 (23):4533–4539
58. Hunt JD, Jackson KA (1966) Nucleation of solid in an undercooled liquid by cavitation. J Appl Phys 17(1):254–257
59. Zhang X, Inada T, Tezuka A (2003) Ultrasonic-induced nucleation of ice in water containing air bubbles. Ultrason Sonochem 10(2):71–76
60. Nakagawa K, Hottot A, Vessot S, Andrieu J (2006) Influence of controlled nucleation by ultrasounds on ice morphology of frozen formulations for pharmaceutical proteins freeze-drying. Chem Eng Process 45(9):783–791
61. Hottot A, Nakagawa K, Andrieu J (2008) Effect of ultrasound-controlled nucleation on structural and morphological properties of freeze-dried mannitol solutions. Chem Eng Res Des 86(2):193–200
62. Saclier M, Peczalski R, Andrieu J (2010) Effect of ultrasonically induced nucleation on ice crystal size and shape during freezing in vials. Chem Eng Sci 65(10):3064–3071
63. Acton E, Morris GJ (2004) Method and apparatus for freeze drying material. Patent Application GB 2,400,901 A, 27 Oct 2004
64. Passot S, Tréléa IC, Marin M, Galan M, Morris GJ, Fonseca F (2009) Effect of controlled

ice nucleation on primary drying stage and protein recovery in vials cooled in a modified freeze-dryer. J Biochem Eng 131(7):074511
65. Kanda Y, Aoki M, Kosugi T (1992) Freezing of tofu by pressure shift freezing and its structure. Nippon Shokuhin Kogyo Gakkaishai 39 (7):608–614
66. Martino MN, Otero L, Sanz PD, Zaritzky NE (1998) Size and location of ice crystals in pork frozen by high-pressure-assisted freezing as compared to classical methods. Meat Sci 50 (3):303–313
67. Sanz PD, Otero L, de Elvira C, Carrasco JA (1997) Freezing processes in high-pressure domains. Int J Refrig 20(5):301–307
68. Knorr D, Schlueter O, Heinz V (1998) Impact of high hydrostatic pressure on phase transitions of foods. Food Technol 52 (9):42–45
69. Otero L, Sanz PD (1998) High-pressure shift freezing. Part 1. Amount of ice instantaneously formed in the process. Biotechnol Prog 16(6):1030–1036
70. Fernández PP, Otero L, Guignon B, Sanz PD (2006) High-pressure shift freezing versus high-pressure assisted freezing: effects on the microstructure of a food model. Food Hydrocoll 20(4):510–522
71. Gasteyer TH, Sever RR, Hunek B, Grinter N, Verdone ML (2017) Lyophilization system and method. Patent US 9,651,305 B2, 16 May 2017
72. Gasteyer TH III, Sever RR, Hunek B, Grinter N, Verdone ML (2015) Method of inducing nucleation of a material. Patent US 9,453,675 B2, 25 Sept 2016, Patent EP 1,982,133 B1, 15 Jul 2015
73. Konstantinidis AK, Kuu W, Otten L, Nail SL, Sever RR, Bons V, Debo D, Pikal MJ (2011) Controlled nucleation in freeze-drying: effects on pore size in the dried product layer, mass transfer resistance, and primary drying rate. J Pharm Sci 100(8):3453–3470
74. Geidobler R, Winter G (2013) Controlled ice nucleation in the field of freeze-drying: fundamentals and technology review. Eu J Pharm Biopharm 85(2):214–222
75. McDonald K, Sun D-W (2000) Vacuum cooling technology for the food processing industry: a review. J Food Eng 45(2):55–65
76. Kramer M, Sennhenn B, Lee G (2002) Freeze-drying using vacuum-induced surface freezing. J Pharm Sci 91:433–443
77. Oddone I, Pisano R, Bullich R, Stewart P (2014) Vacuum-induced nucleation as a method for freeze-drying cycle optimization. Ind Eng Chem Res 53:18236–18244
78. Roy ML, Pikal MJ (1989) Process control in freeze drying: determination of the end point of sublimation drying by an electronic moisture sensor. J Parenter Sci Technol 43 (2):60–66
79. Pisano R, Capozzi LC (2017) Prediction of product morphology of lyophilized drugs in the case of Vacuum Induced Surface Freezing. Chem Eng Res Des 125(1):119–129
80. Oddone I, Van Bockstal P-J, De Beer T, Pisano R (2016) Impact of vacuum-induced surface freezing on inter- and intra-vial heterogeneity. Eu J Pharm Biopharm 103 (1):167–178
81. Oddone I, Fulginiti D, Barresi AA, Grassini S, Pisano R (2015) Non-invasive temperature monitoring in freeze drying: control of freezing as a case study. Drying Technol 33 (13):1621–1630
82. Kim AI, Akers MJ, Nail SL (1998) The physical state of mannitol after freeze-drying: effects of mannitol concentration, freezing rate, and a noncrystallizing cosolute. J Pharm Sci 87(8):931–935
83. Cavatur RK, Vemuri NM, Pyne A, Chrzan Z, Toledo-Velasquez D, Suryanarayanan R (2002) Crystallization behavior of mannitol in frozen aqueous solutions. Pharm Res 19 (6):894–900
84. Izutsu K, Yoshioka S, Kojima S (1994) Physical stability and protein stability of freeze-dried cakes during storage at elevated temperatures. Pharm Res 45(1):5–8
85. Liao X, Krishnamurthy R, Suryanarayanan R (2007) Influence of processing conditions on the physical state of mannitol - implications in freeze-drying. Pharm Res 24(2):370–376
86. Barresi AA, Ghio S, Fissore D, Pisano R (2009) Freeze drying of pharmaceutical excipients close to collapse temperature: influence of the process conditions on process time and product quality. Drying Technol 27 (6):805–816
87. Webb SD, Cleland JL, Carpenter JF, Randolph TW (2003) Effects of annealing lyophilized and spray-lyophilized formulations of recombinant human interferon-γ. J Pharm Sci 92(4):715–729
88. Kasper JC, Friess W (2011) The freezing step in lyophilization: physico-chemical fundamentals, freezing methods and consequences on process performance and quality attributes of biopharmaceuticals. Eu J Pharm Biopharm 78(2):248–263
89. Kuu WY, O'Bryan KR, Hardwick LM, Paul TW (2011) Product mass transfer resistance directly determined during freeze-drying

cycle runs using tunable diode laser absorption spectroscopy (TDLAS) and pore diffusion model. Pharm Dev Technol 16 (4):343–357
90. Pisano R, Barresi AA, Capozzi LC, Novajra G, Oddone I, Vitale-Brovarone C (2017) Characterization of the mass transfer of lyophilized products based on X-ray micro-computed tomography images. Drying Technol 35 (8):933–938
91. Velardi SA, Barresi A (2008) Development of simplified models for the freeze-drying process and investigation of the optimal operating conditions. Chem Eng Res Des 86 (1A):9–22
92. Franks F, Auffret T (eds) (2007) Freeze-drying of pharmaceuticals and biopharmaceuticals. RSC Publishing, Cambridge
93. Pisano R, Fissore D, Barresi AA (2011) Freeze-drying cycle optimization using model predictive control techniques. Ind Eng Chem Res 50(12):7363–7379
94. Hottot A, Vessot S, Andrieu J (2004) A direct characterization method of the ice morphology. Relationship between mean crystalsize and primary drying times of freeze-drying processes. Drying Technol 22 (8):2009–2021
95. Bursac R, Sever R, Hunek B (2009) A practical method for resolving the nucleation problem in lyophilization. Bioprocess Int:66–72
96. Pikal MJ (1999) Heat and mass transfer in low pressure gases: applications to freeze drying. In: Amidon G, Lee P, Topp L (eds) Transport process in pharmaceutical systems, 1st edn. Marcel Dekker, New York, NY, pp 611–686
97. Pikal MJ, Shah S, Roy ML, Putman R (1990) The secondary drying stage of freeze drying: drying kinetics as a function of temperature and chamber. Int J Pharm 60(3):203–217
98. Pisano R, Fissore D, Barresi AA (2012) Quality by design in the secondary drying step of a freeze-drying process. Drying Technol 30 (11-12):1307–1316
99. Fissore D, Pisano R, Barresi AA (2011) Monitoring of the secondary drying in freeze-drying of pharmaceuticals. J Pharm Sci 100 (2):732–742
100. Oddone I, Pisano R, Barresi AA (2017) Influence of controlled ice nucleation on the freeze-drying of pharmaceutical products: the secondary drying step. Int J Pharm 524 (1-2):134–140
101. Tang X, Nail SL, Pikal MJ (2005) Freeze-drying process design by manometric temperature measurement: design of a smart freeze-dryer. Pharm Res 22(4):685–700
102. Patel SM, Doen T, Pikal MJ (2010) Determination of end point of primary drying in freeze-drying process control. AAPS PharSciTech 11(1):73–84
103. Strambini GB, Gabellieri E (1996) Proteins in frozen solutions: evidence of ice-induced partial unfolding. Biophys J 70(2I):971–976
104. Wang W (2000) Lyophilization and development of solid protein pharmaceuticals. Int J Pharm 203(1):1–60
105. Chang BS, Kendrick BS, Carpenter JF (1996) Surface-induced denaturation of proteins during freezing and its inhibition by surfactants. J Pharm Sci 85(12):1325–1330
106. Eckhardt BM, Oeswein JQ, Bewley TA (1991) Effect of freezing on aggregation of human growth hormone. Pharm Res 8 (11):1360–1363
107. Sarciaux JM, Mansour S, Hageman MJ, Nail SL (1999) Effects of buffer composition and processing conditions on aggregation of bovine IgG during freeze-drying. J Pharm Sci 88(12):1354–1361
108. Siew A (2013) Controlling ice nucleation during the freezing step of lyophilization. Pharm Technol 37(5):36–40
109. Umbach M (2017) Freeze drying plant. Patent EP 3,093,597 B1, 27 Dec 2017
110. Ling W (2014) Controlled nucleation during freezing step of freeze drying cycle using pressure differential ice crystals distribution from condensed frost. Patent US 8,875,413 B2, 4 November 2014
111. GEA. Inducing nucleation in industrial freeze dryers. Manufacturing Chemist 2017 (22 Nov). Available at https://www.manufacturingchemist.com/news/article_page/Inducing_nucleation_in_industrial_freeze_dryers/136511
112. Brower J, Lee R, Wexler E, Finley S, Caldwell M, Studer P (2015) New developments in controlled nucleation: commercializing VERISEQ® nucleation technology. In: Varshney D, Singh M (eds) Lyophilized biologics and vaccines. Springer, New York, NY, pp 73–90
113. Chakravarty P, Lee RC (2013) Method for freeze drying. Patent US 8,549,768 B2, 8 Oct 2013
114. Lee RC, Chakravarty P (2013) Freeze drying method. Patent EP 2,478,313 B1, 25 Oct 2013
115. Azzarella J, Mudhivarthi VK, Wexler E, Ganguly A (2017) Increasing vial to vial homogeneity: an analysis of VERISEQ® nucleation on production scale freeze dryers. BioPharm Int 29(12):36–41

116. Rampersad BM, Sever RR, Humek B, Gasteyer TH III (2012) Freeze-dryer and method of controlling the same. Patent US 8,240,065 B2, 14 Aug 2012
117. Awotwe-Otoo D, Agarabi C, Read EK, Lute S, Brorson KA, Khan MA, Shah RB (2013) Impact of controlled ice nucleation on process performance and quality attributes of a lyophilized monoclonal antibody. Int J Pharm 450(1-2):70–78
118. Sennhenn B, Kramer M (2004) Lyophilization method. Patent US 6,684,524 B1, 3 Feb 2004
119. Arsiccio A, Barresi A, De Beer T, Oddone I, Van Bockstal P-J, Pisano R (2018) Vacuum Induced Surface Freezing as an effective method for improved inter- and intra-vial product homogeneity. Eu J Pharm Biopharm 128(1):210–219
120. Wexler E, Brower J (2015) New developments in controlled nucleation. Pharm Manufactur 2015:26–29 https://www.pharmamanufacturing.com/articles/2015/new-developments-in-controlled-nucleation/

Chapter 5

Tunable Diode Laser Absorption Spectroscopy in Lyophilization

William J. Kessler and Emily Gong

Abstract

Chapter 5 provides a description of a tunable diode laser absorption spectroscopy-based sensor that provides real-time, non-contact measurements of the gas temperature, water vapor concentration, and gas flow velocity in the duct connecting the lyophilizer product chamber and condenser. These measurements are used to calculate the water vapor mass flow rate throughout the primary and secondary drying phases of freeze-drying. The instantaneous mass flow values are integrated to provide a continuous determination of the total amount of water removed during the lyophilization process. Permanent sensor calibration is performed using an interferometric technique leveraging the wave characteristics of light. The sensor calibration is verified using ice slab sublimation tests with direct comparisons of the integrated measurements to gravimetric determinations of total water removed. Direct use of the measured values and the calculated mass flow rate combined with a heat and mass transfer model of vial based freeze-drying have been used to demonstrate numerous applications that will be described in this chapter.

Key words Tunable diode laser absorption spectroscopy, Water vapor mass flow, Freeze drying, Lyophilization, Heat and mass transfer model, Quality by design process development

1 Introduction

Many biopharmaceuticals are labile in solution and must be stabilized for storage, distribution, and patient use. Lyophilization or freeze drying is a frequently used method employing low temperature processing and dehydration to achieve stabilization [1, 2]. While there is some interest in alternative drying systems within the pharmaceutical industry, the level of interest is limited. It is important to recognize that despite some of these methods being promoted for many decades, freeze drying remains the drying method of choice for parenterals. Freeze drying produces stable drug products that can be stored and reconstituted at the time of patient use.

Over the past few decades, lyophilization has been transformed from an art into a science-based process with researchers

Kevin R. Ward and Paul Matejtschuk (eds.), *Lyophilization of Pharmaceuticals and Biologicals: New Technologies and Approaches*, Methods in Pharmacology and Toxicology, https://doi.org/10.1007/978-1-4939-8928-7_5,

developing process monitoring strategies and freeze-drying mathematical models to aid in the development of optimized freeze-drying cycles. The process monitoring tools enable both batch average and vial-specific measurement techniques which, when combined, can provide a nearly complete set of data that can be used to predict and monitor drying behavior [3, 4]. Included among those tools is Tunable Diode Laser Absorption Spectroscopy (TDLAS) [5, 6] which was first applied to freeze drying in 2003. A TDLAS sensor can be used to provide real-time, non-intrusive monitoring of the water vapor mass flow exiting the lyophilizer product chamber, and these continuous measurements can be integrated to provide an indication of total water removed throughout the drying process [7]. Most importantly, the measurement of water vapor mass flow, dm/dt, can be used as an input to heat and mass flow models of freeze drying [8] to enable prediction of key process parameters, including the product temperature during lyophilization, which has a direct impact on product quality [9]. This has led to numerous application demonstrations by both academic and industrial researchers [10–16]. In this chapter, we describe the physics behind the TDLAS-based measurements, the linkage of the measurements to the heat and mass transfer model of lyophilization in vials, and the application of this dual technology approach to process monitoring and cycle development. In addition, an example of a new application of the TDLAS measurement technology is provided which enables development of a freeze-drying process recipe in a single experiment for any product formulation and can be applied to all scale freeze dryers.

2 TDLAS Measurement Principles

A batch average tunable diode laser absorption spectroscopy (TDLAS) sensor measures the water vapor concentration and flow velocity in the flow duct connecting the freeze dryer chamber and condenser (Fig. 1) to enable the determination of water vapor mass flow rates. TDLAS sensors use Beer's Law, well-known spectroscopic principles, and sensitive detection techniques to continuously measure trace concentrations of selected gases. For water vapor detection, the laser wavelength is often tuned to a well-separated absorption lineshape at 1392.5 nm [17]. The Gaussian lineshape from the low pressure measurement environment is analyzed to provide a determination of the gas temperature (from the lineshape full width at half maximum, FWHM) which is used to calculate the absorption linestrength. The linestrength and the integrated area under the absorption lineshape are used to determine the water vapor number density or concentration (molecules cm^{-3}).

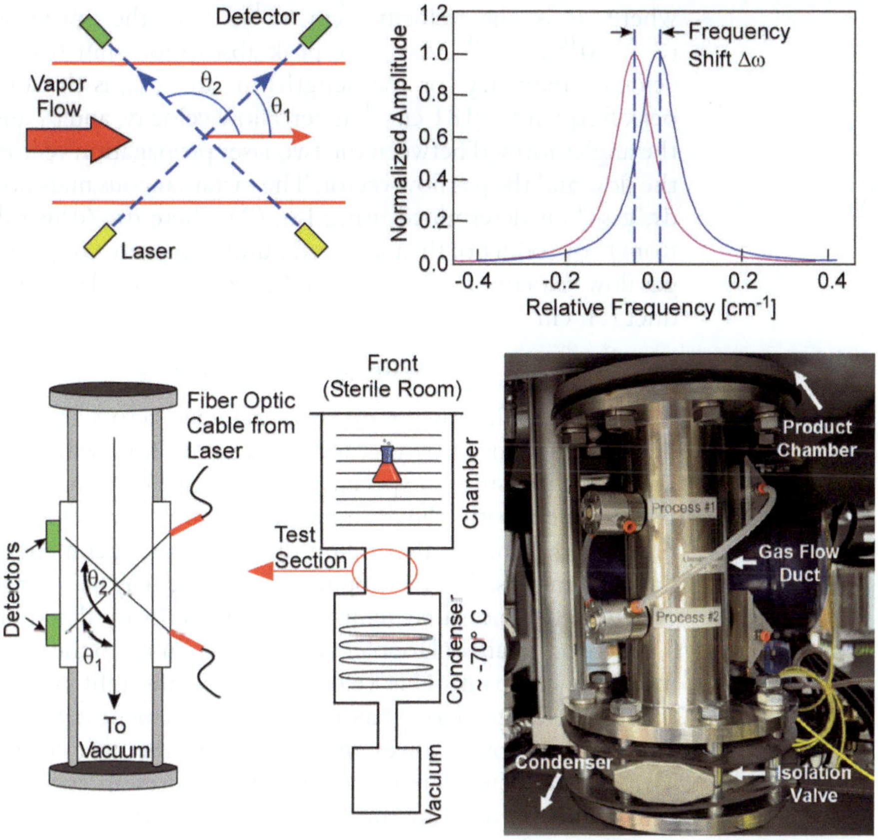

Fig. 1 Illustration and hardware implementation of the velocity measurement concept in the freeze dryer spool, resulting Doppler shifted absorption spectrum

The determination of mass flow also requires the measurement of the gas flow velocity in addition to water vapor density in the measurement volume [18]. The velocity measurement concept is based upon Doppler-shifted absorption measurements as schematically shown in Fig. 1. The velocity is determined from the Doppler-shifted absorption spectrum of water vapor resulting from the laser propagation vector directed at a known angle, θ, to the gas flow velocity vector, u. The absorption spectrum is shifted in wavelength or frequency with respect to the absorption wavelength of a static gas sample by an amount related to the velocity of the gas, u, and the angle between u and the probe laser beam propagation vector. Using two line-of-sight measurements across the spool connecting the freeze dryer chamber and condenser, the frequency shift of one measurement path is compared to the second path within the spool and described by Eq. (1):

$$u = \frac{c \cdot \Delta \nu}{\nu_o \cdot (\cos \theta_1 - \cos \theta_2)} \tag{1}$$

where u is the velocity (cm s^{-1}), c is the speed of light (3×10^{10} cm s^{-1}), $\Delta\nu$ is the peak absorption shift from its zero velocity frequency (or wavelength) in cm^{-1}, ν_o is the absorption peak frequency, 7181 cm^{-1} at zero flow velocity, and θ_1 and θ_2 are the angles formed between the two laser propagation vectors across the flow and the gas flow vector. The instantaneous mass flow (dm/dt, g s^{-1}) is determined using Eq. (2) where dm/dt is calculated from the product of the measured number density (N, g cm^{-3}), the gas flow velocity (u, cm s^{-1}), and the cross-sectional area of the flow duct (A, cm^2):

$$dm/dt\ (g/s) = N \times u \times A \tag{2}$$

Line-of-sight absorption measurements across the lyophilizer duct are influenced by the developing fluid flow within the pipe. While the pressure is expected to be relatively uniform across the measurement path, the gas temperature and flow velocity profiles may not be uniform depending upon the duct geometry and the flow parameters. The developing flow profile may have a significant effect on the measured temperature and velocity determinations. The sensor obtains a Doppler velocity pertaining to the line of sight measurement path. This velocity may be thought of as a radial segment average velocity along the measurement path, while the desired mass flow involves an integral over the duct cross section. To precisely determine the mass flow requires an estimate of the velocity profile to relate the Doppler velocity to the mass flow.

The gas flow may be approximated as a laminar entrance flow in a straight circular pipe within the lyophilizer. The top hat entrance velocity profile evolves into a parabolic profile in the fully developed limit. A uniform velocity core persists at intermediate stations, although the core flow is accelerated above the average velocity. The absorption line shape at any radial position in the flow is a function of both the temperature and velocity at each radial position described by the developing profile. These latter quantities will have changing values across the flow (with the exception of plug flow), and thus the observed absorption lineshapes are essentially averages over these velocity and temperature profiles. Therefore, for all flows more developed than plug flow, the measured velocity is always larger than the average velocity with the difference increasing as the temperature deficit between centerline and outer radial positions becomes larger. This is because the velocities near the center line of the flow tend to be higher than the average velocity and the number densities are also higher than the average (due to the lower temperature). Thus, these values are weighted more toward values nearer the wall. As the flow distribution becomes more parabolic (toward fully developed flow) this effect becomes more pronounced, thus a larger correction is required to determine the line-of-sight average flow velocity.

As described above, the measured temperature is determined from the measured water absorption linewidth. The predicted behavior of the temperature ratio (compared to the average) is more complex than that of the velocity ratio because the measured temperature is affected by two competing phenomena. First, the density is highest on the center line where the temperature is lowest, thus the absorption at center radial positions is weighted more than that near the wall. This makes the measured temperature appear cooler than the line-of-sight average temperature. Alternatively, the effect of the velocity distribution is to make the absorption line shape appear broader, due to the variation in the frequency position of the peak line shifts. This latter effect makes the measured temperature appear warmer than the average temperature.

Following the calculation of the average line-of-sight gas temperature, water vapor number density, and velocity, the water vapor mass flow rate may be calculated using Eq. (2). The resulting mass flow rate does not account for developing velocity flow profile. The line-of-sight average mass flow rate "over-weights" the centerline radial positions, which subtend smaller cross-sectional areas of the duct as compared to outer radial positions. To correct the calculated mass flow rate, a mass scaling factor is continuously determined and used to provide the average mass flow rate.

The total amount of water removed (grams) is determined by integrating the instantaneous mass flow rate measurements. The dual line of sight configuration using a 10-cm diameter duct provides water density and velocity measurement sensitivity of better than ~5×10^{13} molecules cm^{-3} and ~1 m s^{-1}, respectively, and a mass flow sensitivity of better than 10 μg s^{-1}. Measurements of the water sublimation rate, dm/dt (g/s), may be combined with a steady state model of freeze drying [19, 20] to determine a number of key process parameters including the vial heat transfer coefficient, K_v, product resistance to drying, R_p, product temperature, T_b (at the vial bottom), and T_0 (sublimation interface)

2.1 System Requirements

There are a number of lyophilizer system requirements needed for the application of the batch average TDLAS measurement system. The primary requirements include:

- Spool piece connecting the product chamber and condenser of adequate length to enable 45° and 135° optical measurements with respect to the gas flow vector
- Spool outfitted with four optical ports enabling two line-of-sight measurements
- Spool entrance and interior clear of any objects that would create a perturbation in the gas flow

- Isolation valve located downstream of the optical measurement locations
- Nominal spool length of approximately 1.4 × (spool diameter in inches) + 7 (inches)

2.2 System Calibration and Verification of Measurement Accuracy

A calibration factor (quantifying the laser tuning rate) is used for the determination of the gas temperature, water density, and the gas flow velocity. The tunable diode laser wavelength or frequency scan rate (nm/data point, MHz/point or cm^{-1}/point) is determined by launching the fiber coupled diode laser output into a Fabry-Perot Interferometer (FPI). An FPI is an optical cavity formed by two highly reflecting mirrors aligned to oscillate optical radiation between the two mirrors. The FPI may be formed by either flat or concave mirrors. The measurement principle and an experimental schematic of the calibration technique are illustrated in Fig. 2.

The laser light is transmitted through the mirrored cavity only when cavity conditions and the laser wavelength or frequency result in constructive interference of the oscillating light waves within the FPI cavity. The transmission maxima for a cavity constructed of flat mirrors occur separated in frequency by $\Delta\bar{\nu}$ (Free Spectral Range, FSR) described by Eq. (3).

$$\frac{1}{2nL} = \Delta\bar{\nu}(\mathrm{cm}^{-1}) \tag{3}$$

where n is the index of refraction of the medium between the two cavity mirrors ($n = 1$ for air) and L is the separation between the mirrors M_1 and M_2. Figure 3 shows both a water vapor absorption lineshape and a Fabry-Perot Interferometer (FPI) fringe spectrum for a typical diode laser used in the TDLAS sensor.

The diode laser scan rate is dependent upon the laser operating conditions and the sensor is calibrated under each of the anticipated operating conditions. The peak locations in the upper left plot of Fig. 3 are determined and a plot of relative frequency (or wavelength) scanned is plotted in the lower left plot as a function of diode laser injection current (mA). The frequency

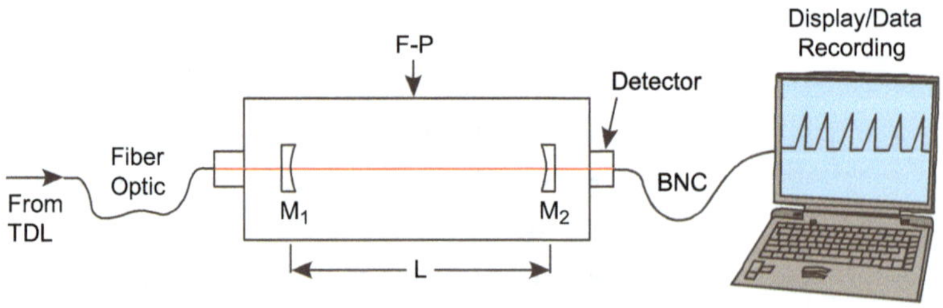

Fig. 2 Schematic diagram of the experimental setup used to calibrate the tunable diode laser frequency scan rate (cm^{-1}/mA)

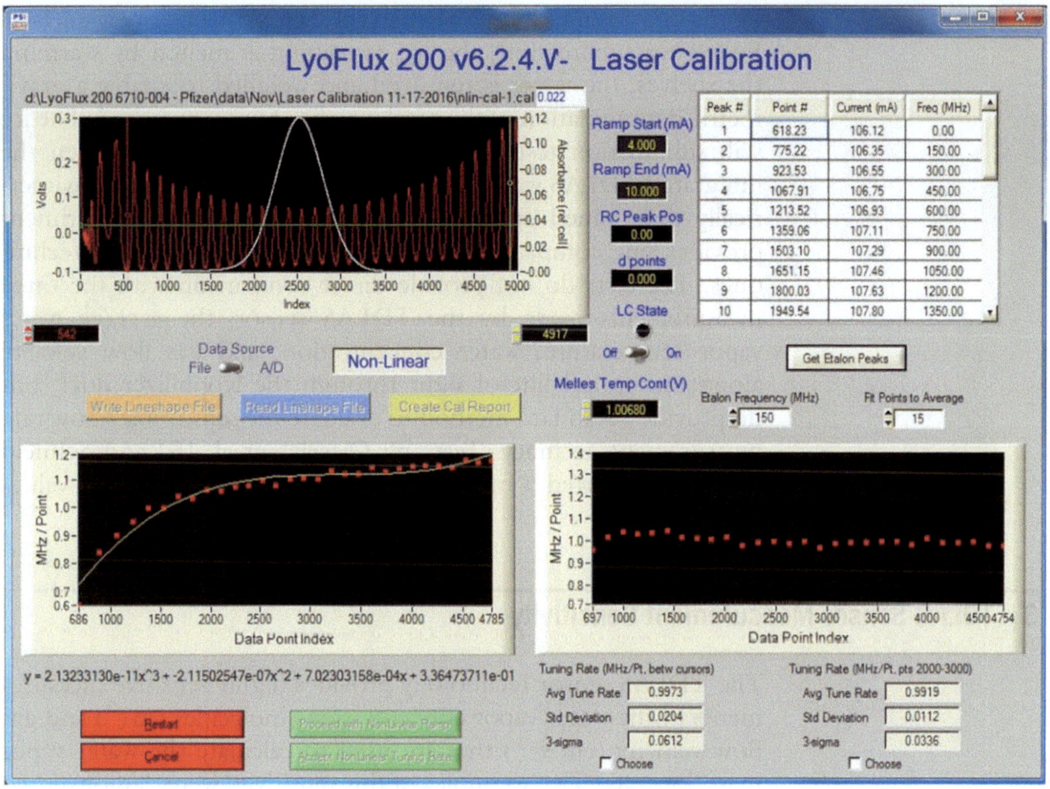

Fig. 3 TDLAS software Laser Calibration GUI screen used to capture and analyze laser wavelength scan calibration data. The upper graph displays a water vapor absorption spectrum and a Fabry-Perot interferometer fringe spectrum for the diode laser used to determine the diode laser wavelength scan rate as a function of injection current. The F-P air gap interferometer mirror separation provides a 150 MHz spacing between transmission maxima

between each of the peaks shown in Fig. 3 is equal to the Free Spectral Range (FSR) of the interferometer. In this case, the FPI used to calibrate the sensor laser has an FSR of 150 MHz. The diode laser current ramp is first scanned using a linear current ramp to determine its nonlinear tuning characteristics. The ramp is then scanned using a nonlinear injection current to achieve a linear frequency tuning rate shown in the lower right plot. A typical laser tuning rate is ~1 MHz/data point.

Assessment of the sensor measurement accuracy is performed using ice slab sublimation tests. "Bottomless trays" are formed by attaching thin black plastic (~0.003 cm thickness) to the stainless steel vial tray frames (using paper clips) typically used to arrange vials on the freeze dryer shelves [7]. Known weights of water are added to the bottomless trays, frozen by cooling the freeze dryer shelf temperature and sublimed under typical lyophilization operating conditions. Typically up to 30% of the ice is sublimed under steady state conditions. Subliming additional ice often results in the ice losing good thermal contact with the shelf surface. Following sublimation, the ice remaining is melted by warming the shelves, the water is removed and weighed to enable a gravimetric determination of the total weight of water removed. The ice slab sublimation tests provide a direct comparison between the integrated TDLAS water mass flow rate ($\mathrm{d}m/\mathrm{d}t$) and the gravimetrically determined amount of water removed. One experiment provides one comparison between the two measurement techniques. The tests do not provide direct comparison with the three measurements made by the TDLAS sensor, the average water vapor temperature, water concentration, and gas flow velocity along the optical line-of-sight through the lyophilizer duct, but do provide a standard method to evaluate the sensor mass flow rate measurement accuracy. Tests by Gieseler et al. [5] and Schneid et al. [9] reported a measurement error $\leq$7% with typical values $\leq$5%.

3 TDLAS Sensor Measurement Sensitivity

The TDLAS sensor technology provides highly sensitive measurements of the water vapor concentration (molecules cm^{-3}) and gas flow velocity (cm s^{-1}) that are used to calculate the water vapor mass flow rate. Two examples of this sensitivity were demonstrated by subliming ice from six 20 mL vials placed on the middle shelf of a Lyostar 3 freeze dryer (SP Scientific, Stone Ridge, NY, USA) during one experiment and one 20 mL vial placed on the middle shelf in a second experiment. During the six vial experiment 10 mL of deionized (DI) water was filled into each vial. At atmospheric pressure the freeze dryer shelf temperature was lowered to −40 °C to freeze the water and sublimation was carried out at a −25 °C shelf temperature and a chamber pressure of 100 mTorr. A plot of the water vapor mass flow rate and the integrated amount of water removed as a function of process time are shown in Fig. 4. At the start of the experiment during vacuum pump down of the chamber, when the chamber pressure approaches the 100 mTorr setpoint and when heat is initially applied to raise the shelf temperature above −40 °C, the frost that formed on the cold shelf heat transfer lines and the shelves begins to flash off. This "flash off" is observed as the spike in the mass flow rate data near process time of <1 h. The integrated water mass flow rate curve shows that the weight of water removed during flash off was ~0.7 g. The source of the water which formed the frost was a combination of water vapor present in the chamber just before vial loading and water vapor from the vials which increases the chamber relative humidity and is dependent upon the vial liquid water temperature and the amount of time before the water in the vials freezes. When only a few vials are dried it is likely that most of the flash off originated from the air

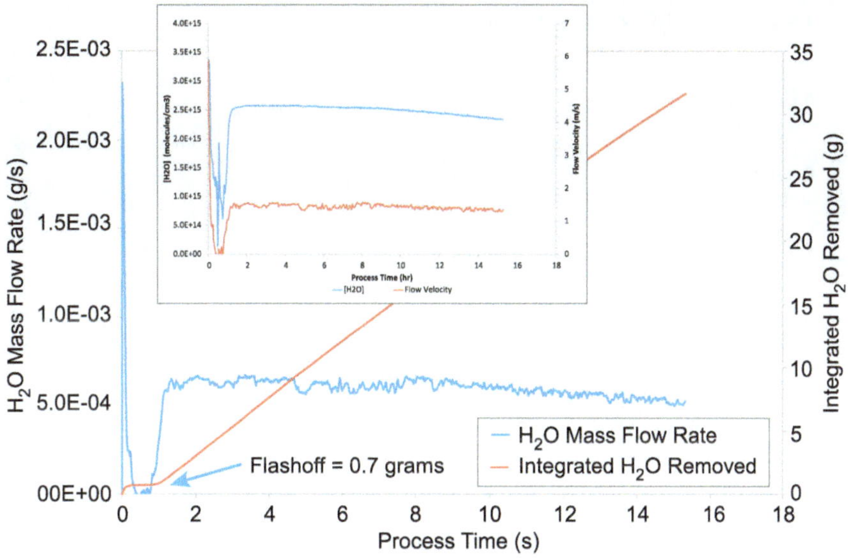

Fig. 4 TDLAS sensor data recorded during a six 20 mL vial DI water sublimation experiment demonstrating the sensor measurement sensitivity. The TDLAS measurement accuracy error in determining the total amount of water removed was ~5.4% compared to the gravimetric determination of total water removed

present in the freeze drying chamber before the filled vials were added, warranting the assumption that none of the flash off was from the vials. Figure 4 shows the average mass flow rate during the experiment to be ~6×10^{-4} g s^{-1}. The insert plot of the water vapor concentration and gas flow velocity as a function of process time shows an average flow velocity of ~1.5 m s^{-1}. The total amount of water removed (subtracting the flash off) as measured by the TDLAS sensor was 30.94 g. The total amount of water removed measured gravimetrically was 32.72 g. The ratio of TDLAS/Gravimetric measurements was 0.946, or a 5.4% under prediction of total water removed measured by the TDLAS sensor.

A similar experiment was performed using a single vial filled with 10 mL of DI water. During this experiment the ice sublimation occurred at shelf temperatures of −20 °C and +70 °C. Figure 5 shows the TDLAS sensor data (similar to Fig. 4) with the average water vapor mass flow rate of ~1.1×10^{-4} (−20 °C shelf temperature) and ~7.5×10^{-4} g s^{-1} (+70 °C shelf temperature). At process times longer than 2.5 h the mass flow rate drops due to more than ~30% of the ice being removed. The ice recedes away from the vial inner surfaces, lowering the heat transfer for sublimation. The average gas flow velocities were ~0.7 m s^{-1} and ~1.7 m s^{-1} respectively. The TDLAS measured total amount of water removed (subtracting the ~1 g of flash off) was 5.79 g while the gravimetric measurement was 5.74 g, resulting in a TDLAS/Gravimetric ratio of 1.009. This corresponds to a TDLAS over prediction of total water removed of 0.9%. Thus, both experiments demonstrate the

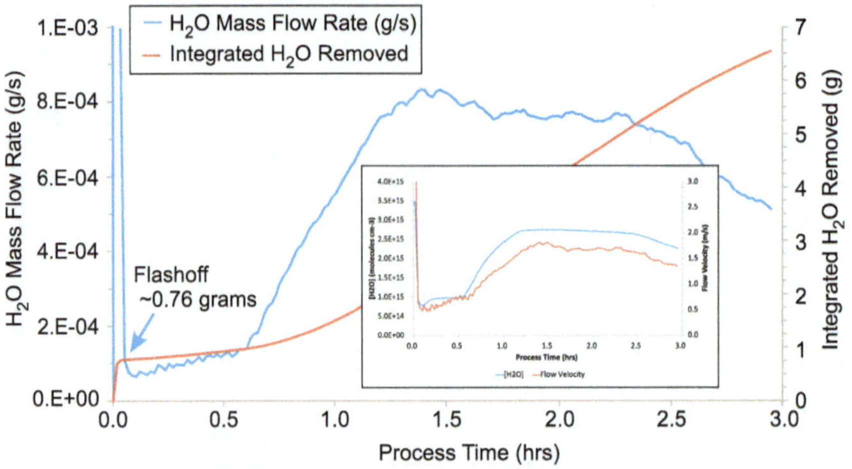

Fig. 5 TDLAS sensor data recorded during a one 20 mL vial DI water sublimation experiment demonstrating the sensor measurement sensitivity. The TDLAS measurement accuracy error in determining the total amount of water removed was ~0.9% compared to the gravimetric determination of total water removed

high measurement sensitivity of the TDLAS measurement technique and the excellent measurement accuracy, even at low mass flow rates resulting from small ice surface areas undergoing sublimation.

4 TDLAS Measurement Applications

There have been numerous demonstrations of application of the batch average TDLAS water vapor mass flow rate sensor for developing, monitoring, and controlling pharmaceutical freeze drying processes. These include determination of: (1) primary and secondary drying endpoints [4, 16]; (2) vial heat transfer coefficients, K_v [9, 10, 21]; (3) product temperature at the vial bottom, T_b [9]; (4) product temperature at the sublimation interface, T_o; and (5) product resistance to drying, R_p [13]. The most advanced use of the sensor has been in the development of primary drying process knowledge and design spaces. The combination of the sensor data, a heat and mass transfer model of vial-based freeze drying, and a procedure for developing freeze-drying processes enables process engineers to create a complete understanding of the pharmaceutical lyophilization process. This includes how the product and freeze dryer will respond to process deviations. This information enables rapid, knowledge-based disposition of highly valuable product following any process deviations. In the remainder of this chapter some of these sensor applications will be described. The reader is encouraged to refer to the peer-reviewed references describing the detailed application of the TDLAS sensor.

4.1 Determination of Primary and Secondary Drying Endpoints

Precise determination of the end of the primary drying phase is important both during the design of the processes as well as for monitoring and controlling of commercial manufacturing. Lyophilization cycles are currently operated using a fixed process design, including fixed time for both the primary and secondary phases of drying. Advancement to secondary drying with the rise in the lyophilizer shelf temperature without the completion of ice sublimation jeopardizes the quality attributes of the product. The TDLAS sensor has been used to monitor drying of numerous "product" drying cycles including mannitol, lactose, trehalose, sucrose, dextran, glycine, PVP and BSA formulations [5, 9]. Measurements and monitoring of the water concentration and mass flow during the primary drying phase using TDLAS enable the determination of the endpoint of primary drying. As the sublimation of ice nears completion, the composition of the gas in the product chamber changes from nearly all water vapor to nearly all nitrogen, and a sharp drop in the TDLAS water concentration curve can be observed. The inflection point of the curve, or when it plateaus, can be used as an indicator of the endpoint of primary drying. Low level, plateaued measurements of the mass flow rate may also be used to indicate the end of primary drying. Figures 4 and 5 demonstrate the capability of the sensor to detect water mass flow even when a very small number of vials are still undergoing sublimation.

The determination of primary and secondary drying endpoints is illustrated in Fig. 6. During this experiment, one shelf of 112 20 mL vials was filled with 3 mL of 5% sucrose formulation undergoing drying. The cycle was driven by the Manometric

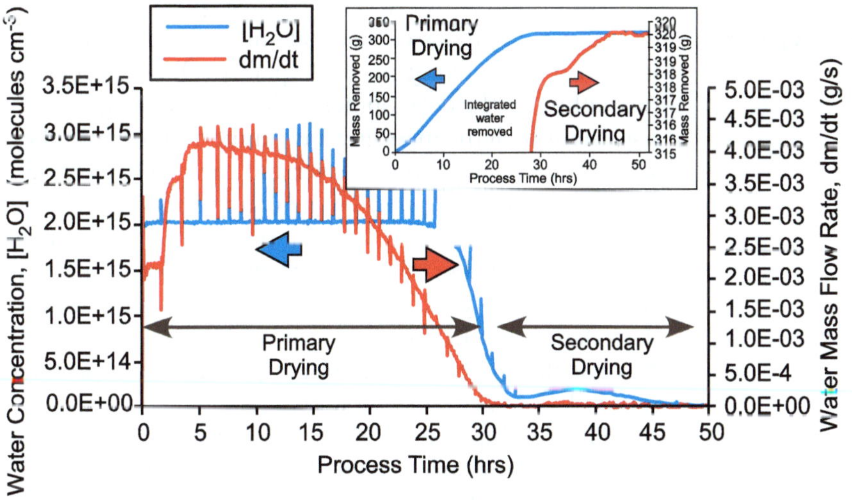

Fig. 6 TDLAS sensor data recorded during drying of (112) 20 mL vials containing 3 mL of 5% sucrose formulation in a Lyostar 3 freeze dryer. Primary and secondary drying endpoints are clearly indicated by the water vapor concentration, water mass flow rate, and the integrated amount of water removed

Temperature Measurement (MTM) based SMART™ Freeze Dryer technology, controlling the process parameters and changing the shelf temperature set points at a constant chamber pressure of 57 mTorr. The spikes in the TDLAS data correspond to isolation valve closure events and increase in the chamber pressure during ~25 s time periods used to determine the MTM product temperature and to control the shelf temperature set points. During primary drying, the water vapor concentration remains constant while the velocity—and thus the mass flow rate shown in Fig. 6—varies with shelf temperature before plateauing and dropping due to increased product resistance to drying and edge vials completing primary drying (prior to center vials) reducing the ice surface area undergoing drying. At the end of primary drying, both the water vapor concentration and the water vapor mass flow rate have dropped to substantially lower values. During secondary drying, the shelf temperature is raised (to +40 °C) and the unfrozen water within the frozen product matrix is driven off. During this time, the water concentration rises with a small increase in the water mass flow rate. The insert graph shows the integrated amount of water removed on both *y*-axes with different scales. The expanded scale curve of the integrated total amount of water removed clearly shows the primary and secondary drying endpoints and the capability of using the TDLAS sensor for monitoring the progression of the lyophilization process. The endpoint determinations made using the TDLAS sensor have been found to be comparable to determinations made from comparative pressure measurements, mass spectrometry, or cold plasma devices [4, 16, 20, 22].

4.2 Determination of Lyophilizer Equipment Capability Limits

Pharmaceutical companies are highly motivated by economic and regulatory forces to develop robust product formulations and lyophilization processes that maximize product throughput consistent with maintaining product quality. One aspect of maximizing throughput is the development of efficient drying processes that are consistent with the mass flow rate limitations of both the laboratory scale process development dryer and the manufacturing scale dryer that will be used to produce the drug product [23]. The development of a process that can be transferred between lyophilizers requires knowledge of the maximum supported rate of mass transfer between the lyophilizer product chamber and the condenser and the relationship between the ice sublimation rate (g s^{-1}) and the dryer shelf temperature, chamber pressure, and product temperature [11, 23, 24].

The development of a sublimation rate curve versus the product chamber pressure is needed to define the lyophilizer operational limitations. Traditionally, this information was gathered through a series of ice slab sublimation tests with each steady state test providing a single data point at a single shelf temperature and pressure. The gravimetric determination of total water removed provided the average sublimation rate during one steady state experiment. Thus, a complete maximum mass flow rate versus pressure curve would require numerous experiments and a large investment of time and labor resources.

The TDLAS sensor technology enables the efficient development of the required data set and the determination of choked flow conditions [11, 24]. A simple method of performing the TDLAS-based experiment is to form 2 cm thick ice slabs on all of the freeze dryer shelves, covering the entire surface area of the shelves. The chamber pressure set point is defined at a very low, unachievable level (e.g., 20 mTorr) even when the ice slabs are maintained at −40 °C. The shelf temperature is then ramped to a starting set point (e.g., −25 °C) and the pressure set point is kept the same. The freeze dryer pressure equilibrates to the lowest achievable value defined by the mass flow rate and the equipment capability. The shelf temperature is maintained at the first set point value until the product temperature equilibrates resulting in a nearly steady state water vapor mass flow rate measured by the TDLAS sensor. The process of raising the shelf temperature set point is then repeated with the chamber pressure and mass flow rate settling to new equilibrium values. Each of these new equilibrium points defines a maximum equipment mass flow rate supported at the equilibrium pressure. The experiment can be continued as long as <30% of the ice has been removed (to maintain good thermal contact between the ice and freeze dryer shelves) and until the maximum equipment capability over the entire pressure range of interest has been defined. Example data showing the freeze dryer pressure and TDLAS measured water vapor mass flow rate data as a function of process time is shown in Fig. 7. Figure 8 shows a plot of the

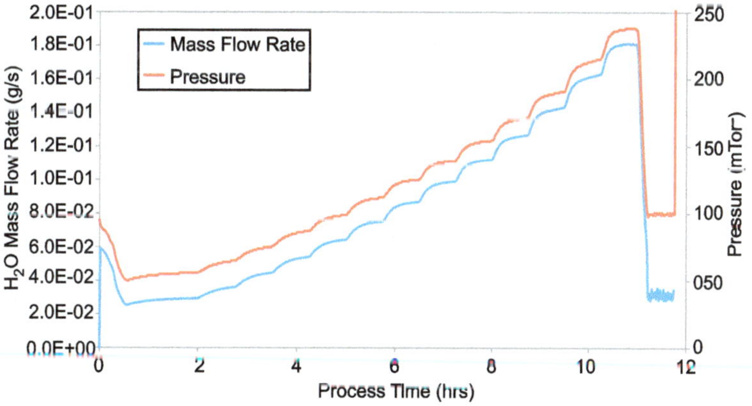

Fig. 7 Water vapor mass flow rate and lyophilizer product chamber pressure measurements recorded during an equipment capability measurement ice slab sublimation experiment. Each pair of equilibrium mass flow rate and pressure measurements defines points on the maximum mass flow rate equipment capability limit curve

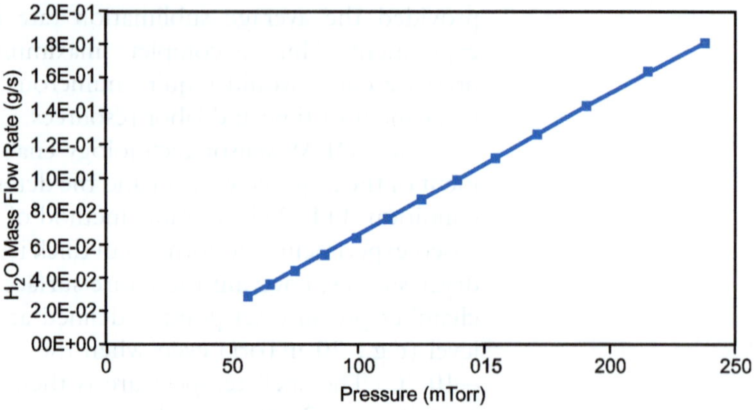

Fig. 8 Maximum supported mass flow rate equipment capability limit curve for a SP Scientific Lyostar 3 freeze dryer defined by the data shown in Fig. 7

equilibrium mass flow rate values as a function of the lyophilizer equilibrium pressures, defining the equipment capability limit. Using the TDLAS sensor and this experimental procedure enables the lyophilizer maximum supported water mass flow rate to be defined in a single day rather than weeks, dramatically saving time and money.

4.3 Determination of Vial Heat Transfer Coefficients, Product Temperature, and Product Resistance

Heat and Mass Transfer Model of Freeze Drying: Heat transfer during vial-based lyophilization can be described in terms of thermal barriers and temperature gradients [19]. Heat is supplied to the frozen product from the drying chamber shelves through the bottom of the glass vials to compensate for the heat removed by sublimation. The mechanisms for heat transfer from the shelf to the bottom of the vial include direct physical contact, gas conduction, and radiation. Radiative heat input can also be supplied to edge and near edge vials from the metal band surrounding the vial array and/or the relatively warm lyophilizer walls and door. Heat flow from the shelves to the product is described by Eq. (4).

$$\frac{dQ}{dt} = A_v \times K_v(T_s - T_b) \tag{4}$$

where dQ/dt is the heat flow (cal s^{-1} or J s^{-1}) to the product; A_v is the cross sectional area of the vial calculated from the vial outer diameter; K_v is the vial heat transfer coefficient (for a specific vial type at a specific pressure and a specific vial configuration); T_s is the temperature of the shelf surface; and T_b is the temperature of the frozen product at the bottom center of the vial. K_v is nearly independent of shelf temperature [19].

In steady state, the heat flow (dQ/dt) can be related to mass flow (dm/dt) by using the heat of ice sublimation, ΔH_s (Eq. 5):

$$\frac{dQ}{dt} = \Delta H_s \frac{dm}{dt} \tag{5}$$

where ΔH_s is 660 cal g^{-1}. Equations (4) and (5) can be combined and rearranged to provide the product temperature at the bottom of the vial, T_b (Eq. 6) or the vial heat transfer coefficient, K_v (Eq. 7).

$$T_b = T_s - \frac{\Delta H_s * {}^{dm}/_{dt}}{A_v \times K_v} \tag{6}$$

K_v can be determined using a DI water experiment during which dm/dt is measured using the TDLAS sensor and the average temperature difference ($T_s - T_b$), can be determined using thermocouples in selected vials (bottom center) as well as adhesive thermocouples on the shelf surface [10, 19, 25].

$$K_v = \frac{\Delta H_s * ({}^{dm}/_{dt})}{A_v * (T_s - T_b)} \tag{7}$$

In the laboratory, the temperature bias between vials containing thermocouples and vials not containing thermocouples is usually very small due to particulate contamination in the product fluid used to fill the vials. This would not be the case in an aseptic, low particle manufacturing environment. The vial cross-sectional area, A_v, is easily determined by measurement or from the vial engineering data. Prior to the introduction of the TDLAS measurement sensor for monitoring lyophilization, the mass flow rate was determined gravimetrically from the known initial mass of water and the remaining mass of water after a predefined time interval of sublimation [19]. This required that a steady state pressure experiment was performed at each pressure of interest, resulting in many days of experiments. Using the TDLAS sensor, all of the pressure-dependent data can be collected within a single experiment. During product drying operations, knowledge of K_v can be combined with dm/dt to provide real-time determinations of batch average product temperature without the use of thermocouples inserted into vials.

Additional analysis allows the determination of the product temperature at the sublimation interface, T_o, for product runs by using Eq. (8) where L_{ice} is the ice thickness, A_p is the cross-sectional area of the product, and K_I is the thermal conductivity of ice. A thermal conductivity of ice of 20.52 (cal h^{-1} cm^{-2} K^{-1}) can be used [19].

$$T_o = T_b - \frac{{}^{dQ}/_{dt} \times L_{ice}}{A_p \times K_I} \tag{8}$$

L_{ice} may be instantaneously calculated from the integrated TDLAS mass removed and the initial mass of water using Eq. (9) [19]:

$$L_{ice} = \frac{m_o - m(t)}{\rho_{ice} \times A_p \times \varepsilon} \tag{9}$$

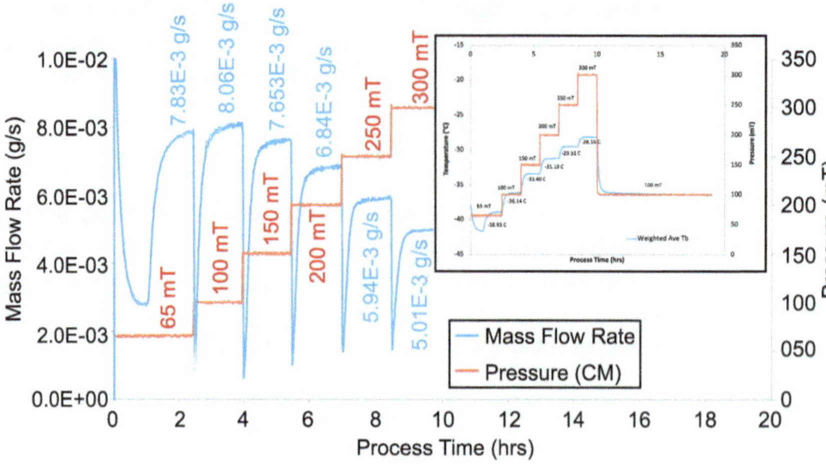

Fig. 9 Mass flow, pressure, and product temperature readings as a function of process time recorded during a DI water sublimation experiment used to determine the vial heat transfer coefficient

where m_o is the initial mass of water, $m(t)$ is the mass of water removed at time t, ρ_{ice} is the density of ice, and ε is the volume fraction of ice.

Product resistance to drying offered by the dry porous solid and the stopper, R_{ps}, may be calculated using Eq. (10):

$$R_{ps} = \frac{A_p(P_{ice} - P_c)}{{}^{dm}/_{dt\,vial}} \tag{10}$$

where A_p is the area of the product undergoing drying, P_{ice} is the vapor pressure of water over the ice at temperature T_o, P_c is the drying chamber vapor pressure, and dm/dt_{vial} is the sublimation rate per vial. P_{ice} (in Torr) is calculated using Eq. (11).

$$P_{ice} = e^{\left(\frac{-6144.96}{T_o} + 24.01849\right)} \tag{11}$$

Determination of vial heat transfer coefficients: Figure 9 shows water vapor mass flow rate and pressure data collected during a TDLAS-based vial heat transfer, K_v, experiment. One hundred twelve 20 mL vials were filled with 10 mL of DI water. Thermocouples were positioned into selected edge and center vials. The DI water was frozen to −40 °C and the chamber pressure was initially reduced to 65 mTorr. The shelf temperature was then raised to −25 °C and held constant at this value throughout the experiment. The pressure was held at the set point value until the product temperature and mass flow rate readings came to equilibrium. The pressure set point was then raised and the system was allowed to equilibrate. This procedure is repeated for each pressure of interest as long as <30% of the ice was sublimed. Using Eq. (8), the product temperature and the TDLAS mass flow rate measurements, the pressure dependent vial heat transfer coefficients were

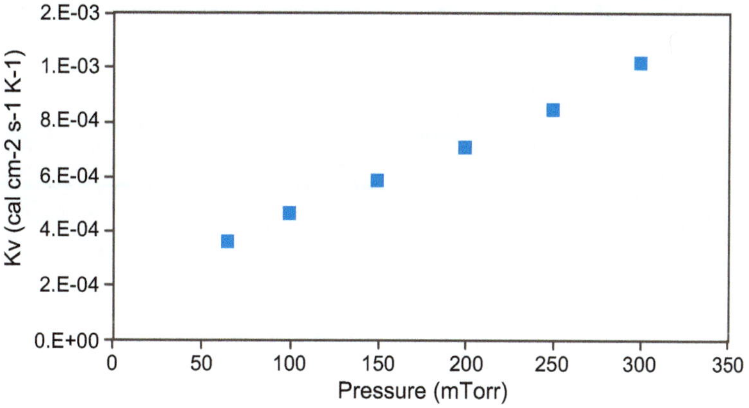

Fig. 10 Weighted batch average vial heat transfer coefficient as a function of pressure calculated from the data shown in Fig. 9. Use of the TDLAS sensor enabled the determination of these values within a single freeze drying experiment

calculated and plotted in Fig. 10. Numerous reports of the use of this technique can be found in the peer-reviewed technical literature [9, 10, 21] including comparisons showing good agreement between batch average TDLAS and gravimetric-based K_v determinations. As with the determination of the equipment capability limit curve, using the TDLAS sensor and this experimental procedure enables the determination of the batch average vial heat transfer coefficients as a function of pressure in a single day rather than weeks, dramatically saving time and money.

Determination of product temperature: Once the vial heat transfer coefficient is determined, batch average product temperatures can be calculated from TDLAS mass flow rates by using Eq. (6). Additional inputs include thermocouple-based shelf temperature measurements, the vial cross-sectional area, and the heat of sublimation of water. Schneid et al. have reported extensively on the validity of TDLAS determined product temperatures in a variety of formulations including 10% glycine, 7.5% mannitol, and 5% sucrose [9]. For all formulations, TDLAS determined product temperatures were within 1–2 °C of thermocouple measured product temperatures of center vials [26].

Figure 11 shows TDLAS and thermocouple probe product temperature data for a 5% sucrose + 5% BSA formulation. In this experiment, 112 20 mL vials were filled with 3 mL of the product solution and were dried in a LyoStar 3 freeze dryer (SP Scientific, Stone Ridge, NY, USA). Thermocouple probes were placed in the bottom center of select vials for comparison to the TDLAS-determined product temperatures. Product temperatures measured by thermocouples show that center vial temperatures run cooler than edge vial temperatures due to radiation from the warm dryer walls and door heating the edge vials. Initially, TDLAS-determined batch average

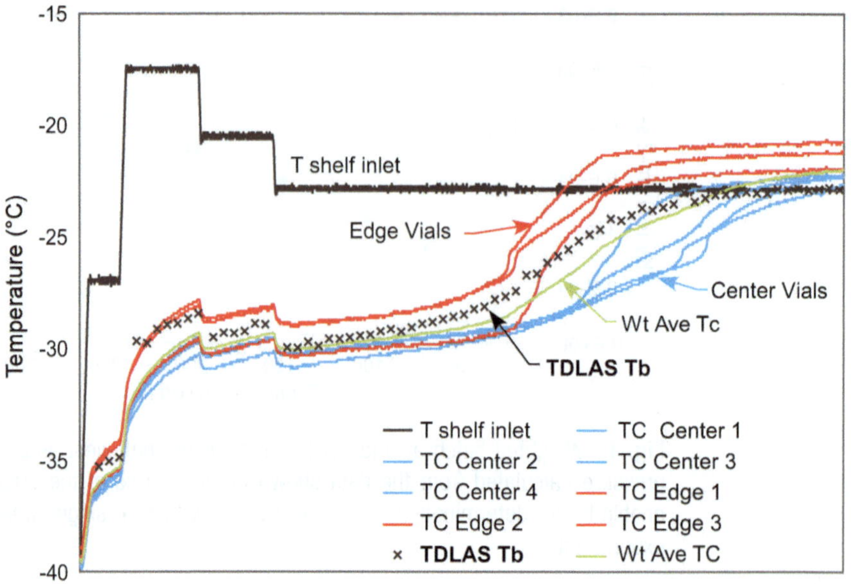

Fig. 11 Product temperature temporal profile for 5% sucrose + 5% BSA during primary drying as determined using thermocouples and TDLAS measurement techniques

product temperatures are biased to edge vial thermocouple measurements. However, for the remainder of primary drying, the TDLAS sensor determined batch average product temperatures closely match the average product temperature between edge and center vials.

Determination of Product Resistance: Determining the product resistance to drying (R_p) is important to inform product formulation, process development, and scale-up to production-scale manufacturing. It is desirable to select excipients and their concentrations in the formulation such that product resistance is minimized to enable the development of an efficient drying process (short cycle time). For process development, R_p values are a critical input needed to develop process knowledge and design space (discussed below) to generate optimized freeze-drying cycles. For process scale-up, product resistance varies between laboratory and GMP manufacturing environments due to the low particle loading in the manufacturing environment. Fewer particulates result in increased supercooling during the freezing step. Increased supercooling results in smaller crystal/pore sizes and higher product resistance to mass transfer through the drying cake.

TDLAS can be utilized to determine the product resistance using Eq. (10) and the measured mass flow rate as described above. Schneid et al. utilized TDLAS-determined R_p to study the contribution to product resistance of common excipients throughout primary drying. During this study, the TDLAS R_p data were compared to MTM R_p data. They concluded that

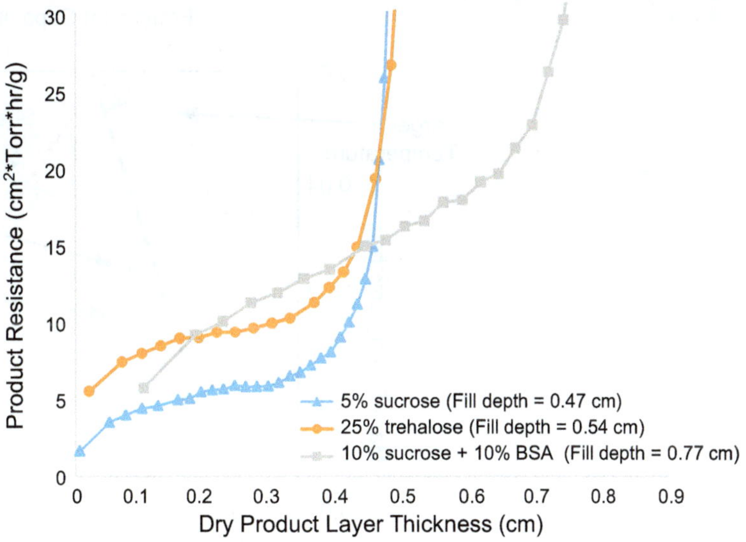

Fig. 12 Product resistance as a function of dry product layer thickness determined by TDLAS water vapor mass flow measurements for 5% sucrose, 25% trehalose, and 10% sucrose + 10% BSA

TDLAS-determined R_p is in good agreement with MTM data early in primary drying. A TDLAS-determined R_p profile for three formulations is shown in Fig. 12. The R_p data display a number of important characteristics including (1) increasing values with increasing dry layer thickness, (2) formulation dependent R_p values with increasing resistance correlated with increasing solid content, and (3) non-physical behavior when approximately 2/3 of the total amount of water from the batch has been removed due to edge vials drying faster than center vials, completing drying and leading to decreasing total ice surface area undergoing sublimation. The ice surface area is an input for calculating R_p, however the decreasing surface area in the calculation remains constant, causing inaccurate R_p calculations late in primary drying. Sharma et al. [26] showed that a linear extrapolation of the R_p curve from the data prior to the sharp rise near the end of primary drying can be used to estimate the number of vials that have completed primary drying and correct the R_p curve.

5 Quality by Design Lyophilization Cycle Development

The development of knowledge and design spaces using the steady state heat and mass transfer equations as described by Pikal [19, 20] was first reported by Chang and Fisher [23]. The approach for generating the process design space has been thoroughly discussed in the literature [24, 27, 28]. Figure 13 shows a graph of the sublimation rate as a function of chamber pressure (P_c) used to

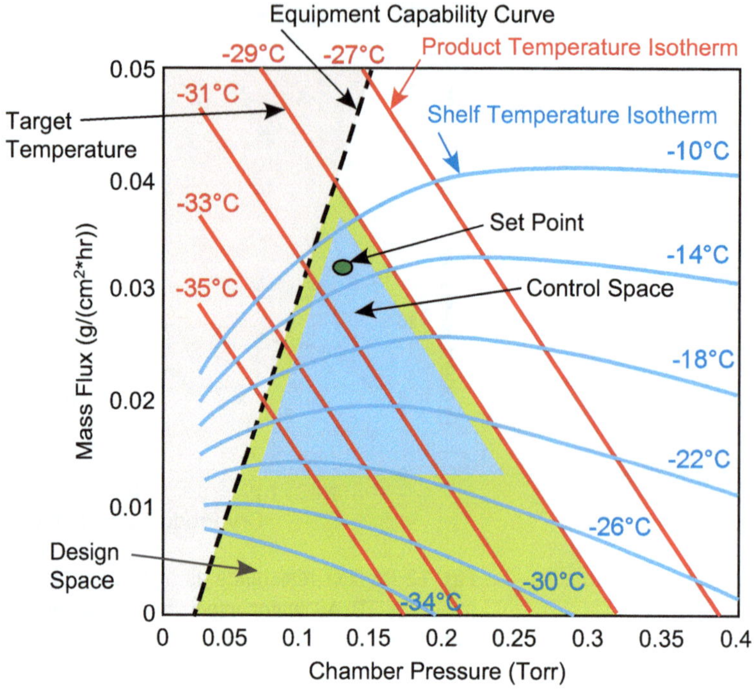

Fig. 13 Example lyophilization process knowledge and design spaces calculated using batch average TDLAS water vapor mass flow rate measurements and a heat and mass transfer model of freeze drying

construct the knowledge and design space for the primary drying stage of freeze drying. There are five steps that are carried out to create the knowledge and design spaces:

1. Measure the product formulation collapse (T_c) or eutectic melt temperature (T_{eu}).
2. Establish the relationship between process variables the user can control (T_s and P_c) and the key parameter not controlled, product temperature at the sublimation interface, T_o.
   (a) Experiment: Measure the vial heat transfer coefficient, K_v, as a function of P_c
   (b) Experiment: Measure the product resistance to drying, R_p
3. Calculate the design space including the sublimation rate vs. chamber pressure for shelf temperature isotherms and for product temperature isotherms using steady state heat and mass transfer theory.
4. Experiment: Determine the lyophilizer equipment capability limit [11].
5. Graph the process knowledge space and define the process design space (Fig. 13).

The design space is further bound by product temperature constraints (<collapse temperature any other temperature related

behavior associated with poor stability or other poor product performance).

Step 1 is accomplished by performing Differential Scanning Calorimetry (DSC) and freeze drying microscopy measurements to determine the glass transition temperature of the maximally concentrated solute, T_g', and the collapse or eutectic melt temperature. This is discussed in detail in Chap. 1 of this volume. Step 2 is completed by using the TDLAS sensor (or gravimetric measurements) to determine the vial heat transfer coefficient, K_v, as a function of the process chamber pressure and the product resistance to drying, R_p. R_p can be continuously determined using the TDLAS dm/dt measurements during a conservative product drying experiment until approximately 2/3 of the way through primary drying when some of the edge vials complete drying and the total ice surface undergoing drying is no longer known. This results in the R_p curve rapidly and non-physically rising. The R_p value just prior to this rapid increase should be used for subsequent calculations in Step 3. In Step 3 arbitrary values of T_s and P_c are chosen and used to iteratively calculate T_b using Eq. (12) [28]:

$$\{\Delta H_s \times A_p[2.698 \times 10^{10} \times \exp(-6144.96/T_b) - P_c]\}/R_p = K_v \times A_v(T_s - T_b) \quad (12)$$

The calculated values of T_b are used to calculate the pressure dependent mass flow rate using Eq. (13):

$$dm/dt = K_v A_v(T_s - T_b) \quad (13)$$

This process is repeated choosing new values of P_c at the same T_s to create the data for one shelf temperature isotherm curve. The calculations are then repeated to create a family of shelf temperature isotherm curves. Also during Step 3 product temperature isotherm curves are calculated using Eq. (14) [27]:

$$dm/dt = A_p\left[2.698 \times 10^{10}\exp(-6144.96/T_b) - P_c\right]/R_p \quad (14)$$

Arbitrary values of the product temperature, T_b, and the chamber pressure, P_c, are used in combination with the product resistance to drying, R_p, determined during Step 2 to calculate the mass flow rate, dm/dt, as a function of pressure at a constant T_b value to create one product temperature isotherm curve. This process is then repeated for a different value of T_b to create a family of product temperature isotherm curves of dm/dt as a function of pressure. Step 4 is then carried out by performing a TDLAS monitored ice slab sublimation experiment to determine the equipment capability curve as described above.

In Step 5, the shelf temperature and product temperature isotherm curves are combined with the equipment capability curve to create the graphical knowledge and design spaces shown in Fig. 13.

The freeze drying process cannot be run in the pink shaded area above the maximum mass flux line because the mass flow rates are not supported by the lyophilizer. The design space shaded in green must be below both the equipment capability limit and below the target product temperature which is typically 3–5 °C below the product formulation collapse or eutectic melt temperature. The blue shaded area indicates an example process control space and the red oval represents an example target set of operating conditions within the control space. The target is a compromise between the most efficient process possible and a set of conditions that provides flexibility to handle potential process deviations while still maintaining the product below the critical temperature. The development and usage of the process knowledge, design and control spaces is consistent with Quality by Design (QbD) principles and it enables the rapid disposition of product following a process deviation, because it allows the operators to accurately predict if the deviation resulted in the product temperature exceeding the critical temperature during primary drying.

6 TDLAS-Based SMART™ Freeze Dryer

As outlined above, developing a fully characterized process knowledge and design space is a robust method for process development. This procedure generates optimum cycles and can be used to determine the impacts of process deviations on product quality. However, the complexity of this method may be prohibitive, especially for companies that have limited institutional knowledge of lyophilization. SMART™ freeze drying technology was developed to enable rapid process design that requires a lower level of effort. The SMART™ software (SP Scientific, Stone Ridge, NY, USA) automatically generates a freeze drying cycle based on user inputs of product characteristics and vial dimensions combined with in-process product temperature measurements and a pseudo-steady state heat and mass transfer model of freeze drying in vials. Case studies have shown a potential saving of $40k per cycle and a reduction in development time by 78% using SMART™ freeze drying technology to develop new freeze-drying cycles [29].

SMART™ Freeze Dryer Algorithm: To initiate a SMART™ Freeze Dryer cycle, the user inputs parameters related to the product thermal characteristics (collapse temperature), type (amorphous or crystalline, protein or small molecule), and concentration. Additional inputs include vial dimensions. The software then uses the SMART™ Freeze Dryer algorithm to automatically develop a process including freezing and primary and secondary drying. Freezing includes two separate recipes depending on whether the product is amorphous or crystalline. The user can modify the freezing step based on their product thermal characteristics and whether or not

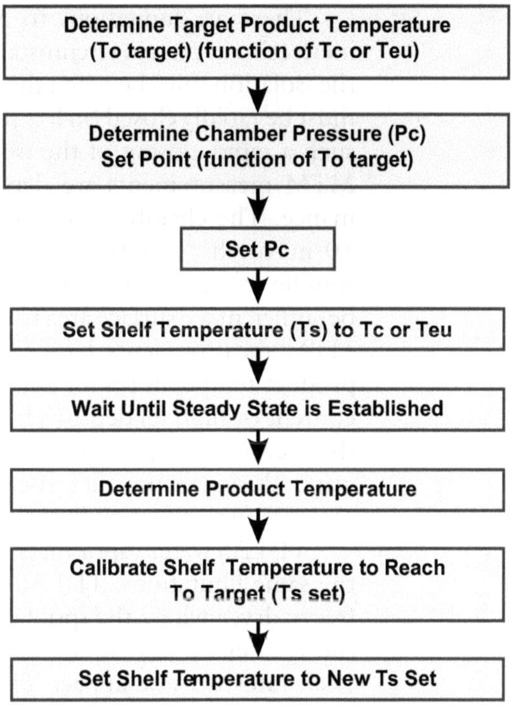

Fig. 14 Simplified schematic of the SMART™ Freeze Dryer algorithm during primary drying

additional annealing steps must be included. During primary drying, the algorithm calculates and implements shelf temperature changes required to maintain the product at a target temperature as shown in Fig. 14. The end of primary drying is determined either by manometric temperature measurements (MTM) or the difference between the Pirani gauge and the capacitance manometer. The algorithm progresses the cycle to secondary drying once the end of primary drying is detected.

During primary drying, the SMART™ freeze dryer algorithm relies on process analytical technologies capable of determining the product temperature during the freeze-drying cycle. The SMART™ algorithm was initially established around manometric temperature measurements for determining the product temperature. The development of the SMART™ Freeze Dryer utilizing MTM-based product temperature measurements is described in detail by Tang et al. [30]. MTM determines the product temperature by collecting and analyzing the transient pressure response when the isolation valve between the product chamber and condenser is quickly closed during primary drying. Sublimation of water causes the pressure in the chamber to rise, and this pressure rise is fitted to an equation to determine the product temperature. A thorough discussion of the application of the MTM-based SMART™ Freeze Dryer technology has been reported by Gieseler et al. [31].

There are limitations to MTM measurements that render it ineffective in certain circumstances. First, for MTM measurements, the isolation valve between the product chamber and the condenser must be rapidly closed (in less than 1 s). For large-scale freeze dryers, such a rapid closing of the isolation valve is not feasible. Second, MTM measurements are dependent on the freeze dryer performance. The chamber leak rate must be sufficiently low (less than 30 mTorr h^{-1} for the SP Scientific LyoStar 3 freeze dryer) and roughly constant throughout the pressure rise. Third, there must be sufficient ice surface area to support MTM measurements. Lastly, MTM measurements have limited ability to accurately calculate product temperatures for amorphous formulations with high solid content or high fill depth. The dry product layer that forms during the freeze-drying process increases over time and will reabsorb water during a pressure rise test. This will lead to a decreased pressure rise and an under-calculation of the product temperature.

TDLAS water vapor mass flow measurements are not subject to the same limitations. TDLAS can be implemented on any scale of freeze dryer where the spool connecting the product chamber and the condenser has sufficient length for the optical components. Leak rates do not impact TDLAS measurements, and as shown above, TDLAS can accurately measure water sublimation from even a single vial placed in a LyoStar 3. TDLAS measurements are agnostic of product and are applicable to all formulations where water is the solvent. For TDLAS-based SMART™ freeze-drying cycles, TDLAS-determined product temperatures are used to calculate the shelf temperatures required to keep the product at the target product temperature. Communication between the freeze dryer and TDLAS system enables the transfer of information necessary to control the process.

Experimental Results: TDLAS-based SMART™ has been implemented on both a lab-scale freeze dryer (LyoStar 3) and a pilot-scale freeze dryer (LyoConstellation S20, SP Scientific, Stone Ridge, NY, USA) for a variety of product formulations including those where MTM product temperature measurements have been shown to be inaccurate. Formulations of common excipients and model proteins were chosen to test the TDLAS-based SMART™ algorithm with relevant compounds. The formulations tested were 5% sucrose, 25% trehalose, 10% sucrose + 10% bovine serum albumin (BSA). High solid content formulations were included because they are challenging for the MTM-based SMART™ freeze dryer. Table 1 summarizes the cycles developed for the formulations tested in the lab-scale LyoStar 3. Maintaining the product temperature below the collapse temperature is crucial for maintaining product quality. Figure 15 shows product temperature data during the first 2/3 of primary drying for 5% sucrose dried in a LyoStar 3 dryer. TDLAS-calculated product temperatures closely match

Table 1
Primary drying conditions defined using the SMART™ Freeze Dryer in the lab-scale LyoStar 3 for 5% sucrose in two vial types (I and II), 25% trehalose and 10% sucrose + 10% BSA

Product, Number of vials, Fill volume	Primary drying recipe			
	Step #1	Step #2	Step #3	Step #4
5% sucrose, 112 × 20 mL vials (I) 3 mL	T_s: −34 °C t: 103 min P_c: 57 mTorr	T_s: −27.4 °C t: 286 min P_c: 57 mTorr	T_s: −29.9 °C t: 704 min P_c: 57 mTorr	T_s: −32 °C t: 1856 min P_c: 57 mTorr
5% sucrose, 112 × 20 mL vials (II) 3 mL	T_s: −34 °C t: 103 min P_c: 57 mTorr	T_s: −25.1 °C t: 290 min P_c: 57 mTorr	T_s: −28.9 °C t: 1937 min P_c: 57 mTorr	–
25% trehalose 112 × 20 mL vials (I) 3 mL	T_s: −28 °C t: 115 min P_c: 74 mTorr	T_s: −21 °C t: 646 min P_c: 74 mTorr	T_s: −23 °C t: 1048 min P_c: 74 mTorr	–
10% sucrose + 10% BSA, 160 × 20 mL vials (II) 3 mL	T_s: −22 °C t: 126 min P_c: 97 mTorr	T_s: −10.4 °C t: 418 min P_c: 97 mTorr	T_s: −14.4 °C t: 2104 min P_c: 97 mTorr	–

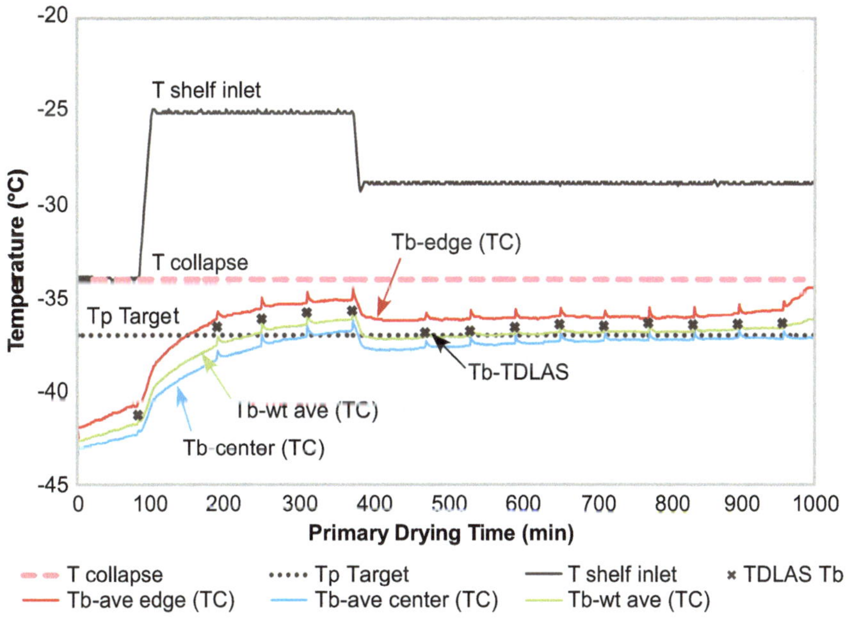

Fig. 15 SMART™ Freeze Dryer cycle of 5% Sucrose in the lab-scale LyoStar 3 dryer. First 2/3 of primary drying

product temperatures measured with thermocouple probes, and the freeze-drying cycle maintained the product temperatures below collapse during the first 2/3 of primary drying. After approximately 2/3 of the total primary drying time when some edge vials have completed drying, no shelf temperature changes are made.

Table 2
Primary drying conditions defined using the SMART™ Freeze Dryer in the pilot-scale LyOrion for 5% sucrose and 10% sucrose + 10% BSA

Product (Cycle #), Number of vials, Fill volume	Primary drying recipe			
	Step #1	Step #2	Step #3	Step #4
5% sucrose, 382 × 20 mL vials (II) 3 mL	T_s: −34 °C t: 103 min P_c: 57 mTorr	T_s: −23.9 °C t: 370 min P_c: 57 mTorr	T_s: −28.1 °C t: 1678 min P_c: 57 mTorr	–
10% sucrose + 10% BSA, 480 × 20 mL vials (II) 5 mL	T_s: −22 °C t: 127 min P_c: 97 mTorr	T_s: −10.6 °C t: 329 min P_c: 97 mTorr	T_s: −14.2 °C t: 340 min P_c: 97 mTorr	T_s: −17.9 °C t: 1799 min P_c: 57 mTorr

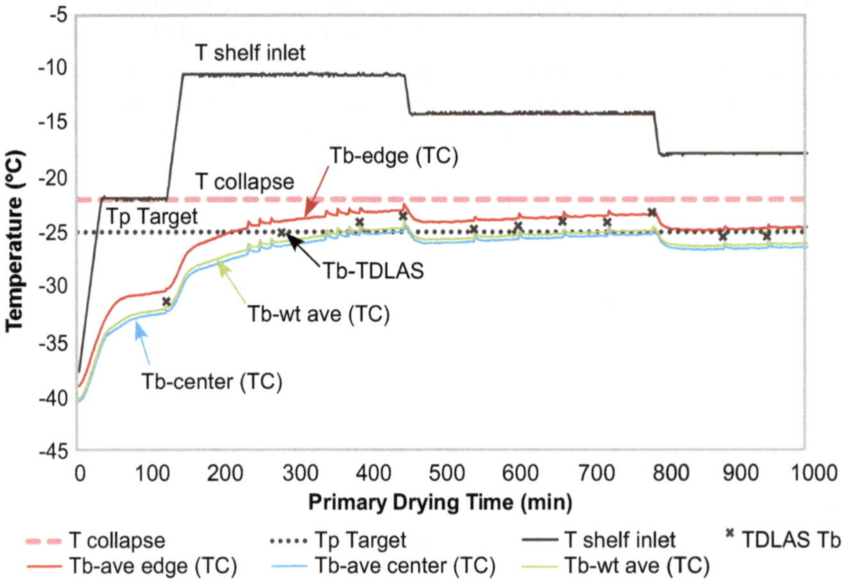

Fig. 16 SMART™ Freeze Dryer cycle of 10% sucrose + 10% BSA in the pilot-scale LyoConstellation S20. First 2/3 of primary drying

Two formulations, 5% sucrose and 10% sucrose + 10% BSA, were also tested in the pilot-scale LyoConstellation S20 freeze dryer. Table 2 summarizes the cycles developed. Figure 16 shows product temperature data during the first 2/3 of primary drying for 10% sucrose + 10% BSA dried in the LyoConstellation S20. Again, TDLAS-calculated product temperatures closely match product temperatures measured with thermocouple probes, and the freeze-drying cycle maintained the product temperatures below collapse during the first 2/3 of primary drying.

Additional tests were performed with solutions of polyvinylpyrrolidone (PVP). PVP is not commonly used in lyophilized formulations; however, it is a useful test case as it is a highly

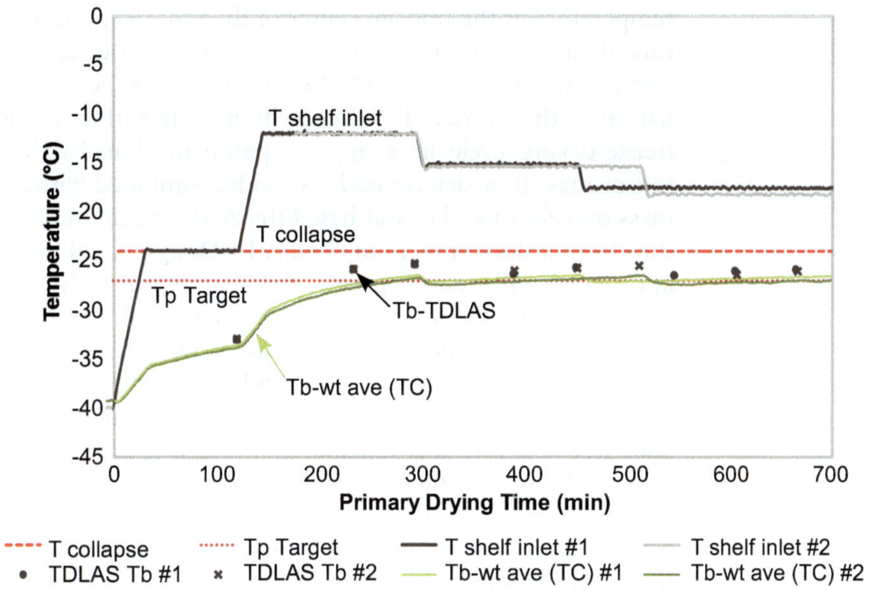

Fig. 17 Two SMART™ Freeze Dryer cycles of 10% PVP in the lab-scale LyoStar 3. First 2/3 of primary drying

hygroscopic polymer that readily reabsorbs water in the dried product layer. MTM-calculated product temperatures have been shown to fail with PVP solutions very early in the cycle [31]. TDLAS-based SMART™ was used to develop a cycle for a 10% PVP solution with 112 20 mL vials with a 3 mL fill. As shown in Fig. 17, TDLAS-calculated product temperatures closely match product temperatures measured with thermocouple probes for two consecutive cycles. The freeze-drying cycle developed by the TDLAS-based SMART™ algorithm maintained the product temperatures below collapse during the first 2/3 of primary drying. Additionally, the SMART™ cycles were repeatable, with only minor differences observed between the two cycles.

7 Summary

The development and application of a unique tunable diode laser absorption spectroscopy (TDLAS) water vapor mass flow rate sensor has been described. The TDLAS sensor installed in the duct connecting the lyophilizer chamber and condenser enables non-contact, continuous determinations of the ice sublimation rate, possessing a mass flow measurement sensitivity better than 10 μg s^{-1}. The sensor has been demonstrated on laboratory, pilot and production scale freeze dryers. Sensor applications have included the determination of the: (1) primary and secondary freeze-drying endpoints, (2) maximum supported lyophilizer ice sublimation rate, (3) vial heat transfer coefficients, (4) product temperature at the bottom center of the vial, (5) product temperature at the ice sublimation interface, and (6) product resistance to drying. In addition, the TDLAS sensor can also be used in combination with a SMART™ freeze-drying algorithm to develop a freeze-drying cycle in a single experiment. Finally, the TDLAS sensor mass flow determinations can be combined with a heat and mass transfer model of vial-based freeze drying and used to enable the efficient development of Quality by Design based freeze-drying knowledge and design spaces. This data is not only valuable for process development, but also for efficient disposition of product batches following process deviations. New measurement applications and automation of existing applications are continuing while use of the sensor technology on larger pilot and manufacturing scale freeze dryers is advancing. Continued application and widespread adoption of the TDLAS sensor for process monitoring and control will result in improved product quality and lead to improved process efficiency and lower production costs for lyophilized drug therapies.

References

1. Pikal M (2002) Lyophilization. In: Swarbrick J, Boylan JC (eds) Encyclopedia of pharmaceutical technology, vol 6. Marcel Dekker, New York, NY, pp 991299–991326
2. Franks F (1990) Freeze-drying: from empiricism to predictability. CryoLetters 11:93–110
3. Jameel F, Kessler WJ (2011) Real-time monitoring and controlling of lyophilization process parameters through process analytical technology tools. In: Undey C, Low D, Menezes JC, Koch M (eds) PAT applied in biopharmaceutical process development and manufacturing, vol 33., 978-1-4398-2945-5. CRC Press, Boca Raton, FL
4. Patel SM, Pikal M (2009) Process analytical technologies (PAT) in freeze-drying of parenteral products. Pharm Dev Technol 14(6):567–587
5. Gieseler H, Kessler WJ, Finson MF et al (2007) Evaluation of tunable diode laser absorption spectroscopy for in-process water vapor mass flux measurements during freeze-drying. J Pharm Sci 96(7):1776–1793
6. Schneid S, Gieseler H (2009) Process analytical technology (PAT) in freeze drying: tunable diode laser absorption spectroscopy as an evolving tool for cycle monitoring. Eur Pharm Rev 6:18–25
7. Schneid S, Gieseler H, Kessler W, Pikal MJ (2006) Process analytical technology in freeze drying: accuracy of mass balance determination using tunable diode laser absorption spectroscopy (TDLAS). Proceeding of AAPS Annual Meeting and Exposition, San Antonio, TX, Oct. 29–Nov. 2
8. Kuu WY, Nail SL, Sacha G (2009) Rapid freeze-drying cycle optimization using computer programs developed based on heat and mass transfer models and facilitated by tunable diode laser absorption spectroscopy (TDLAS). J Pharm Sci 98(9):3469–3482
9. Schneid S, Gieseler H, Kessler WJ, Pikal MJ (2009) Non-invasive product temperature determination during primary drying using tunable diode laser absorption spectroscopy. J Pharm Sci 98(9):3401–3418
10. Kuu WY, Nail SL, Sacha G (2009) Rapid determination of vial heat transfer parameters using tunable diode laser absorption spectroscopy (TDLAS) in response to step-changes in pressure set-point during freeze-drying. J Pharm Sci 98(3):1136–1154
11. Patel SM, Chaudhuri S, Pikal MJ (2008) Choked flow and importance of Mach I in freeze-drying process design. Proceedings of Freeze Drying of Pharmaceuticals and Biologicals Conference, Breckenridge, CO
12. Patel SM, Chaudhuri S, Pikal MJ (2010) Choked flow and importance of mach I in freeze-drying process design. Chem Eng Sci 65:5716–5727
13. Kuu WY, O'Bryan KR, Hardwick LM, Paul TW (2011) Product mass transfer resistance directly determined during freeze-drying cycle runs using tunable diode laser absorption

spectroscopy (TDLAS) and pore diffusion model. Pharm DevTechnol 16(4):343–357

14. Awotwe-Otoo D, Agarabi C, Khan MA (2014) An integrated process analytical technology (PAT) approach to monitoring the effect of supercooling on lyophilization product and process parameters of model monoclonal antibody formulations. J Pharm Sci 103(7):2042–2052
15. Schneid S, Gieseler H, Kessler WJ, Luthra SA, Pikal MJ (2011) Optimization of the secondary drying step in freeze drying using TDLAS technology. PharmSciTech 12(1):379–387
16. Nail S, Tchessalov et al (2017) Recommended best practices for process monitoring instrumentation in pharmaceutical freeze drying – 2017. AAPS PharmSciTech 18(7):2379–2393
17. Rothman LS, Gamache RR, Goldman A et al (1994) The HITRAN database: 1986 edition. Appl Optics 33(21):4851–4867
18. Miller MF, Kessler WJ, Allen MG (1996) Diode laser-based air mass flux sensor for subsonic aeropropulsion inlets. Appl Optics 35 (24):4905–4912
19. Pikal MJ (1985) Use of laboratory data in freeze drying process design: heat and mass transfer coefficients and the computer simulation of freeze drying. J Parenter Sci Technol 39:115–138
20. Milton N, Pikal MJ, Roy ML, Nail SL (1997) Evaluation of manometric temperature measurement as a method of monitoring product temperature during lyophilization. PDA J PharmSciTech 51:7–16
21. Schneid S, Gieseler H, Kessler W, Pikal MJ (2006) Position dependent vial heat transfer coefficient: a comparison of tunable diode laser absorption spectroscopy and gravimetric measurements. Proc. CPPR Freeze-Drying of Pharmaceuticals and Biologicals, Garmisch-Partenkirchen, Germany
22. Patel SM, Doen T, Schneid S, Pikal MJ (2007) Determination of the end point of primary drying in freeze-drying process control. Proceedings of AAPS Annual Meeting and Exposition, San Diego, CA
23. Chang BS, Fisher NL (1995) Development of an efficient single-step freeze-drying cycle for protein formulations. Pharm Res 12:831–837
24. Nail SL, Searles JA (2008) Elements of quality by design in development and scale-up of freeze-dried parenterals. Int Bio Pharm 21:44
25. Lupo K, Kessler WJ, Pikal MJ (2016) Application of tunable diode laser absorption spectroscopy mass flow rate sensor for monitoring vial drying heterogeneity: single vial TDLAS. Proceedings of Freeze Drying of Pharmaceuticals and Biologicals Conference, Breckenridge, CO
26. Sharma P, Kessler WJ, Bogner R, Thakur M, Pikal M (2018) Applications of tunable diode laser absorption spectroscopy (TDLAS): In-process estimation of primary drying heterogeneity and product temperature during lyophilization, J Pharm Sci [Epub ahead of print] https://doi.org/10.1016/j.xphs.2018.07.031
27. Nail SL, Kessler WJ (2010) Experience with tunable diode laser absorption spectroscopy at laboratory and production scales. Proceedings of Freeze Drying of Pharmaceuticals and Biologicals Conference, Garmisch-Partenkirchen, Germany
28. Wegiel L, Nail S, Ganguly A (2014) A primary drying optimization using a three-dimensional design space. Proceedings of Freeze Drying of Pharmaceuticals and Biologicals Conference, Garmisch-Partenkirchen, Germany
29. Sesholtz D, Mather L (2007) 'Smart' freeze-drying. Innov Pharm Technol
30. Tang C, Nail SL, Pikal MJ (2005) Freeze-drying process design by manometric temperature measurement: design of a smart freeze-dryer. Pharm Res 22(4):685–700
31. Gieseler H, Kramer T, Pikal MJ (2007) Use of manometric temperature measurement (MTM) and SMART™ freeze dryer technology for development of an optimized freeze-drying cycle. J Pharm Sci 96(12):3402–3418

Chapter 6

Containment Options for the Freeze-Drying of Biological Entities and Potent Materials

Chris Cherry

Abstract

This chapter examines the characteristics and use of containment systems to perform various applications of freeze-drying. Specific consideration is given to containment system design, effects on mass and heat transfer, containment of microorganisms, and recommendations for the future application of containment options.

An assessment is made of previously characterized containment systems developed for freeze-drying which include a reusable aluminum box and the disposable Gore Lyoguard. Common design features of both were determined and a suitable, cost-effective, off the shelf alternative identified in the form of sterilization pouches. Further consideration is given to previous studies that have characterized and compared the effects on mass and heat transfer that barriers cause by increasing resistance to water vapor movement. In addition, the subsequent increases to heat transfer brought about by resistance to mass transfer are also further considered.

Key words Containment, Lyophilization, Sterile processing, Contamination, Culture, Disposables

1 Introduction

In general, freeze-dried biological products can be placed into one of four groups. The first comprises aqueous solutions of biological products which pose no risk to health and need no protection from potential environmental contamination, such as monoclonal antibodies for diagnostic reagents or immunoassay. This category of products can be freeze-dried in a non-sterile facility and do not require special conditions to protect the environment and staff.

Group two consists of non-hazardous products that need to be protected from contaminating microorganisms. Examples would be therapeutic proteins, of which there are many [1], and are intended for systemic administration. These products are manufactured aseptically following strict agency guidelines and as described by Trappler [2], Snowman [3], and Akers [4] are processed in a

Kevin R. Ward and Paul Matejtschuk (eds.), *Lyophilization of Pharmaceuticals and Biologicals: New Technologies and Approaches*, Methods in Pharmacology and Toxicology, https://doi.org/10.1007/978-1-4939-8928-7_6,

sterile environment during filling, transfer, and freeze-drying until the stoppered vials are crimped.

The third group is categorized by products that require both protection from environmental contaminants but are, themselves, potentially hazardous and cannot, therefore, be allowed to contaminate the environment. Examples include microbial standards or biological samples which may contain pathogens. When freeze-drying large numbers of viruses and bacteria they can be entrained in the sublimating water vapor, termed ablation, which can lead to severe contamination of the freeze-drier and potentially operators and environment. Such products can be filled into vials in a contained area. However, their freeze-drying must take place in a contained facility, such as a negative pressure isolator or room, followed by rigorous decontamination of the freeze-drier and the facility. In a multiproduct facility this can cause considerable downtime between products leading to inefficiencies.

The fourth and final category comprises potentially hazardous products that must also be protected from contamination. Their freeze-drying combines the need for sterility, followed by thorough decontamination. An example is the freeze-drying of cytotoxic drugs. Again, their freeze-drying must take place in a contained facility, followed by rigorous decontamination of the freeze-drier and plant.

This chapter is concerned with the application of containment systems that prevent movement of microorganisms. These barriers are porous enough to allow passage of water vapor and small molecules but are able to exclude microorganisms and large molecules such as proteins, specifically, products that fall into group two and group three of this classification. Products in group four fall outside the scope of consideration as small molecule cytotoxic compounds would unlikely be retained or excluded by the containment systems studied. Indeed, it is considered that these types of compounds can only be contained effectively using isolators [5].

2 Freeze-Drying Containment Systems

The concept of sterile freeze-drying in an unclean environment was first investigated by Taylor et al. [6] using an aluminum box incorporating a system for vial stoppering and vapor exchange. An adapted gas mask filter system allowed exchange of water vapor during freeze-drying of serum where an increase in product temperature of 4 °C (compared to conventionally freeze-dried serum) was reported. In addition, the filter was shown to exclude microorganisms when challenged with aerosolized *Serratia marscesens*. More recently W. L. Gore & Associates, Inc. developed the Gore Lyoguard which utilizes an ePTFE membrane allowing water vapor movement during freeze-drying. Gassler and Rey [7] demonstrated this membrane was able to retain 1 μm latex beads and also prevented contamination of nutrient rich media contained within the apparatus when externally challenged with *Bacillus subtilis* var. *niger*. The Lyoguard was also found to provide faster and more uniform heat transfer *vis a vis* stainless steel trays. Again, higher product temperatures were recorded which were attributed to mass transfer resistance.

When considering the aluminum box and the Gore Lyoguard, common design features become apparent. Any freeze-drying containment system must have a bacterially retentive barrier that also allows the free passage of water vapor. The materials of construction should have excellent heat transfer properties and be sufficiently inert not to contaminate parenteral products. However, neither the aluminum box nor the Gore Lyoguard are able to perform both bulk and vial freeze-drying. Therefore, this study sought a design that would satisfy the previous criteria but also be versatile enough to perform both bulk and vial freeze-drying.

An envelope type design was considered to be a versatile, economic, and simple system that met all of the required design features. The design would be easy to manufacture from layers of material to allow passage of water vapor. Trays of vials could be sealed inside the envelope and the flexibility of the envelope would allow shelf stoppering of vials (Fig. 1). Furthermore, trays of bulk product could also be sealed into envelopes to perform bulk freeze-drying.

It was straightforward to find a product that met these design features. Chevron style self-sealing sterilization pouches were already available from most laboratory suppliers in a range of

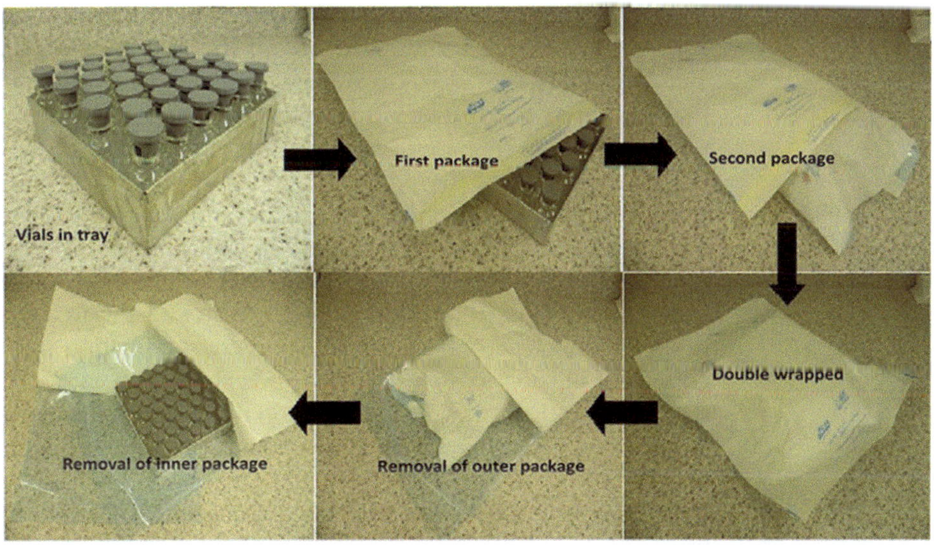

Fig. 1 Method used to double wrap trays of vials in sterilization pouch

sizes. These pouches are designed for the sterilization of medical devices [8] or equipment using super-heated steam in an autoclave or by ethylene oxide gas [9]. They consist of one side, a clear polymer film that would not unnecessarily interfere with heat transfer and the other a gas permeable layer that allows mass transfer but also excludes microorganisms [10]. Moreover, these items were already designed for use in the pharmaceutical industry and were manufactured from compliant materials.

Two types of chevron style self-seal sterilization pouches were used, one formed from latex impregnated medical grade paper with a laminated polyester base and the second made from Tyvek 1073B [11] with an identical laminated polyester base. Although specifically treated with a latex coat, paper can also still shed particles and particle shedding is critically monitored during pharmaceutical manufacture to prevent product contaminant, however, it was not assessed during this study.

3 Barrier Effects on Mass and Heat Transfer

Both Taylor et al. [6] and Gassler and Rey [7] studies showed that a bacterially retentive media allowed the passage of water vapor during the primary and secondary drying stages of freeze-drying but that these media increase product temperature. However, only Gassler and Rey mentioned that primary drying time was increased [7]. As Pikal states "*The theoretical description of primary drying is a problem in coupled mass and heat transfer*" [12] and in the author's previous work experiments were designed to investigate the effect barriers had upon coupled mass and heat transfer during sublimation, their effect on structure and function of an antibody, and their ability to prevent microbial contamination of nutrient rich media [13]. By modifying techniques used in the literature, paper, and Tyvek pouches, Gore Lyoguard, partially-stoppered vials, and protein dry layer were investigated to understand how resistance to water vapor movement effected heat transfer and how this is manifested during freeze-drying.

It was found that containment in a double layer of either paper or Tyvek pouches caused an increase in the sublimation time and, therefore, a decrease in sublimation rate when compared with non-contained partially-stoppered vials. Water filled vials contained in Tyvek pouches took longer to complete sublimation than vials contained in paper pouches whether at a shelf temperature (Ts) of 0 °C or at −10 °C (Fig. 2). Sublimation times were 12.5% longer in paper and 25% longer in Tyvek when compared to non-contained vials at Ts 0 °C. At Ts −10 °C sublimation times were 27% longer in paper and 43% longer in Tyvek when compared to non-contained vials.

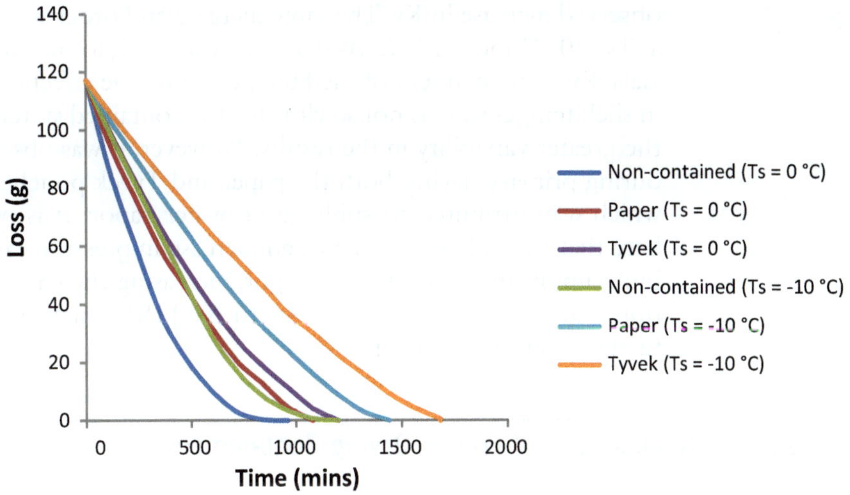

Fig. 2 Effect of barriers on sublimation time using pure water

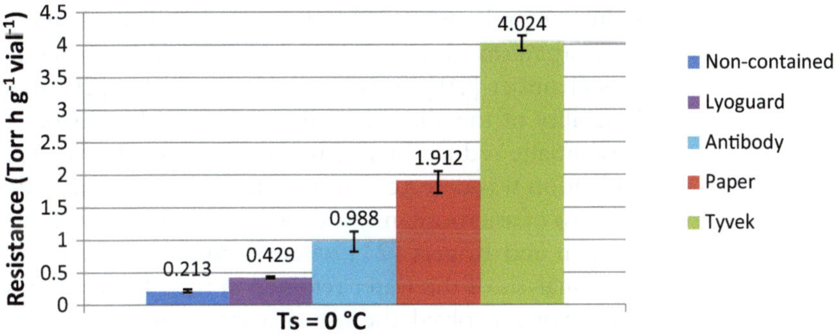

Fig. 3 Comparison of resistance to sublimation presented by the different barriers to water vapor flow

In addition, product temperature (Tp) increased when subliming pure water and also when freeze-drying crystalline (mannitol) and amorphous (trehalose) antibody formulations using paper and Tyvek pouches. During these tests it was observed that paper increased Tp for both antibody formulations by 8–9 °C and Tyvek by around 10–15 °C although shelf temperature had to be lowered for the amorphous formulation to prevent collapse.

Dry layer resistance for many protein products is important and is reported extensively in the literature [14–17]. It was determined that dry layer resistance was found to be greater than the resistance offered by a vented stopper and interestingly also the Lyoguard ePTFE membrane. However, dry layer resistance of the amorphous antibody formulation is considerably less than that of the paper or Tyvek barriers as shown in Fig. 3.

For different containment systems the vial heat transfer coefficient (Kv) was determined and compared to non-contained vials. Non-contained vials had the lowest Kv and Tyvek had the largest observed increase in Kv. The same increase and order was observed at Ts = 0 °C and −10 °C. As would be expected, for non-contained vials, Kv is independent of shelf temperature. The effect of a change in shelf temperature is not so clear for the contained systems due to the greater variability in the results. However, it was observed that during primary drying both the paper and Tyvek pouches inflated which was attributed to sublimating water vapor. It is postulated here that the inflation is due to an increase in pressure caused by a build-up of sublimating water vapor, increasing the gas concentration and the contribution of Kg to Kv [18] which is discussed further later in this chapter.

4 Microbiological Applications of Freeze-Drying Containment

Loss of substrate by ablation can occur when preserving microorganisms by freeze-drying and there exists a paucity of studies detailing methods for containment of microorganisms during freeze-drying. A preliminary study by Adams indicated that ablation of microorganisms during freeze-drying could be contained within a glass chamber [19]. Another study by Adams [20] demonstrated the ability of the aluminum box described by Taylor et al. [6] to substantially reduce loss of microorganisms; however, some contamination was detected around the seals after freeze-drying.

Loss of microorganisms during freeze-drying was first reported by Stein and Rogers [21] when *Bacillus anthracis* was recovered upon analysis of the water retained in their freeze-drier condenser. Their work involved the use of pathogenic organisms and highlighted the need to protect workers from accidental infection. Following this Reitman et al. [22] and Busby [23] showed that the presence of inline cotton filters between the drying microorganism and the condenser prevented carryover and recovery of microorganism in the condenser. Thus, the inclusion of a crude filter went some way to prevent accidental infection of personnel and provides an early justification for the adoption of containment for this type of work. During a more recent study Barbaree and Sanchez [24] freeze-dried two different bacterial cultures of *Pseudomonas aeruginosa* and *Proteus mirabilis* together in the same freeze-drier. When the dried cultures were reconstituted and cultured, growth of the *Pseudomonas* was detected contaminating vials that originally contained only *Proteus* and *vice versa*. They concluded that during the drying process organism had ablated, cross contaminating vials in the freeze-drier chamber. In addition, Cammack and Adams [25] also described the loss of virus titer when freeze-drying vaccines.

Escherichia coli has been used as a trace organism to investigate ablation during preservation by freeze-drying [19]. In that study *E. coli* was cultivated, harvested, and resuspended at high cell densities before being freeze-dried in a vial inside what was termed a "mini-chamber." After freeze-drying the vials were sealed and the mini chamber rinsed and then cultured indicating that considerable numbers of microorganisms had ablated from the dried product. As Adams suggests, protective containment devices could prevent ablation of attenuated vaccines during freeze-drying and it was postulated that the pouches could contain microorganisms during the freeze-drying process [26].

5 Containment of Microorganism Ablation During Freeze-Drying of *Escherichia coli*

The mini chamber designed by Adams [19] was a larger vial cut into two that could be sealed to contain a smaller vial containing suspensions of *E. coli.* A known amount of organism in differing suspending mediums was added to the smaller vial and freeze-dried inside the mini chamber. To determine the extent of ablation, debris was recovered and enumerated to determine the amounts of microorganism present. It was found that varying amounts of organism could be recovered depending upon the formulation used and also that semi-stoppering reduced the losses of bacteria during drying. This approach was duplicated by Cherry et al. [27] and vials containing *E. coli* JM 109 were double wrapped in either paper or Tyvek pouches (Fig. 1).

Importantly, the *E. coli* was deliberately suspended in 0.9% sodium chloride for freeze-drying and the cycle intentionally designed so that the product temperature would exceed the eutectic temperature of sodium chloride, thus causing the formulation to boil under vacuum and consequently lead to blow out from the vial neck. This blow out causes debris to be ejected from the neck of the vial subsequently contaminating the local area. Furthermore, if the filled vials were not semi-stoppered maximum ejection of ablated microorganism could be achieved. This was demonstrated where blowout from the vials can be seen coating the shelf above with debris (Fig. 4). During this experiment a Ts of 4 °C was used yielding an initial Tp of −28 °C that slowly increased until the completion of drying (taken as Tp = Ts) with a total drying time of 9 h. The experiment was then repeated double wrapping the trays in paper and using the lower Ts of 0 °C. Similar results were observed with debris covering the inner layer of the inner pouch. Importantly Tp was around −28 °C and total drying time was 9 h indicating the vials had experienced the same conditions as during the previous experiment. Repeating the experiment with Tyvek pouches, Ts was dropped to −5 °C, and again blowout was observed, Tp was around −26 °C, and drying time was around 9 h. Thus, a consistent freeze-drying process yielding observable blowout with paper (Ts of 0 °C) and Tyvek (Ts of −5 °C) pouches was obtained.

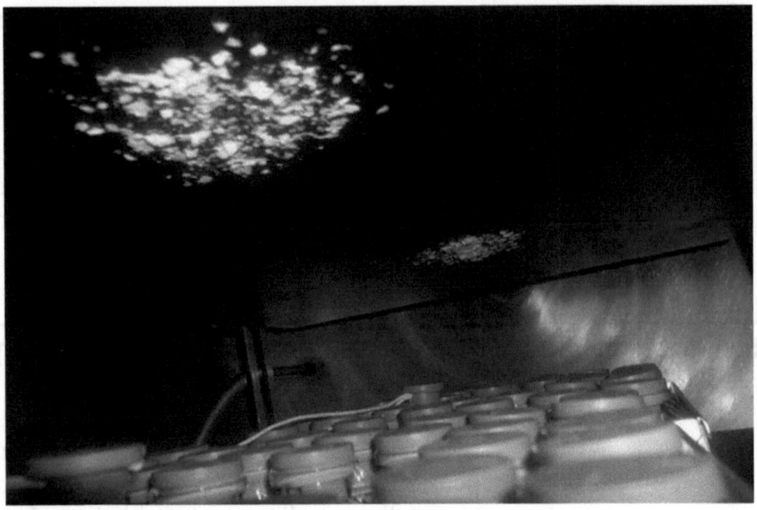

Fig. 4 Blow-out coating the upper shelf observed when freeze-drying 0.9% saline

6 Discussion and Conclusions

All previous work on containment for freeze-drying reported an increase in product temperature during primary drying suggesting that the barrier is affecting the steady state. Resistance was partially investigated by Gassler and Rey [7] who demonstrated that the Lyoguard PTFE membrane provided 10–15% more resistance to mass transfer during sublimation. The importance of understanding this was highlighted more recently by Patel and Pikal who discuss the relative benefits of the use of the Gore Lyoguard and highlight the importance of the "quantitative characterization" of mass and heat transfer using the Lyoguard trays [28]. With consideration to these aspects, the effects that pouches had on mass and heat transfer during freeze-drying were compared to stopper resistance, product dry-layer resistance, and the Gore Lyoguard membrane resistance to derive an overall analysis.

It has been determined that the resistance of the barrier to sublimating water vapor is the most important factor affecting mass transfer. The restriction of sublimating water, slowing the sublimation process, reduces the cooling effects due to the latent heat losses from sublimation. Therefore, without appropriate reduction in Ts to compensate for this increase in Tp product collapse could potentially occur. This study has experimentally defined a ranking whereby increasing resistance to water vapor movement during freeze-drying, imposed by a barrier, has been found to decrease the sublimation rate and subsequently increase product temperature and process time. The resistance imposed by the Lyoguard membrane was low and comparable to stopper resistance as hypothesized by Patel and Pikal [28]. It was also less than the product dry layer resistance as Gassler and Rey [7] confirmed. Pouches made of paper and Tyvek imposed a greater resistance than that of the dry product layer but still allowed sublimation to proceed, albeit at a slightly slower rate. Previously the dry product layer has been the highest reported resistance encountered by water vapor during freeze-drying. The greatest resistance is imposed by the Tyvek pouches and is four times the dry product layer resistance. Thus, it is possible to impose a far greater resistance to mass transfer than dry product layer and still freeze-dry. Furthermore, previous testing of the Lyoguard by Mayeresse et al. determined the physical effects that a protein would be subjected to, but not how a protein would behave [29]. Subsequently, it has been demonstrated that reduced mass transfer rate has no deleterious effect on the activity or structure of a model pharmaceutical protein [13].

The resistance of the barrier also increased the heat transfer coefficient of the system with higher resistance increasing the heat transfer coefficient. It is postulated that observed bag inflation within the chamber indicates increasing pressure around the system. The higher the resistance, the higher pressure imposed and the larger the increase in heat transfer coefficient. This suggests that gas conduction (Kg) is the dominant heat transfer factor being affected since it is the only factor that is pressure dependent. To investigate the effects that pouches have on the heat transfer coefficient, in particular the pressure increases that their resistance causes, further data analysis has been performed. The application of Eq. (1) taken from Pikal [12] has enabled the determination of the pressure inside the pouches (Table 1) using experimental data [30].

$$\frac{\mathrm{Rb}}{\mathrm{Rs}+\mathrm{Rb}}=\frac{(\mathrm{Pp}-\mathrm{Pc})}{(\mathrm{Po}-\mathrm{Pc})} \tag{1}$$

where Rb is barrier resistance, Rs is stopper resistance, Pp is the pressure inside the pouch, Pc is the chamber pressure, and Po is the vapor pressure of ice.

Table 1
Values determined from experimental data for actual pressures inside the pouches or containment system, demonstrating that increasing resistance increases internal pressure

Barrier material	Pp (pressure inside pouch) Torr
Tyvek	1.047
Paper	0.578
Lyoguard	0.08

Table 1 shows that it is possible to derive the pressure inside the pouch during freeze-drying and confirms the experimental observation where pouches expanded due to the resistance to water vapor passage. This caused an increase in pressure inside the pouch causing inflation. These pressures are greater than the chamber pressures for each experiment but less than the vapor pressure of sublimating ice. With some further work to determine the separation distance between the vial base and the surface upon it rests these pressures could be used to determine Kg using equations detailed by Pikal [12]. Furthermore, if the emissivity of the pouches is determined, radiative heat transfer contributions can also be calculated and combined with contact terms to provide a complete view of heat transfer effects. These expressions could then be combined, as Kv = Kg + Kr + Kc, and compared to values calculated earlier for Kv.

With this understanding of containment it would seem appropriate that containment of trays can only be considered applicable to the processing of small scale batches of orphan and niche biopharmaceutical products where Ts can be reduced to prevent collapse of protein products with the trade-off of longer processing times, depending upon the porosity of the barrier. However, the importance of freeze-drying containment to industry must be considered objectively. It has been 35 years since the concept of sterile freeze-drying in a non-sterile environment was first tested and since then only the Gore Lyoguard has been developed. If such an apparatus was of major importance to the pharmaceutical industry then it is reasonable to suppose that further research would have been undertaken. Moreover, the pharmaceutical industry tends to be risk averse and the adoption of new technology can be slow, unless the financial rewards are great, due to the extra regulatory scrutiny and justification the introduction of a new process demands. Thus the main interest in the use of sterilization pouches for contained freeze-drying would initially seem limited to small volume products or to academia. However, potential bio-safety applications offer exciting alternative applications that could be more relevant industrially.

The contamination of the freeze-drier and environment, attributable to ablation, is well documented and shown to be prevented by the Gore Lyoguard membrane [7]. It has been demonstrated that pouches can prevent contamination of the freeze-drier and environment by ablation when freeze-drying high initial concentrations of *E. coli* JM 109 deliberately formulated to induce collapse (representing the worst case for microorganism ablation). To achieve this, results indicated that a double layer of pouches are required for absolute containment. It is hoped that this will stimulate other laboratories to investigate the use of pouches to freeze-dry a range of microorganisms varying in size and pathogenicity. For example, DNA plasmid could be formulated and freeze-dried and ablation assayed for using PCR. In terms of relative sizes, this could be considered a virus model for a freeze-drying process and would address the requirement Adams highlights [26] for a containment device to prevent ablation of attenuated vaccine. Here, the need for such a system is suggested when describing a hypothetical processing chain for a bio-hazardous product. Thus the product could be filled into vials and could "*be contained within filter boxes designed to reduce ablation and spillage*" before being loaded into the freeze-drier.

7 Future Options

It has been demonstrated that the factor governing mass and heat transfer during freeze-drying when using barriers to water vapor is the resistance of that barrier to water vapor movement. It has been shown that there are materials available, for example the ePTFE of the Gore Lyoguard, which provides minimal resistance to water vapor movement and, subsequently, minimal effects on mass and heat transfer. To limit excursions from established cycles the ideal next generation freeze-drying pouch would be made of a material that has exceptionally low resistance to water vapor movement and, therefore, less impact on the freeze-drying process but also has the strength and tear resistance of paper or Tyvek. Materials to be used for the porous layers of freeze-drying pouches can be considered simply as filtration media and many types of filtration media are available from suppliers. To investigate the variety of filter materials available, an apparatus could be developed to perform a thorough survey of the behavior of filter materials. These data can then be used to select the best type of filter media for inclusion into specialist freeze-drying containment pouches or envelopes. This could also potentially be coupled to computer simulation where the experimental observation correlated to a computer model could provide information as to surface area requirements in relation to throughputs of the barrier layer and could be used to predict effective surface area requirements. Therefore, if a membrane material existed that provided little or no resistance to water vapor it could be sized appropriately. Pouches could then be designed with small windows containing the exact surface area of required material. Here, it is proposed that fragile membranes are incorporated into a flexible pouch and protected by an inert cage system preventing accidental rupture.

Finally, the use of pouches for contained freeze-drying is thought to be appropriate for the preservation of tissue samples for transplant. Amniotic membrane has been shown to be effective in the treatment of pterygium by Nakamura et al. [31] and for the re-construction of the ocular surface by Libera et al. [32]. Both of these researchers used amniotic membrane preserved by freeze-drying. Human amniotic membrane was obtained from donors undergoing Caesarean section, washed with buffer and antibiotics, freeze-dried, and then gamma irradiated. According to Nakamura et al. the material preserves well and readily rehydrates [31]. It is postulated that these samples could be collected and washed in the same way but packaged under the clean conditions of the operating theater into freeze-drying containment pouches. These samples could then be freeze-dried in the laboratory and then stored within the same packages until required. Bone allografts are another tissue used for transplants that are preserved by freeze-drying. Jackson et al. detail methods for this procedure [33] but again it would seem plausible that samples could be packaged in freeze-drying containment pouches under clean conditions, freeze-dried in the laboratory, and stored until required.

In conclusion, during freeze-drying, barriers provide resistance to water vapor movement causing a lowering of sublimation rate (mass transfer), increased process time, an increase in product temperature, and an increase in heat transfer coefficient. However, these changes are shown to have no effect on the structure and function of a protein. It is also evident that pouches prevent contamination of a sterile product, allowing sterile freeze-drying to be performed in a normal laboratory environment and indicating that it is possible to perform sterile freeze-drying of pharmaceutical products using pouches. In addition, it has been demonstrated that pouches are able to contain ablation of microorganisms during a freeze-drying process. Previous studies have found potentially dangerous contamination of the freeze-drier and condenser when preserving microbes by freeze-drying caused by particles ablating from vials. The use of pouches as barriers contains the ablated microorganisms, thereby preventing contamination.

References

1. Wang W (2000) Lyophilisation and development of solid protein pharmaceuticals. Int J Pharm 203:1–60
2. Trappler E (1995) Lyophilisation. In: Groves MJ, Murty R (eds) Aseptic pharmaceutical manufacturing II applications for the 1990s. Interpharm Press Incorporated, Buffalo Grove, IL
3. Snowman JW (1995) Lyophilisation under barrier technology. In: Groves MJ, Murty R (eds) Aseptic pharmaceutical manufacturing II applications for the 1990s. Interpharm Press Incorporated, Buffalo Grove, IL
4. Akers MJ (2010) Freeze-dry (lyophilisation) processing. In: Sterile drug products formulation, packaging, manufacturing and quality. Informa Healthcare, New York, NY
5. Suzuki O, Tanaka K, Watanabe N, Takeda M (2003) Design criteria and containment evaluation for pharmaceutical containment systems in aseptic dosage form manufacturing facilities. Pharm Technol 27:24–31
6. Taylor R, Boardman CFB, Wallis RG (1978) Sterile freeze-drying in an unclean environment. J Appl Chem Biotechnol 28:213–216
7. Gassler M, Rey L (2004) Development of a new concept for bulk freeze-drying: lyoguard freeze-dry packaging. In: Rey L, May JC (eds) Freeze-drying/lyophilization of pharmaceutical and biological products. 2nd edition, Informa Healthcare, New York, NY
8. Dunkelberg H, Rohmann S (2006) Test to determine sterile integrity of wrapped medical products at a probability of recontamination of

1:1,000,000. Infect Control Hosp Epidemiol 27(4):367–371

9. Nolan PJ (2004) Sterile medical device package development. In: Standard handbook of biomedical engineering and design. McGraw-Hill, New York, NY
10. Dunkelberg H, Schmelz U (2009) Determination of the efficacy of sterile barrier systems against microbial challenges during transport and storage. Infect Control Hosp Epidemiol 30(2):179–183
11. DuPont (2009) DuPont medical packaging guide technical reference guide
12. Pikal MJ (1985) Use of laboratory data in freeze-drying process design: heat and mass transfer coefficients and the computer simulation of freeze-drying. J Parenter Sci Technol 39:115–138
13. Cherry CLA, Millward H, Cooper R, Landon J (2014) A novel approach to sterile pharmaceutical freeze-drying. Pharm Dev Technol 19 (1):73–81
14. Konstantinidis AK, Kuu W, Otten L, Nail SL, Sever RR (2011) Controlled nucleation in freeze-drying: effects on pore size in the dried product layer, mass transfer resistance, and primary drying rate. J Pharm Sci 100 (8):3453–3470
15. Kuu WY, Hardwick LM, Akers MJ (2006) Rapid determination of dry layer mass transfer resistance for various pharmaceutical formulations during primary drying using product temperature profiles. Int J Pharm 313:99–113
16. Tang X, Nail SL, Pikal MJ (2006) Evaluation of manometric temperature measurement, a process analytical tool for freeze-drying: Part II measurement of dry layer resistance. AAPS PharmSciTech 7(4):E77
17. Lu X, Pikal MJ (2004) Freeze-drying of mannitol-trehalose-sodium chloride based formulations: the impact of annealing on dry layer resistance to mass transfer and cake structure. Pharm Dev Technol 9(1):85–95
18. Patel SM, Pikal MJ (2010) Freeze-drying in novel container systems: characterisation of heat and mass transfer in glass syringes. J Pharm Sci 99(7):3188–3204
19. Adams GDJ (1991) The loss of substrate from a vial during freeze-drying using *Escherichia coli* as a trace organism. J Chem Technol Biotechnol 52:511–518
20. Adams GDJ (1994) Freeze-drying of biohazardous products. In: Hambleton P, Melling J, Salusbury T (eds) Biosafety in industrial biotechnology. Chapman and Hall, London
21. Stein CD, Rogers H (1950) Recovery of viable microorganisms and viruses from vapors removed from frozen suspensions of biologic material during lyophilisation. Am J Vet Res 11:339–344
22. Reitman M, Moss ML, Bruce Harstad J, Alg RL, Gross NH (1954) Potential infectious hazards of laboratory techniques. J Bacteriol 65(5):541–544
23. Busby D (1959) Contamination of apparatus during freeze-drying. J Hyg (London) 57:403–406
24. Barbaree JM, Sanchez A (1982) Cross contamination during lyophilisation. Cryobiology 19:443–447
25. Cammack KA, Adams GDJ (1985) Formulation and storage. In: Spier RE, Griffiths JB (eds) Animal cell biotechnology, vol 2. Academic Press Inc. Ltd., London
26. Adams GDJ (1996) Lyophilisation of vaccines. In: Robinson A, Farrar G, Wiblin C (eds) Methods in molecular medicine: vaccine protocols. Humana Press Inc., Totowa, NJ
27. Cherry CLA, Cooper R, Millward H, Landon J (2015) Proof of concept: containment systems that prevent freeze-dryer contamination when lyophilizing Escherichia coli (JM 109). Drying Technol 33(4):466–470
28. Patel SM, Pikal MJ (2011) Emerging freeze-drying process development and scale-up issues. AAPS PharmSciTech 12(1):372
29. Mayeresse Y, de Cupere V, Veillon R, Brendle J (2009) Considerations for transferring a bulk freeze-drying process from a glass container to a tray. Pharm Eng 29:36
30. Cherry CLA (2013) Development of novel containment systems for freeze-drying. Doctoral dissertation, Cardiff Metropolitan University
31. Nakamura T, Inatomi T, Sekiyama E, Ang LPK, Yokoi N, Kinoshita S (2006) Novel clinical application of sterilised, freeze-dried amniotic membrane to treat patients with pterygium. Acta Ophthalmol Scand 84:401–405
32. Libera RD, Barreto de Melo B, Lima A, Haapalainen EF, Cristovam P, Gomes JAP (2008) Assessment of the use of cryopreserved freeze-dried amniotic membrane (AM) for the reconstruction of ocular surface in rabbit model. Arq Bras Oftalmol 71 (5):669–673
33. Jackson DW, Grood ES, Wilcox P, Butler DL, Simon TM, Holden JP (1988) The effects of processing techniques on the mechanical properties of bone-anterior cruciate ligament-bone allografts. Am J Sports Med 16(2):101–105

Chapter 7

Freeze-Drying Systems: Freeze Dryer Interface Design Requirements and Automatic Loading and Unloading Systems (ALUS™)

Maik Guttzeit, Carolin Wolf, Johannes Selch, and Thomas Beutler

Abstract

The requirements for manufacturing pharmaceutical products are increasing constantly, especially for aseptic and/or products. In the same time there is a clear tendency towards more complex and multi-purpose equipment. In liquid container (mainly vial or syringes) lines the handling of the critical and more often expensive product must be safe and reliable. If the lines are combined with freeze dryers, the interface between the liquid handling parts (filler, container transport, capping), the interface to the freeze dryer has to be observed sensitively. This is because of the different conditions between the 2 sections. While the liquid handling parts are now in most applications covered by isolator technology or Restricted Access Barrier Systems (RABS), which facilitates decontamination cycles and laminar air flow, the freeze dryer has no directional air flow and is equipment which is usually sterilized by saturated steam. These differences have to be taken into consideration during the design and manufacturing process. Additionally there will be increased future vial handling requirements like tracking of the pharmaceutical product.

Key words Automated loading unloading systems (ALUS), Good manufacturing practice, Isolators, Restricted access barrier systems (RABS), Process flow, Combined systems

1 Introduction

In aseptic pharmaceutical processes, freeze-drying is used to increase the shelf-life of products that are often filled in single containers such as vials or syringes. The entire manufacturing process—including filling, loading, and unloading of freeze dryer—usually takes place in Grade A (EU GMP-Guideline Annex 1 [1]) conditions. To reduce the risk of cross-contamination and minimize the cost of implementing expensive Grade A areas, barrier systems are frequently used.

Barrier systems can be divided into RABS (restricted area barrier systems) and isolators. Both systems have different subcategories and designs. This article will focus on isolators installed

Kevin R. Ward and Paul Matejtschuk (eds.), *Lyophilization of Pharmaceuticals and Biologicals: New Technologies and Approaches*, Methods in Pharmacology and Toxicology, https://doi.org/10.1007/978-1-4939-8928-7_7,

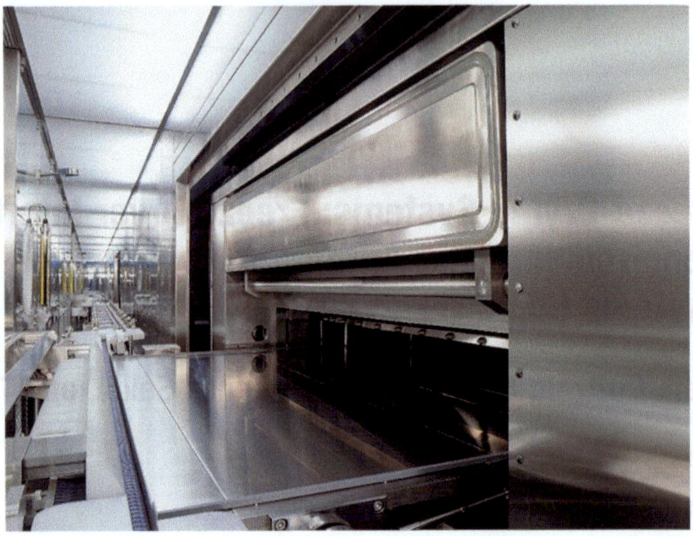

Fig. 1 A loading and unloading door, including a connection plate to a loading and unloading system

around the loading and unloading device of a freeze dryer (Fig. 1) as well as the interface between the freeze dryer and the isolator.

The latter requires special attention as there are two different process areas operating under different aseptic conditions: first, there is the isolator, usually classified as Grade A because of its laminar airflow. Second, there is the interior of the freeze dryer; although this can be considered a sterile surface; it is not equipped with a controlled airflow. Design considerations will be described below.

2 The Freeze Dryer-Filling Line Interface

The outer side of the freeze dryer is not generally regarded as a process contact surface (as defined in ASME BPE 2016 [2]). However, the area leading into the isolator should be carefully considered during the design phase (note: neither the freeze dryer nor the isolator[s] are considered to be product contact surfaces according to the lyophilization section of ASME BPE). The same requirements that are applicable to other isolator interiors do, though, apply to this area, for parameters such as surface roughness, welding requirements, materials, and the absence of gaps and non-cleanable spots. As there is a door between the isolator and the freeze dryer, there will also be mechanical movement. This comes with the usual associated risks, such as interference with the laminar airflow, movement above the vials, and/or the abrasion of moving and closing parts.

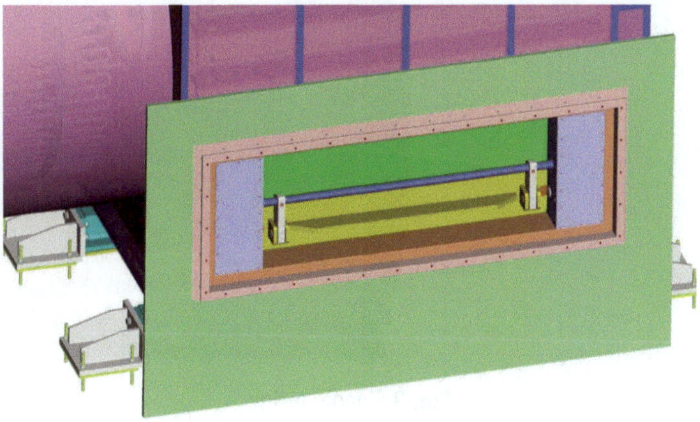

Fig. 2 Slot/pizza door design

The size of the loading and unloading door—often called a pizza door or slot door—is reduced to a minimum to minimize the interaction between the two areas (Fig. 2). There are different concepts for the door movement: the loading and unloading door either opens upward, downward or operates as a slot door. Opening should only be possible if there is no risk of contamination of either the isolator or the freeze dryer.

Despite the above-mentioned aspect that moving parts might have negative impact in general, there are also advantages and disadvantages for the best solution of door movement direction. The door might open as a swing door to the upper or lower part of the opening. If it swings open upward, it may have interference with the laminar flow, if the door swings downward, the inner part of the door is exposed to the mechanism which docks to the shelves and all potential particles will be collected on the door surface and brought into the freeze dryer during closing. A slot door which slides up or down is very difficult to clean and difficult to decontaminate/sterilize. If the door moves into an uncontrolled area, this is an absolutely unacceptable approach. The chosen concept has to be evaluated as part of the related risk assessment. The most challenging aspect might be the swing door which opens upward, but there is no statistical data available.

As the loading and unloading door serves as the boundary of both critical systems (freeze dryer and isolator), the design must be adapted to fulfill both requirements. The door might be operated by electrical or hydraulic drives which have to be suitably covered, but must also have access for maintenance and replacement. The door locking concept must also meet different design aspects, both equipment parts have to be separated completely to maintain desired conditions and the door must be able to withstand the pressure within the freeze dryer during SIP (Fig. 3).

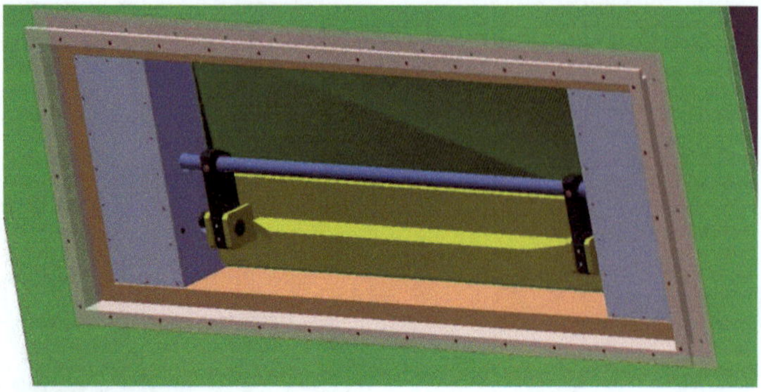

Fig. 3 Flange design

3 Good Manufacturing Process (GMP) Considerations

During freeze dryer operation, conditions can be extreme (low vacuum during freeze-drying and high pressure during steam sterilization (~1.5 bar)); this requires the loading and unloading door to be tightly sealed. The door opens frequently, which should also be considered during the design phase. The seal must both withstand the intense operating conditions, comply with Good Manufacturing Practice (Code of Federal Regulations CFR 21 CFR § 177.2600) [3] requirements, and facilitate easy replacement during maintenance. In some applications, two different sets of seals are used. While one is engaged under vacuum, the other—often designed as an inflatable seal—is employed during sterilization. The usage of double seal concepts must be very carefully considered for loading doors. While the service door opens into the machine area only, the loading door's surrounding is also a clean room area and the grooves of a deflated second seal ring might be difficult to clean and decontaminate as part of isolator routine.

The opening of the isolator must be larger than that of the loading and unloading door to enable a full range of movement. The loading and unloading door mechanism, which is covered by cladding, must be accessible. Yet, this flange must also be sufficiently tight (as defined by ISO 10648-1, Containment enclosures).

The freeze dryer must not be accessible using isolator gloves during normal operation. All intended activities, such as replacing the loading and unloading door seal, should be done while the isolator doors are open. Manual cleaning should also be done with open doors; if specific risks are associated with the product; washdown procedures should be considered prior to opening the door.

ISO 13408-6 (Isolator Systems) suggests the use of automated clean-in-place (CIP) processes, which should be designed in. There are, however, no specific requirements regarding the manual or automatic cleaning of the freeze dryer/isolator interface.

All process contact surfaces must be accessible to the cleaning agent and be sufficiently robust to withstand the cleaning process.

The same requirements also apply to the decontamination cycle. All the outside parts of the freeze dryer must be compatible with those of the isolator. Most often, hydrogen peroxide gas is used for the decontamination process and, at the end of a cycle, it must be verified that the remaining hydrogen peroxide level has no impact on the next product [4]. The decontamination cycle must also be done within a defined temperature range to achieve the required level of bio reduction. The freeze dryer often operates at very low or very high temperatures; so, if it is not possible to keep the isolator-exposed surfaces of the freeze dryer within the desired range, the decontamination cycle should be delayed until a more suitable temperature is achieved.

Depending on the specific requirements of the owner/user, the leak tightness of the entire isolator should be Class 2 or 3, according to ISO 10648-2:1994. In reality, no connection is 100% tight, so the system leak rate is always a sum of its parts (doors, ports, glove ports, sensors, interior connections, interfaces with upstream/downstream equipment, and the freeze dryer flange). As such, the leak rates for every single opening within the freeze-drying system should be much lower (i.e., leak rate door ~1×10^{-3} mbar L s^{-1}). As the freeze dryer—as a pressure vessel—and the isolator are often sourced from different suppliers or made using different manufacturing processes, the connections should be leak tested prior to integration. This is a key risk reduction step as access is very limited when the freeze dryer and isolator are installed.

Any installation within the isolator has a negative impact on the laminar airflow and the impact must be validated. This applies to the movement of the loading and unloading door through the laminar airflow, the flow condition when the loading and unloading door is open and the plate docking to the shelf. As this plate covers a particularly large area, it has a significant impact on the laminar airflow.

Liquid formulations can be extremely temperature sensitive. Therefore, such products need to be cooled as fast as possible. Given that the temperature control of conveyor belts is not possible, the product containers must be brought immediately into the freeze dryer. This requires some design considerations: the shelves should be set to the desired cooling temperature during loading and the rows of vials should be pushed into the freeze dryer as quickly as possible. Whereas other products can be pushed as a complete shelf package in one stroke, vials containing temperature-sensitive product should be pushed in single rows or a few at a time.

If the shelf temperature induces condensation, the isolator should be designed in such a way to reduce the overall moisture content. Otherwise, the condensed moisture (or ice) on the shelves will impact the loading process and the performance of the freeze-drying cycle. Since an isolator has a limited volume, it is easier to facilitate the reduction of moisture content compared to an entire clean room. Nevertheless, due to high air velocity, the amount of dehumidified air is significant. There are different technical solutions available, like absorption/desiccant dehumidification, but in most cases thermal condensation dehumidification is used. The type used depends on the eventual required moisture content as a function of temperature difference between the freeze dryer shelves and the surrounded air. It has to be evaluated if classical mechanical/refrigerative methods are sufficient and probably a combination between mechanical/refrigerative and desiccant methods may lead to best results.

As previously mentioned, conditions within the freeze dryer and isolator are different; this is also true for pressure. To enable a smooth opening process, any pressure difference must be equalized. Because of problematic sterilization issues, there is usually no direct pipe between the freeze dryer and the isolator. As such, pressure equalization should be done "indirectly," ideally using a venting system. As this equilibrates the pressure between the plant room and the isolator, it is necessary to use sterile filters to maintain Grade-A conditions inside the isolator.

It is not possible to open an isolator without breaking the Grade-A condition, therefore the traditional placement of cable-based product sensors inside the freeze dryer is not possible. Wireless sensors may be introduced into the system. They must be placed inside the isolator prior to start of decontamination and must be placed on the conveyor while loading.

The movement of containers in and out of the freeze dryer will influence the required outer dimensions of the isolator. This should also be considered in terms of cleaning and decontamination as well (Fig. 4).

4 Automated Loading Unloading Systems (ALUS)

With regards to a control and operation system, the two machines can be either operated as a single system, or independently using limited signal exchange. Usually, more signal exchange is required between isolators and loading/unloading systems than between an isolator and a freeze dryer. Nevertheless, it must be ensured that no one system contaminates another; therefore, the doors should be interlocked. It is also important to monitor when decontamination cannot be done, such as when the freeze-drying temperature would influence the decontamination result (see above). Not only the freeze dryer, but also the loading and unloading system (ALUS™) needs to comply with certain guidelines.

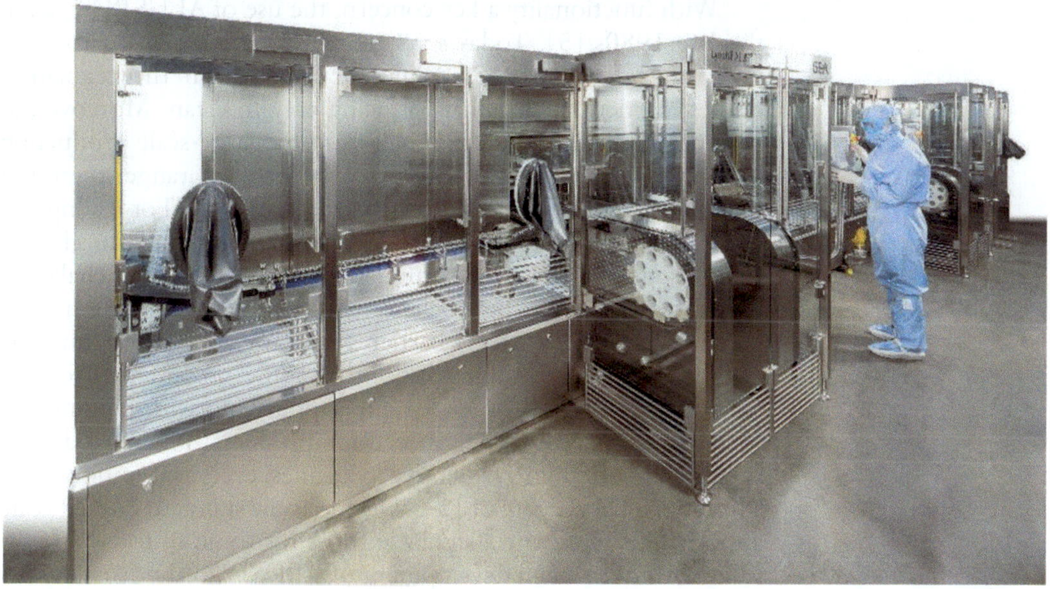

Fig. 4 RABS design with pusher

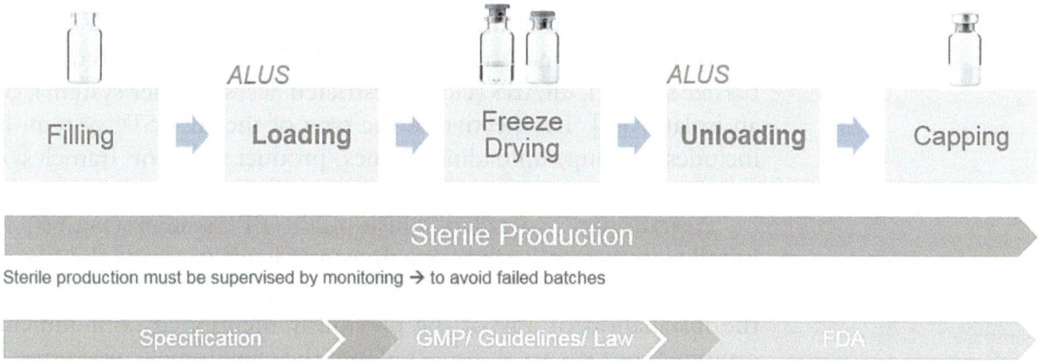

Fig. 5 Sterile Production

Typically, automatic loading and unloading systems are used to load and unload production and pilot-scale freeze dryers to avoid as much human intervention as possible and can prevent product contamination. Sterile production (Fig. 5) begins with filling product into pharmaceutical containers (vials). With ALUS™, liquid or solid product in vials is loaded into and unloaded from the freeze dryer under carefully controlled and monitored conditions, fulfilling the required specifications—US Food and Drug Administration (FDA) requirements and good manufacturing practice (EU GMP-Guideline Annex 1 [1])—for sterile production. The use of ALUS™ also increases production efficiency and minimizes contamination risk by automating the loading/unloading processes before and after freeze-drying (Fig. 5).

With functionality a key concern, the use of ALUS™ began in the late 1980s [5]. Today's systems have been designed to meet increasing (EU GMP-Guideline) demands from the regulatory bodies, particularly in terms of being easy to clean. Moreover, as manufacturers continue to switch from the large-scale production of a single product to a more extensive product range, there is a growing need for multipurpose freeze dryer lines. For example, a company making a nontoxic product may wish to switch to a highly toxic product line in the future. In this situation, the challenge would be to find the best balance between containment (an open or closed restricted access barrier system or an isolator) and the optimum level of productivity both for the present and for the future. That is a tall order for any supplier, notwithstanding the ever-increasing cost of pharmaceutical products. When producing small batches of highly expensive medicines, every vial counts. Even a rejection/fail vial rate of 1%—which was the standard rate 20 years ago—would represent a significant loss for some of today's high-value cytotoxics. The development of ALUS™ in the last 10 years has been driven by the absolute need to minimize rejected vials while maintaining high levels of productivity.

ALUS™ can be divided into stationary and flexible systems. Depending on the individual process and product requirements, the containment method can be an oRABS (open restricted access barrier system), cRABS (closed restricted access barrier system), or an isolator [6]. Irrespective of the type of the ALUS™ system, it includes loading/unloading frames/product trays or frameless/tray-less functionality.

A stationary, so-called "push-pull" (PP) system (Fig. 6) is installed in front of each freeze dryer and loads/unloads the freeze dryer from the same (sterile) side. Using stationary ALUS™ allows the installation of any of the previously mentioned containment options. The vials are transported into the containment area using a conveyor belt from the filling station to a shelf located in front of the freeze dryer slot door; here, they are collected until the desired number of vials for one shelf is reached. During the next step, a pusher moves the vial package inside the freeze dryer to position it on the desired shelf in the vacuum chamber. Once the required batch size is obtained, the freeze dryer is hermetically closed and the lyophilization process is initiated. When the process terminates, the freeze dryer shelves are unloaded by pulling the vials out of the freeze dryer in a row by row manner. The conveyor belt then transports them to the capper station.

An alternative to stationary push-pull systems is the so-called "push-push" system (Fig. 7). All the functional loading parts are installed in front of each freeze dryer as per the push-pull system. It also loads the freeze dryer from one side (usually the sterile side).

The push-pull and push-push systems operate in the same way until the lyophilization process terminates; with a push-push

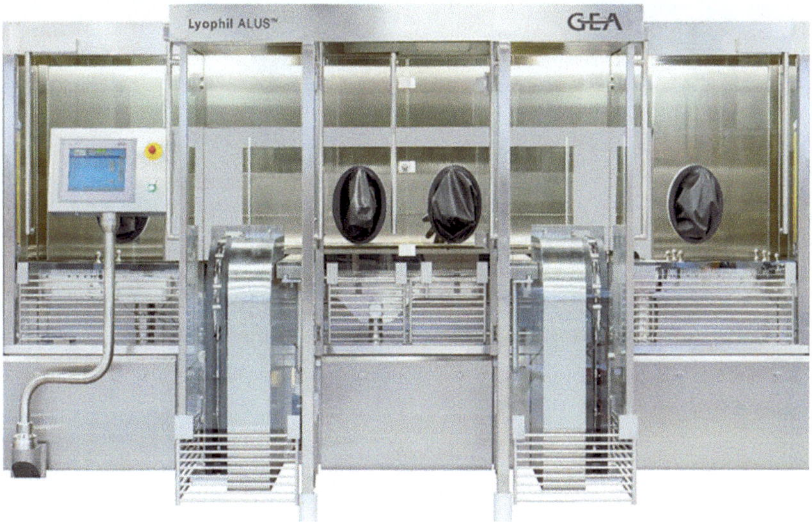

Fig. 6 A stationary push pull ALUS™ system (GEA Group)

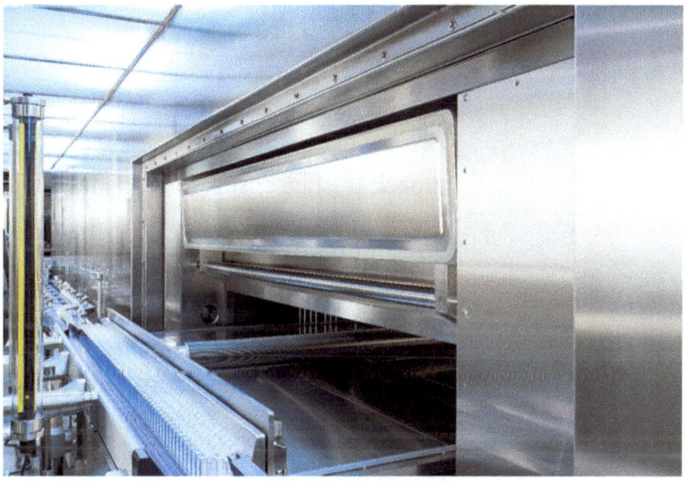

Fig. 7 A stationary push-push ALUS™ (back-pusher system)

system, the freeze dryer shelves are unloaded using a back-pusher device, which is installed on the full-sized door at the back of the freeze dryer. It pushes the vials out of the freeze dryer in a row-by-row manner. The conveyor belt then transports them to the capper station.

All the moveable parts of a back-pusher system (within the freeze dryer chamber) are covered with bellows. These bellows are leak tested before unloading and guarantee the strict separation between the sterile product room (inside the freeze dryer) and the technical room (outside the freeze dryer). The back-pusher is cleaned during the freeze dryer clean-in-place (CIP) cycle. Using

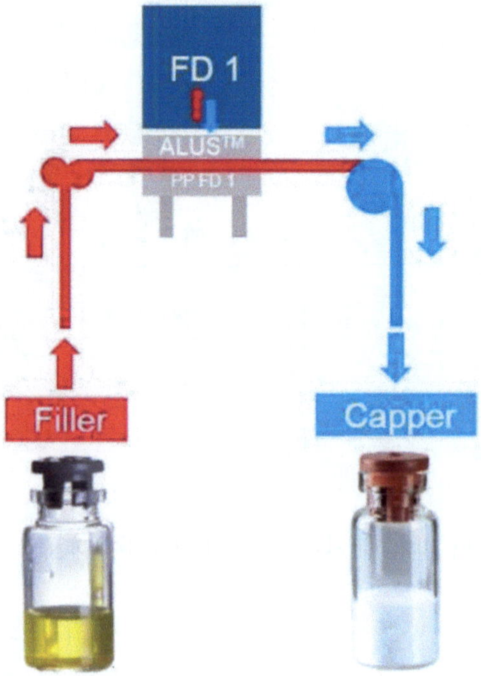

Fig. 8 Production flow: one freeze dryer

a back-pusher ensures compliance with FDA guidelines (no parts moving above the product).

Figures 8, 9, 10, and 11 show production flow examples of stationary ALUS™ systems.

A "transfer cart" (TC) system (Fig. 12) is far more complex in terms of construction, albeit a lot more flexible. This mobile cart system is used when more than two freeze dryers have to be loaded/unloaded. One cart (or multiple carts) move(s) in front of the freeze dryers and loads/unloads the freeze dryer shelf by shelf. Contrary to the stationary system, a flexible ALUS™ can only be implemented with oRABS containment.

5 Process Flow Options

The first step of a loading/unloading process with a flexible ALUS™ constitutes the preparation of a vial package—sized according to the freeze dryer shelf size—on the formatting table (FT). The transfer cart is then positioned in front of the loading table and a pusher moves the vial package onto the transfer cart. The transfer cart moves the vial package to the designated freeze dryer shelf. As such, the freeze dryer shelves are filled with the desired number of vials before the freeze dryer is hermetically closed and the freeze-drying process is induced. Once the

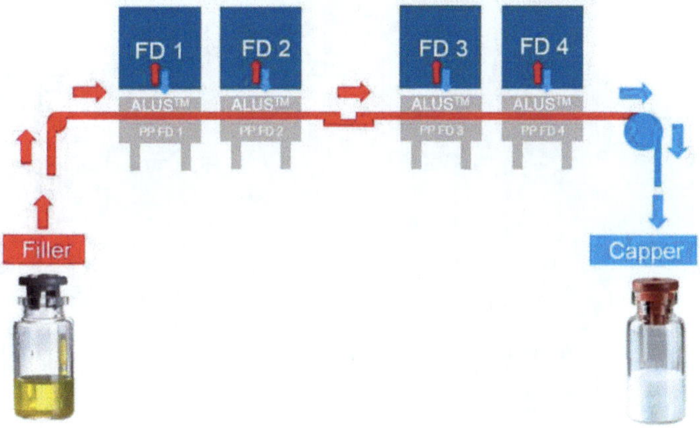

Fig. 9 Production flow: multiple freeze dryers (filler and capper on opposite sides)

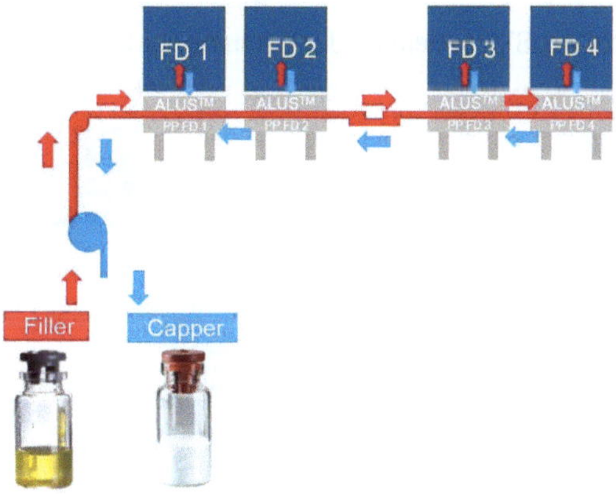

Fig. 10 Production flow: multiple freeze dryers (filler and capper on same side)

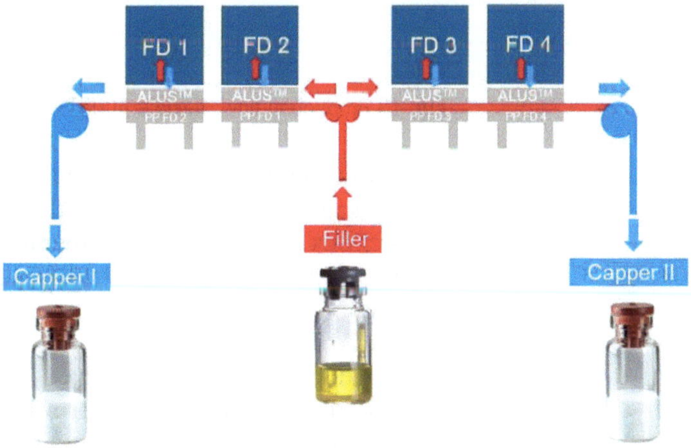

Fig. 11 Production flow: multiple freeze dryer (T-configuration)

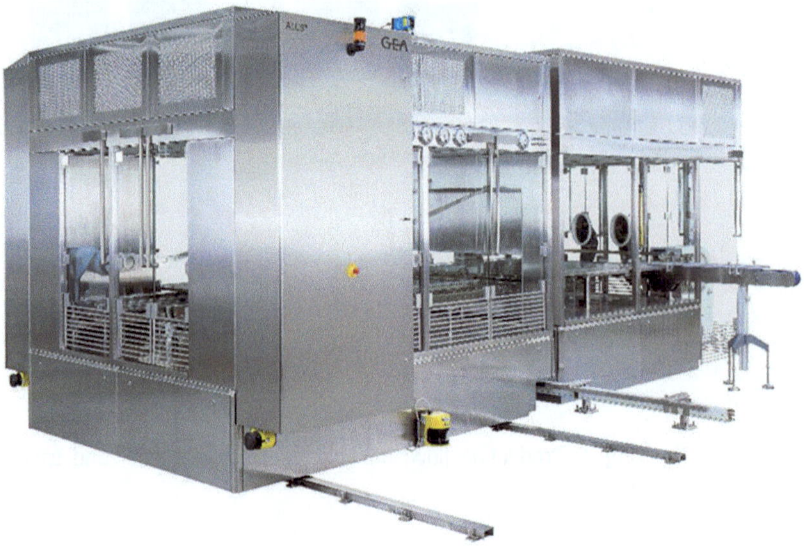

Fig. 12 Flexible ALUS™ system (ALUS™ transfer cart)

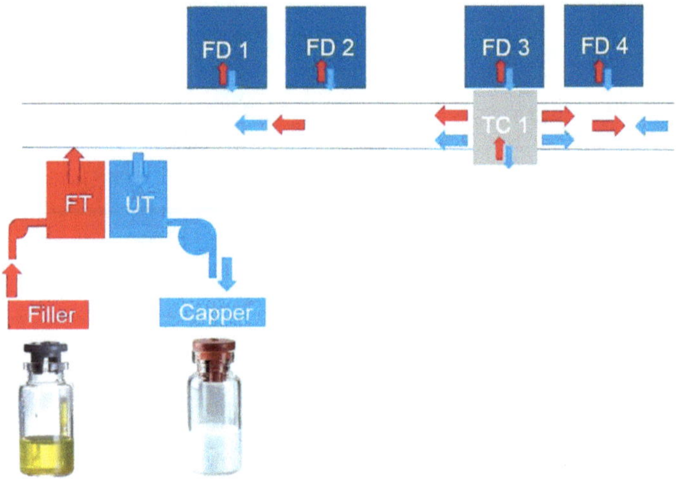

Fig. 13 Production flow: flexible ALUS™ (filler and capper on same side)

lyophilization process finishes, the freeze dryer is unloaded and the vial packages are transported to the unloading table (UT) via the transfer cart and are subsequently moved to the capping station on a conveyor belt.

Figures 13, 14, and 15 show production flow examples using a flexible ALUS™.

Besides the installation of fixed or mobile ALUS units, it is also possible to combine them to provide a solution for almost every conceivable configuration and accommodate a wide range of product flow, flexibility, sterility, and GMP requirements. The combination of PP and TC systems allows for one-sided loading and

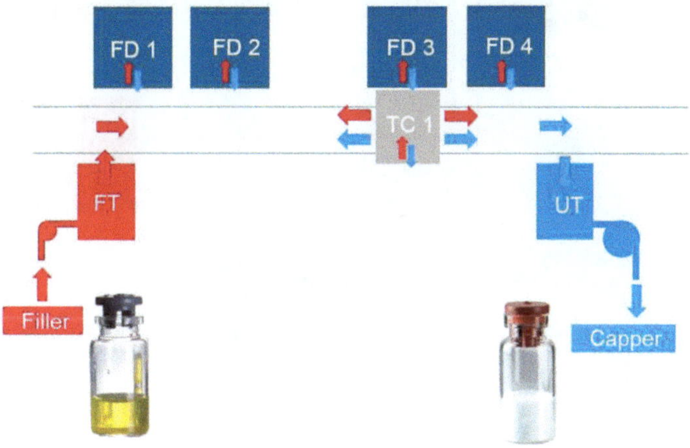

Fig. 14 Production flow: flexible ALUS™ (filler and capper on opposite sides)

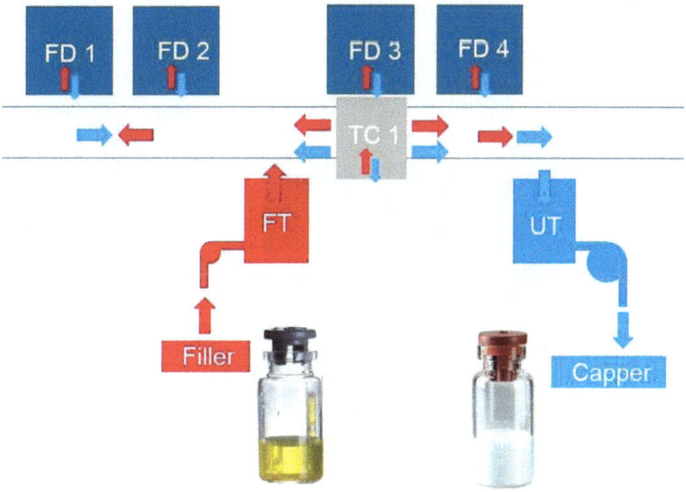

Fig. 15 Production flow: flexible ALUS™ (T-configuration)

unloading of single or multiple freeze dryers, as well as pass-through setups, wherein loading is done out on one side and unloading on the other. Figures 16 and 17 show production flow example combined with flexible and stationary ALUS™.

Additionally, beyond containment and layout, vial transport speed and a compact, easy-to-clean design must be considered when implementing an efficient, safe, and GMP-compliant ALUS™.

The system of choice should be able to achieve a throughput rate of 500 vials min^{-1} when loading and up to 800 vials min^{-1} when unloading. The actual speed of an ALUS™ installation depends on whether loading is done in single- or multiple-row formation. A maximum loading speed of 750 vials min^{-1} is usually possible with a multiple-row setup.

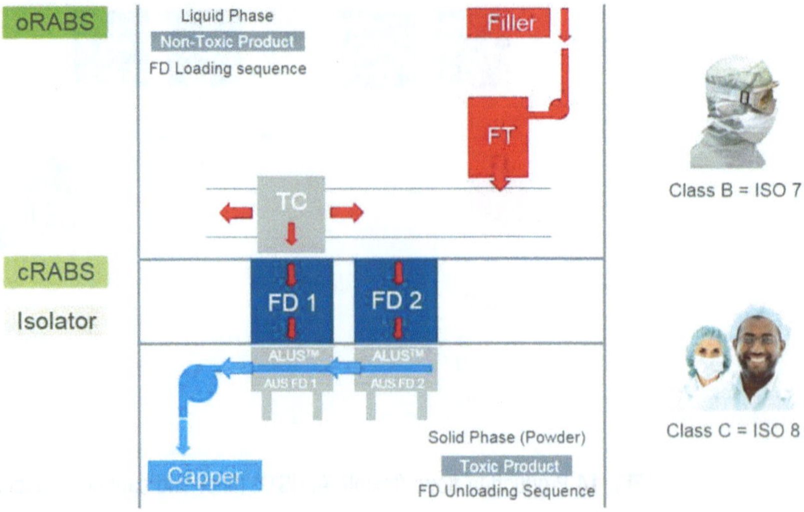

Fig. 16 Production flow: pass-through configuration

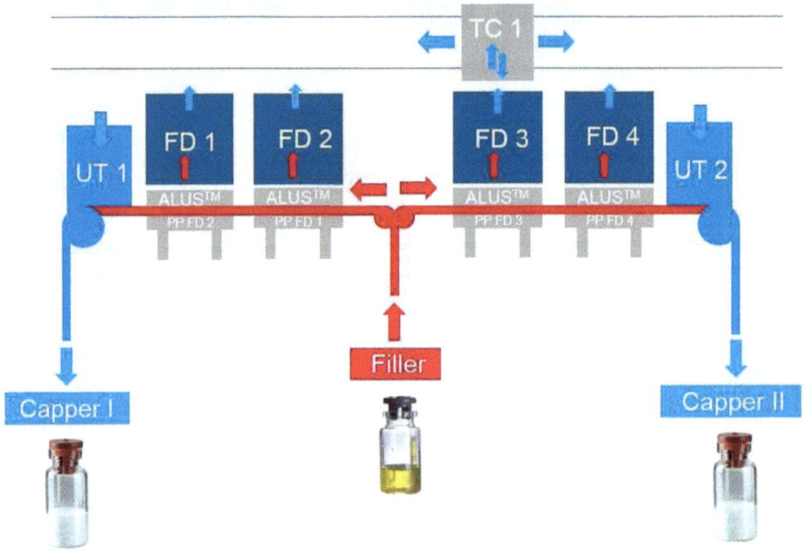

Fig. 17 Production flow: pass-through configuration

To facilitate cleaning and prevent moving part-derived particles from entering the vials, a common solution is to situate any drives that require routine service, as well as any electrical parts, beneath a solid base plate. This sealed and separated area eliminates any risk of contamination. It also makes it possible to service the machine without breaching the sterile production area and guarantees safe and contamination-free operation. Furthermore, excellent laminar flow and H_2O_2 (Vaporized Hydrogen Peroxide)-compatible components inside the production room are required.

6 Future Developments

To further optimize automatic loading and unloading, many optional features have been developed in recent years, such as "cold shelf loading" (loading the vials on precooled shelves for sensitive products).

In the future, an important feature for "high-end" ALUS™ will be the full traceability of individual vials. Vial tracking systems will help the pharmaceutical industry to implement the EU's drug anti-counterfeiting directive (due to come into effect in 2018), safeguard the rights of trademark and patent holders, and thereby protect patients. The legislation will require pharmaceutical manufacturers to provide a unique serial number for every vial—which will be sent to a national database—to ensure that every vial can be verified before reaching the patient.

A fully developed system for the implementation of vial traceability is GEA's LYODATA™ system (Fig. 18). It incorporates a code reading infeed prior to the freeze dryer (after the filling station) and a code reading outfeed prior to the capping station. Each of the vials is marked with an individual data matrix that contains detailed information about time, position, context, partial

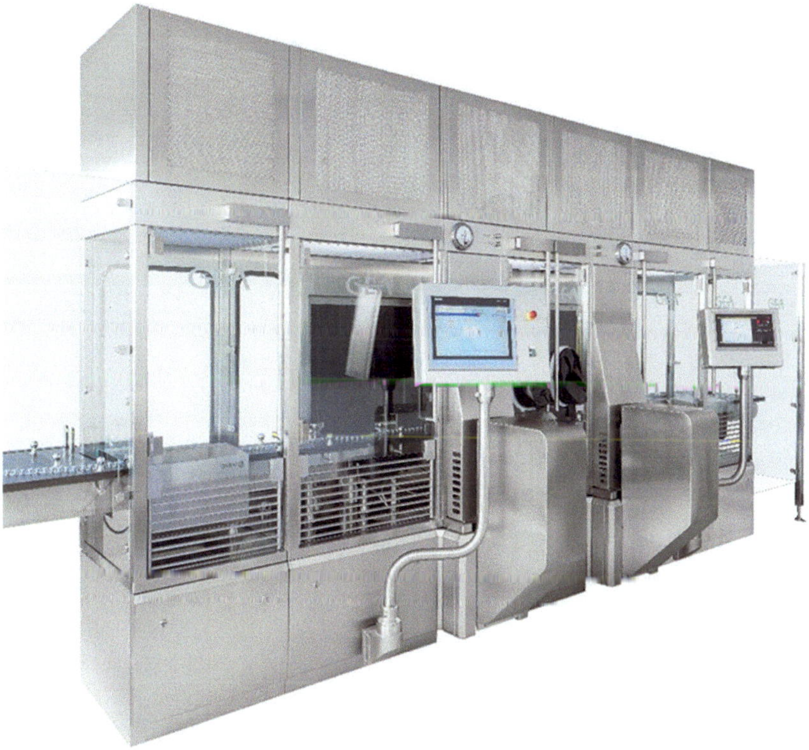

Fig. 18 GEA's LYODATA™ system

weight, etc. The data matrix works with GS1 application identifiers based on ISO/IEC 16022 and GS1 general specifications. The national database gives direct feedback regarding the originality of the product and, for medication verification; it can be scanned by the pharmacist before being prescribed to the patient. The advantages for the pharmaceutical manufacturer, apart from the ability to comply with regulations, include easier line clearance, the prevention of cross-contamination, and improved troubleshooting options. It facilitates secure product monitoring throughout the entire manufacturing process.

References

1. EU GMP guidelines Annex 1. Manufacture of sterile medicinal products (2008) https://ec.europa.eu/health/sites/health/files/files/eudralex/vol-4/2008_11_25_gmp-an1_en.pdf
2. Figure SD-5.4.1.3-1 Lyophilizer Sterile Boundary in ASME BPE (2016) http://files.asme.org/Catalog/Codes/PrintBook/35606.pdf
3. Code of Federal Regulations CFR 21 CFR § 177.2600 https://www.accessdata.fda.gov/scripts/cdrh/cfdocs/cfcfr/CFRSearch.cfm?fr=177.2600
4. PHSS: No.2: "Environmental Contamination Control Practice (2002) https://phss.site-ym.com/store/ViewProduct.aspx?id=1990368
5. Rey L, May JC (eds) (2004) Freeze drying/lyophilization of pharmaceutical and biological products, 2nd edn. Marcel Dekker, New York, NY
6. PHSS Guidance on isolators and RABS – 15: https://phss.site-ym.com/store/ViewProduct.aspx?id=1819470

Chapter 8

Regulatory Aspects of Freeze-Drying

David Awotwe-Otoo and Mansoor Khan

Abstract

Freeze-drying or lyophilization has become an important formulation and stabilization strategy in the pharmaceutical industry for drugs, vaccines, antibodies, and other biological materials, for improving their long-term stability. For biological products whose storage in aqueous solution results in instability, freeze-drying prolongs the shelf-life by inhibiting chemical, physical, and microbiological pathways that occur in the presence of moisture. Due to the complex multi-step processes involved in lyophilization, it is crucial to ensure a robust and efficient cycle, which in turn ensures that high-quality products are consistently manufactured that meet the labelled therapeutic claim over the shelf life of the product. Most lyophilized small molecule drug products are usually very simple formulations containing the active ingredient, water, and in some cases, buffer. Even with these simple formulations, a number of post-approval manufacturing process changes occur occasionally due to their failure to consistently meet desirable target qualities such as reconstitution time, low moisture content, and stability. In most cases, the root causes for such failure are identified as poor lyophilization cycles or a lack of operator training.

An overall understanding of the lyophilization process, as well as use of optimum lyophilization process parameters, would provide the Agency with a greater level of knowledge and help with the approval process. This will also facilitate a greater understanding between the FDA and industrial sponsors on the regulatory aspects of lyophilized drug products.

This chapter provides an overview of the application of risk analysis to defining and measuring the critical parameters of lyophilization, for which a specific level of scrutiny is required, to ensure a robust and controlled process. Particular focus will be on the key steps of risk management through ICH Q9 applied to the freeze-drying process, with specific examples, as applied to the lyophilization of a model monoclonal antibody. The application of various process analytical technology (PAT) tools for monitoring and controlling the various processes, with specific examples, will also be discussed.

Key words Quality by design (QbD), Critical quality attributes (CQA), Process analytical technology (PAT), Regulatory requirements, Freeze-drying process, Optical coherence tomography (OCT)

Disclaimer: The views expressed in this chapter are those of the authors and do not necessarily represent the position of the Agency.

Kevin R. Ward and Paul Matejtschuk (eds.), *Lyophilization of Pharmaceuticals and Biologicals: New Technologies and Approaches*, Methods in Pharmacology and Toxicology, https://doi.org/10.1007/978-1-4939-8928-7_8,

1 Introduction

Freeze-drying or lyophilization is being used for many pharmaceutical and biopharmaceutical products that are unstable in the liquid state for a substantial period of time. Currently, roughly 50% of marketed therapeutic protein products are lyophilized (1). As more new chemical and biological entities are being explored as therapeutic agents, lyophilization has often been used to increase the stability and shelf-life of these products. Many of such new chemical entities (NCEs) also suffer from poor solubility and bioavailability, and therefore preparation of amorphous solid dispersions by lyophilization represents a promising alternative to overcome such challenges, especially in the presence of non-aqueous co-solvents (2).

In 2015, six novel antibody therapeutics were granted first approvals (3). Such antibody therapeutics are lyophilized, so as to improve their long-term stability. In the lyophilized state, the water fraction of the product is significantly reduced through a combination of sublimation and desorption so that chemical and physical degradation reactions are inhibited or sufficiently decelerated, resulting in improved long-term stability of the drug product. The final lyophilized product assumes a very high surface area with a porous cake which enables it to be easily reconstituted quickly when needed for use. This is particularly useful for products such as vaccines, antibodies, and many parenteral drugs.

Lyophilization is a very complex, multi-step process which begins with the freezing of the aqueous formulation in vials below the thermodynamic freezing point of the solution, causing most of the water to form ice crystals and the solutes to become crystallized or transformed into a solid amorphous system. This is followed by the primary drying step, where the ice crystals are removed by sublimation under vacuum and increased shelf-temperature, and then the secondary drying step, where most of the unfrozen water still absorbed in the interstitial region is removed by desorption at elevated shelf temperatures and low chamber pressure to allow the desired low moisture content to be achieved (4, 5). The lyophilization process can therefore result in possible destabilizing effects on the final drug product. For example, for protein-based biopharmaceutical products, the freezing step could result in aggregation due to increased protein-protein interaction (6), pH changes due to crystallization of buffer salts, reduced hydrophobic interactions due to the "dehydration" effect of ice formation, formation of large ice–aqueous interfaces, and increase in ionic strength (5). During the primary drying process, the removal of the hydration shell from proteins in the absence of appropriate stabilizers can cause destabilization of the protein structure (7). In order to achieve a high-quality lyophilized dosage form, a combination of optimal formulation design and freeze-dry cycle design is needed.

The goal of pharmaceutical development, in the twenty-first century, is a shift in paradigm from the traditional, data-driven, and rigorous testing of the final product, to a science-based and risk-based approach, where "critical formulation attributes and process parameters are generally identified through an assessment of the extent to which their variation can impact the quality of the drug product" (8). This shift to the adoption of modern quality techniques seeks to ensure a coordinated operation of the regulatory review, compliance and inspection policies, leading to more knowledge-based submissions of New Drug Applications (NDA), Abbreviated New Drug Applications (ANDA), as well as Biologics License Applications (BLA), where the focus is on sound science and engineering principles for assessing and mitigating risks of poor product and process quality.

This systematic approach to product development is referred to as Quality by Design (QbD), and it begins with predefined objectives and emphasis on product and process understanding, based on sound science and quality risk management. The key factors for QbD are the identification, understanding, and control of critical product and process parameters and ultimately the development of a design space and a control strategy to ensure that good product quality represents an acceptably low risk of failing to achieve the desired clinical attributes (9). The measuring and control of critical product and process parameters require the implementation of process analytical technology (PAT), which is defined as a system for designing, analyzing, and controlling manufacturing through timely measurements of critical quality and performance attributes of raw and in-process materials and processes with the goal of ensuring final product quality (Guidance for Industry—PAT, (10)).

To date, publications and presentations from the FDA indicate the goal of reaching a desired state of "a maximally efficient, agile, flexible pharmaceutical manufacturing sector that reliably produces high-quality drug products without extensive oversight" (11). This has culminated in the roll out of three harmonized guidance, Q8, Q9, and Q10, which integrate the principles of Quality Risk Management (QRM), Process Analytical Technology (PAT), and Quality Systems (QS) (8, 10, 12, 13). These cGMP initiatives are to provide a model for drug product submissions while assisting both industry and the FDA in a move toward a more scientific, risk-based, holistic, and proactive approach to pharmaceutical development (14).

The implementation of QbD has started with many elements embedded in the drug product review program at the Office of Biotechnology Products (OBP). Full implementation has been slowed by the functional and structural complexity of biotechnology products, their manufacturing process, and the inherent difficulty involved in evaluating the impact of each process parameter on each quality attribute and impact of the quality attributes on safety and efficacy.

Lyophilization as a manufacturing process spans other FDA centers besides CDER. As an example, some vaccines are also lyophilized for stability considerations, where the sponsors submit applications to the Center for Biologics Evaluation and Research (CBER).

2 Challenges in Implementing Quality by Design in Lyophilization of Biologics

Achieving the key goals in the QbD paradigm, as applied to lyophilized biologics, requires understanding of the raw materials, excipients, the lyophilization process, and their impact on quality of the final lyophilized drug product. This involves the building of an efficient manufacturing process and a robust lyophilization cycle that will consistently deliver the best quality drug product to meet patient needs and also provide economic benefits in terms of energy, time, and resources, with the best quality cycles. This requires the collaborative efforts among interdisciplinary teams from chemistry, biology, physics and engineering, process engineers, mathematics, statistics and regulatory affairs, and significant investment into developing a fundamental understanding of critical processes and product attributes, establishment of design controls and testing based on product quality and within the limits of scientific understanding. The knowledge gained over the product's life cycle is then applied to operate in an environment of continuous improvement.

A well-implemented QbD benefits both FDA and the industry, in that, it provides for better coordination across the various review disciplines, compliance, and inspection, while also reducing the overall costs of manufacturing by significantly reducing the number of post-approval manufacturing changes.

For small molecule pharmaceuticals, especially generic drugs, the scope and philosophy for the application of QbD are well established because prior knowledge from innovator companies can be leveraged. This is not the same with the application of QbD in the lyophilization of biologics, such as monoclonal antibodies, where its application involves some nuances and complexities, largely due to the unique, sensitive, higher level structures of proteins, as well as challenges associated with their development and manufacturing (15). For example, for small molecules, the term "quality" is defined as "the suitability of either a drug substance or drug product for its intended use, including attributes such as identity, strength, and purity" (8). This definition may not be entirely applicable to lyophilized proteins since for these, the term "quality" may at the first instance be attributed to other physical characteristics such as cake elegance and residual moisture, rather than the stability of the active. Under such circumstances, lyophilized vials with collapsed cake would be routinely rejected from a batch even though the drug product may be stable from a pharmaceutical standpoint. Other factors such as scaling-up, transferring technologies, and results from laboratory to major production units, ensuring homogeneity and compliance with key regulations require a sound understanding of both product and process-related attributes to ensure effective QbD implementation. By implementing QbD in lyophilized biologics, the goal is to be able to identify and control possible interactions that may arise between formulation and process parameters that may have significant effects on the quality attributes of the final products (16).

3 General Steps for Implementing Quality by Design (QbD) in the Lyophilization of Biologics

The following sections describe the various key steps in implementing QbD for lyophilized biologics. While the implementation of QbD would generally vary with product class and complexity, it nonetheless follows a common concept, as outlined in the three harmonized guidance which integrate the principles of Quality Risk Management (QRM), Process Analytical Technology (PAT), and Quality Systems (QS). A general approach to the formulation design and development of a lyophilized drug product using QbD is shown in Fig. 1.

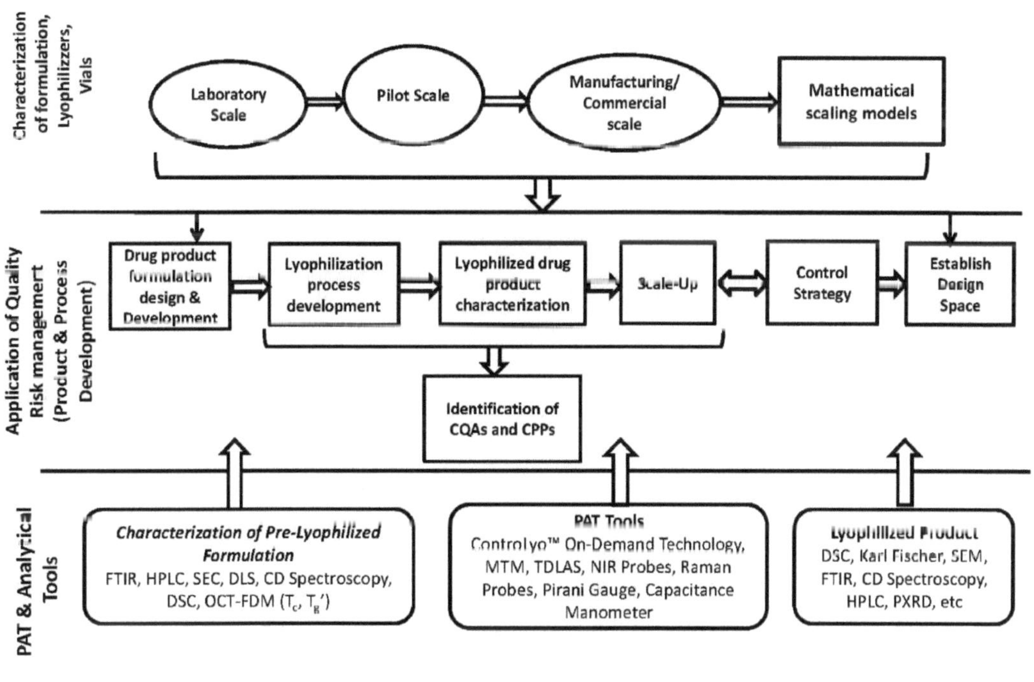

Fig. 1 Simplified outline showing the application of QbD and PAT to the development of a lyophilized drug product

3.1 Defining Quality Target Product Profile (QTPP)

The QTTP serves as the foundation for the product design and development and is defined as the prospective summary of the quality characteristics of a drug product that will be achieved to ensure the desired quality, considering the safety and efficacy of the drug product (8).

QTPP is usually established as soon as a drug is identified as a viable candidate for commercialization. The QTPP comprise several key sections and include the following at a particular time in development: Description—Information relating to the completed/planned studies to support the target with Protocol IDs and submission dates. It should include:

- Detail regarding the treatment or prevention of specific disease
- Indications and Usage
- Dosage and Administration
- Dosage Forms and Strengths
- Contraindications
- Warning and Precautions
- Adverse Reactions
- Drug Interactions
- Clinical Pharmacology
- Use in specific populations
- Drug Abuse and Dependence
- Overdosage
- Nonclinical Toxicology
- Clinical Studies
- References
- How supplied/Storage and handling
- Patient Counseling Information

with each section containing (1) Target, (2) Annotations, and (3) Comments.

It provides the information necessary for an open and constructive communication that will not only ensure that the drug sponsor and the FDA have the same understanding of the risks involved with the proposed labeling but also potentially minimize the risk of late-stage development failures, ensure the safety and efficacy data availability in a timely manner, and improve labeling content, and potentially reduce the total time involved with drug development (9).

For a lyophilized monoclonal antibody formulation, the QTPP should generally include the dosage form, appearance, mode of administration, concentration or content per vial, reconstitution media, reconstitution volume, mode of reconstitution, reconstitution time, post-constitution storage and stability and drug product quality criteria (e.g., sterility and purity) (17).

3.2 Identifying Critical Quality Attributes (CQAs)

Once QTTPs are identified, the next step is to identify preliminary critical quality attributes. The critical quality attributes are physical, chemical, biological, or microbiological properties or characteristics that should be within an appropriate limit, range, or distribution to ensure the desired product quality (8). Not every attribute may be necessarily critical to the quality of the product and so a combination of prior knowledge and/or experience gained from similar biological molecules as well as relevant information from a variety of resources such as literature and accumulated preliminary laboratory experimental data could be used to create the list of preliminary CQAs that relate to or affect the formulation QTTP. These critical attributes are subject to further refinement or updates throughout the product's life cycle. This is usually achieved through risk assessment where the importance of each product attribute is ranked based on its impact on safety and efficacy.

For a model monoclonal antibody formulation, a typical list of CQAs would comprise the freeze-drying properties such as collapse temperature (Tg′ for an amorphous product or Teu for a crystalline product), final cake appearance (color, density, uniformity, absence of meltback, shrinkage, and/or collapse), solution appearance upon reconstitution (completeness, clarity, color), reconstitution time, residual moisture content, protein purity (chemical changes, presence of aggregates, visible and sub-visible particles), and potency (17). A similar list of formulation components such as excipients, buffer components, surfactant, protein concentration, pH, ionic strength, vial configuration, stoppers and fill volumes; freeze-drying process operating parameters such as freezing ramp rate, hold time, primary drying conditions of shelf temperature, chamber pressure and duration, secondary drying conditions (shelf temperature, pressure and duration) and equipment conditions (including the batch size/load and scale effects) are created and the effects of these parameters on CQAs are studied (9).

3.3 Performing Risk Assessment

The application of risk assessment provides a mechanism by which process parameters are studied against quality and process attributes in order to prioritize parameters for experimental studies. It provides an understanding of relationships that exist among formulation parameters, process inputs/material attributes, and product quality attributes and enables the identification of robust process conditions and their acceptable limits.

Risk assessment begins with the systematic use of information such as prior knowledge, historical data, theoretical analyses, and information available in literature to create a list of product CQAs that affect the QTTP. Once CQAs are identified, various methods are applied to analyze and understand the presence or absence of interactions and identify the parameters that significantly impact the CQAs, termed critical process parameters (CPP) (9, 15).

Practical ways of analyzing these factors include the use of risk analysis tools such as Cause and Effect (Ishikawa or Fishbone) diagrams, Cause and Effect Matrices, Failure Mode Effects Analysis (FMEA), Failure Mode Effects and Criticality Analysis (FMECA), Fault Tree Analysis (FTA), and Risk Ranking Analysis (12).

Once the process parameters are identified, these are further characterized using statistical design of experiments (DoE) to determine the degree of impact each parameter has on the CQA. Here, screening experiments such as Plackett-Burman, fractional factorial, and full factorial experimental designs could be used to determine the extent of main effect of process parameters on CQAs. Based on statistical significance in these experiments or Pareto ranking analysis, process parameters that are observed to significantly impact CQAs are categorized as critical process parameters (CPP) while the other parameters that are not statistically significant but are important for consistency of process performance are categorized as key process parameters (KPP). CPPs are further studied using design of experiments involving multivariate combinations and interactions with other parameters to define the optimum operating boundaries. A response surface experimental design, such as Box-Behnken design or Central Composite design, could be used to study main and interaction effects of process parameters on CQAs, depending on the number and levels of the factors selected. Data obtained are to determine the acceptable ranges (upper and lower limits) for the key and critical process parameters within which quality is assured. The validity of the operating boundaries of model can then be confirmed with verification experiments at full scale. This helps to identify robust process conditions and their acceptable limits.

Risk assessment is a continuous process and is performed at various unit operations during development. As additional process information is obtained over the life cycle of the product, it is possible for the criticality of some attributes or parameters to change. In such instances, there is the need to revisit risk assessment since the changes in the prioritization must be demonstrated by data.

3.4 Defining the Design Space

Design space is defined as the "multidimensional combination and interaction of input variables and process parameters that have been demonstrated to provide assurance of quality" (8). Design space defines the acceptable processing conditions that have been shown to provide repeatable, consistent, and provable assurance of product quality (with underlying assumption of patient safety and efficacy) (15).

For lyophilized products, the concept of design space involves a thorough understanding of the criticality of the components of the formulation as well as the selection of the appropriate ranges of the process parameters for lyophilization. The concept of design space is therefore a combination of factors that affect both product and process. It is known that during lyophilization, the product temperature at the sublimation interface (T_p) is a critical parameter which significantly affects the final product quality attributes such as cake elegance and residual moisture content and so must be kept below the collapse temperature (T_c) of the formulation to avoid macroscopic collapse. However, the product temperature at the sublimation interface cannot be directly controlled and is influenced by other processing factors such as shelf temperature and the chamber pressure. The chamber pressure and shelf temperature also have a complex effect on product temperature and sublimation rate of the product. Ideally, increasing the chamber pressure increases the rate of heat transfer to support the sublimation rate by increasing the thermal conductance of gas between the shelf surface and the product vial. However, this has the tendency of causing an increase in the product temperature above the critical collapse temperature of the product, resulting in macroscopic collapse. Macroscopic collapse is a characteristic of predominantly amorphous formulations and it is undesirable and could lead to rejection of an entire batch. Therefore, there is the need to establish limits of chamber pressure, shelf temperature, and product temperature to ensure that a pharmaceutically elegant product is produced. A very efficient lyophilization process is one which operates within the design space at the highest allowable shelf temperature and the lowest chamber pressure that would still maintain the target product temperature during primary drying (5, 18, 19).

The design space is proposed by the applicant and is subject to regulatory assessment and approval. It allows more effective dialogue between industry and the regulatory agency during the application review process in that it provides structured information about product and process development that is well aligned with risk and science-based approach. From a regulatory standpoint, working within the design space is not considered a reportable change. However, working outside of the design space is considered a change that requires a regulatory post-approval change process (15).

3.5 Defining Process Control Strategy

The FDA considers a process as well understood when all critical sources of variability are identified, explained, managed and product quality attributes can be accurately and reliably predicted within the design space. Once a sufficient level of process understanding has been achieved, a control strategy should be developed to ensure that the process remains in control within the normal variation in material attributes and process operating ranges. Control strategy is defined as "a planned set of controls, derived from current product and process understanding that assures process performance and product quality" (10). Process control strategy is a cornerstone of a modern pharmaceutical quality system and can be a combination of parametric and attribute-based controls. It is established via risk assessment and includes material controls (qualification and specifications of raw materials, excipients, drug active, packaging material, etc.), procedural controls (equipment, facility, quality system, etc.), process monitoring and controls (critical and key process parameters), in-process controls, lot release testing, characterization testing, comparability testing, and stability testing (9, 15). Generally, real-time monitoring and control of the process is preferred over relying on end-product-testing. Real-time monitoring and control of critical process parameters integrates a broad spectrum of analytical technologies or tools that are capable of providing in-line and at-line measurements. Such analytical tools are usually interfaced to production plant control networks and assimilated into standard procedures to ensure consistency to the process through improved quality, efficiency through reduction of cycle and prevent batch product rejection.

4 Application of Process Analytical Technology (PAT) in the Lyophilization of Biologics

In the past, most lyophilization process optimization had mainly focused on the primary drying step, since it is the longest step of the entire process. With improved process understanding, the freezing step has been identified as the most important step of the lyophilization process since it significantly impacts both the primary and secondary drying steps, as well as the physical properties of the lyophilized products such as residual moisture content, cake morphology, and reconstitution time (20).

With the shift in paradigm from rigorous testing of the final drug product to a risk-based approach of continuous monitoring and control of critical steps of the manufacturing process, process analytical technology (PAT) has become an integral part of the lyophilization process development. PAT is defined as a system for designing, analyzing, and controlling manufacturing through timely measurements of critical quality and performance attributes of raw and in-process materials and processes with the goal of ensuring final product quality. PAT tools specified by the FDA include multivariate data acquisition and analysis tools such as statistical design of experiment and chemometric tools used to identify and address interactions of product and process variables, process analyzers capable of in-line, at-line and on-line measurement and control of critical process parameters, process and end-point monitoring and control tools to monitor the end-point of each intermediate process step before the next process step is initiated and continuous improvement and management tools (10).

Especially for high-value biopharmaceutical products, it is extremely critical to ensure that the end-points of all intermediate process steps are reached before the next step is initiated since a premature transition could result in unanticipated product deviations and subsequent batch rejection. This is very common in situations where the proper end-point of primary drying is not met in order to ensure that all ice is removed by sublimation before ramping into the secondary drying phase for desorption. The result is product melt-back. Melt-back compromises product quality and is a criterion for rejection, per United States Food and Drug Administration (US FDA) inspection guidelines (21).

4.1 PAT Tools for Characterization of the Bulk Solution

In the design of a lyophilization cycle, it is imperative to know the critical properties of the bulk formulation, such as the macroscopic collapse temperature (T_c), the stability of the drug, and the properties of the excipients used, since these properties ultimately affect the lyophilization process. Traditionally, most lyophilization cycle designs have been driven by the determination of the glass transition temperature of the maximally freeze-concentrated amorphous solution (T_g') or the eutectic temperature (T_{eu}), if solutes are crystallized in the frozen solution, using differential scanning calorimetry. The macroscopic collapse temperature (T_c) is the temperature above which the freeze-dried product loses macroscopic structure and collapses during lyophilization (5). It is therefore the most critical lyophilization parameter, since freeze-drying below T_c is necessary to ensure that the final product has an elegant appearance, low residual moisture content, good storage stability, and reconstitution characteristics. T_c is dictated by the composition of the formulation. Since each pure amorphous excipient used in the formulation has a characteristic T_g' and collapse temperature, the T_c is the mass averaged temperatures of all the components in the amorphous phase. Therefore, accurate measure of T_c is critical to lyophilization process development (5, 22).

While traditional lyophilization cycle designs have relied on the determination of T_g' or T_{eu} using differential scanning calorimetry, as a guideline for setting primary drying temperatures, this has often resulted in significantly lower primary drying temperatures and unnecessarily longer freeze-drying times because T_g' is usually lower than the T_c. The T_c is usually estimated to be 2–3 °C lower than the T_g' for amorphous solutes or equivalent to the eutectic temperature, T_{eu} for crystalline solutes. However, the collapse temperature may be as much as 10 °C higher than the T_g' in formulations with high protein content or low disaccharide content (23). Moreover, the changes in viscous flow associated with the Tg′ may become undetected in some high protein formulations or may overlap with other thermal events, thus making the prediction of the critical process temperature impossible.

Light Transmission-Freeze Dry microscopy (LT-FDM) represents a better option for determining the T_c. It involves placing about 1–2 μL of the liquid formulation between two microscopic cover slips, cooling the liquid to −40 °C or lower to ensure complete freezing, and subjecting the frozen film to vacuum. The temperature is then slowly increased at a ramp rate of 1 °C min^{-1} to bring about sublimation. As the temperature rises, viscous flow results in changes to the structure of the freeze-dried solid which may result in collapse of the freeze-dried cake. The drawback with LT-FDM is that thin films may have different ice nucleation rates, crystallization tendencies for solutes, frozen product structures, and drying rates as compared to bulk products in vials. Thus, current LT-FDM does not always accurately estimate Tc for freeze-drying in a vial. As such the difference in T_c determined using LT-FDM and that observed during freeze-drying in a vial are typically several degrees, with much larger discrepancies observed in some protein formulations (24).

A novel approach, based on time-domain optical coherence tomography (OCT-FDM) allows for real-time, three-dimensional imaging of the formulation in a vial during lyophilization. This technique, which combines high-resolution optical imaging capability of optical coherence tomography and a single vial freeze dryer (SVFD), monitors the structural changes in the product and allows full exploration of the product response to temperature changes in the sample vial during the lyophilization (Fig. 2). This circumvents the issues associated with DSC and LT-FDM and allows the accurate determination of both microscopic and macroscopic collapse of the formulation in the same vial used during production operation. The volumetric micron-level resolution and three-dimensional imaging capabilities of OCT significantly enhance the current capabilities beyond the measurement of T_c to full exploration of the product response to temperature changes and imaging of structural changes and fine features of the freeze-drying process including ice nucleation and the freezing stage of lyophilization (24, 25).

Results of such measurements determine the allowable range for shelf temperature and subsequently the product temperature at the sublimation interface during primary drying and such information is expected to be included in a biologics license application (BLA) or new drug application (NDA) to the FDA.

4.2 PAT Tools for Monitoring and Controlling the Freezing Step

The freezing step is a complex process which involves three steps, namely nucleation, crystallization of the freeze concentrate and for the maximal freeze concentrate, either freeze-separation in eutectic products or concentration in the amorphous products. When liquid drug product formulation is cooled at atmospheric pressure, the product does not freeze spontaneously at its equilibrium freezing point. The formulation solution must usually be cooled down to temperatures that are significantly lower than the equilibrium

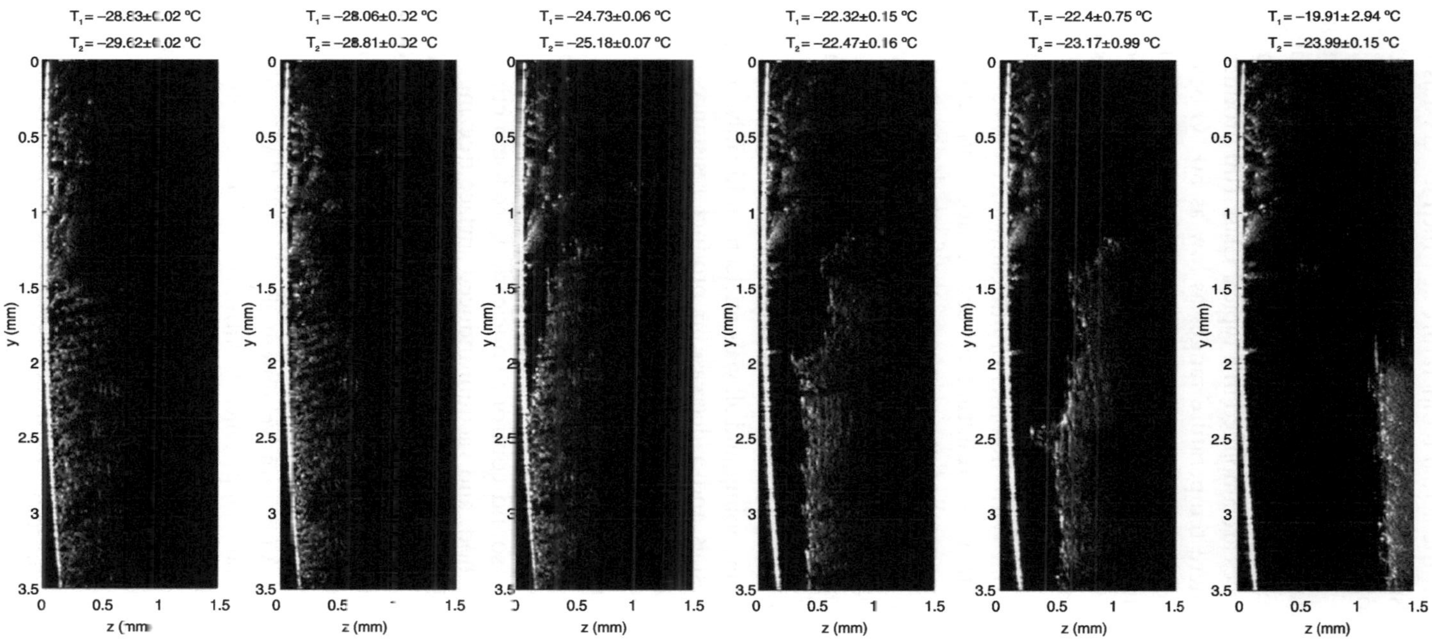

Fig. 2 Representative cross-sectional (y–z plane) OCT images showing the sublimation front, onset of product shrinkage, and macroscopic collapse at different times during OCT-FDM. T_1 and T_2 are the product temperatures measured at the middle and center bottom of the product at different times during the OCT-FDM run (Unpublished data)

freezing point in order to initialize the formation of ice crystals. The difference between the equilibrium ice formation temperature and the actual temperature at which ice crystals first form is called "supercooling." The degree of supercooling is dependent on the solution properties and process conditions (1).

In a laboratory freeze-dryer, the ice nucleation in individual vials occurs randomly and spans a temperature range of 10–17 °C below the thermodynamic freezing point. Such observed differences are amplified in a typical Class 100 production environment, where temperature ranges as low as 30 °C below the thermodynamic freezing point are observed, due to the absence of dust or dirt particles which act as heterogeneous nucleation sites (26). The result is increased manufacturing and energy costs as well as vial-to-vial heterogeneity in the final product attributes.

The first step in the freezing process is the onset of ice nucleation. With the onset of nucleation, ice crystals begin to grow at a certain rate, resulting in freeze-concentration of the solution. In an uncontrolled environment, the formulation must be cooled down to temperatures that are significantly lower than the equilibrium freezing point to initialize ice formation. With a high degree of supercooling, the product vials nucleate at different times, resulting in smaller ice crystals and increased resistance to ice sublimation. When ice nucleation is controlled, it results in a lower degree of supercooling and all vials nucleate uniformly, resulting in larger ice crystals and a decrease in product resistance to ice sublimation during primary drying. Physical properties such as cake structure, residual moisture content, and reconstitution time are also impacted by the degree of supercooling (26).

Various methods that allow for the direct control of the freezing step have been proposed in literature (see Chapter 4), such as ultrasound-controlled nucleation, ice fog method, electro-freezing method, and vacuum-induced surface freezing. While such methods have demonstrated potential success for process improvement at the laboratory and pilot scales, they are invasive methods and their applicability to commercial-scale manufacturing of regulated biopharmaceutical products would seem very difficult to achieve because of the economic as well as the sterility and safety concerns.

A noninvasive, potentially scalable PAT tool for controlling the freezing step, called ControLyo™ Nucleation On-Demand Technology, has been shown to significantly improve both process and product in many experimental systems. This technology works by reducing the product temperature of the vials to a selected temperature value, followed by pressurizing the lyophilization chamber with an inert sterile gas such as argon or nitrogen. When thermal equilibrium has been achieved in all vials, the chamber is rapidly depressurized, causing ice crystals to form at the top of the solution and propagate throughout the vials within seconds. When vials in the chamber nucleate simultaneously at a lower degree of super-

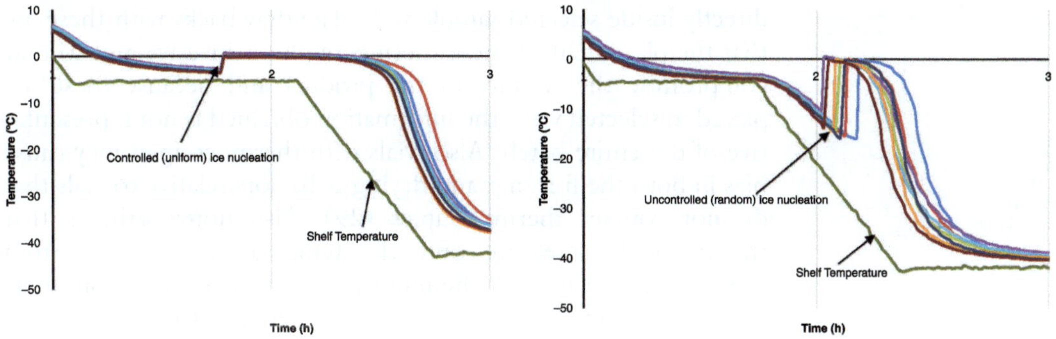

Fig. 3 Product temperature profiles showing the nucleation behavior during the freezing step for controlled ice nucleation and uncontrolled ice nucleation

cooling (Fig. 3), it results in the formation larger ice crystals and larger pores during primary drying due to decreased resistance to mass transfer and a significant decrease in primary drying time. Studies have demonstrated that for every 1 °C increase in the nucleation temperature, primary drying can be reduced by as much as 3–4%. Primary drying cycle reductions of up to 41% have been reported with controlled ice nucleation method (27, 28).

4.3 PAT Tools for Monitoring and Control of the Primary Drying Step

At the completion of freezing step, the chamber pressure is lowered and the shelf temperature is increased to initiate primary drying. This causes the ice sublimation front to move downward through the frozen product, thus causing the water vapor to transit through the channels left by the sublimed ice above. The level of resistance to the mass transfer of water vapor depends on the ice crystal structure formed and this affects the overall primary drying time.

During primary drying, the product temperature at the sublimation interface (T_p) is the most relevant product parameter that must be controlled in order to ensure a robust cycle. Ideally, T_p must be below the "critical" temperature of the product (glass transition temperature (Tg′ or perhaps more usefully, especially at high protein concentrations, T_c) for amorphous and eutectic temperature (T_{eu}) for crystalline products) to avoid macroscopic collapse of the lyophilized cakes. Macroscopic collapse negatively affects final product quality such as product appearance, subvisible particles, residual moisture, and reconstitution time (26).

Therefore, the accurate determination of such critical process parameters such as the sublimation rate (dm/dt), the product mass transfer resistance, and product temperature at the sublimation interface are very critical to the control of the overall lyophilization process as well as the final product quality. T_p cannot be directly controlled but is influenced by the heat input by the shelves and chamber pressure. Various techniques have been proposed to monitor the product temperature, such as the use of thermocouple sensors and electrical resistance detectors (RTD), which are placed directly inside selected sample vials. The drawbacks with these are that the placement of these thermocouples is invasive and so may compromise the sterility of the product and because these are placed in selected vials, the information obtained is not representative of the entire batch. Also, vials with thermocouples may cause bias in both the freezing and drying behaviors relative to vials that do not contain thermocouples (29). Also noteworthy is that thermocouples measure only the temperature at the bottom of the vials (T_b) and not the temperature at the sublimation interface (T_p), which is more critically related to the product macrocollapse.

Various noninvasive PAT tools for monitoring critical process and product parameters, such as Raman and near-infrared (NIR) probes, have been proposed. These act as complimentary PAT tools whereby Raman probes are positioned noninvasively above the vials while NIR probes are placed on the side of the vial to monitor the physical and critical process step changes such as water-to-ice conversion, product crystallization, kinetics of polymorphic transitions, and solid-state characterization. The drawback with these PAT tools is that both water and ice produce very weak Raman signals, while NIR spectra are typically composed of broad overlapping and poorly defined absorption bands because of the effect of physical properties of the sample such as particle size and density. As such, spectra obtained from these probes are multivariate in nature and require chemometric analyses to build a robust prediction model to extract both physical and chemical information on the samples (30).

More reliable, noninvasive PAT tools that provide valuable information in the monitoring and control of the primary drying step include Manometric Temperature Measurement (MTM) and Tunable Diode Laser Absorption Spectroscopy (TDLAS). MTM works by a procedure whereby the product temperature at the sublimation interface is measured by closing the isolation valve between the chamber and the condenser for a short period of time and measuring the pressure versus time data. The MTM equation is then fitted to the pressure rise data and the analysis provides real-time information about important process parameters such as the product resistance, the cake thickness, and sublimation rate. The data obtained provides information to the lyophilization control software, called SMART™, which makes adjustments to shelf temperature in a closed feedback loop. By monitoring and controlling product temperature during processing, critically harmful temperatures can be avoided and scientifically derived drying times can be determined. The information obtained is representative of the entire batch and gives valuable insight into the cake morphology and final product quality attributes (31).

TDLAS is an in-line technology that works on spectroscopic principles and sensitive detection techniques to measure the absorption of radiation of water vapor in real time using a laser beam attached to the spool connecting the chamber and the condenser. The sensors measure the water vapor concentration and vapor flow velocity and the instantaneous measurements can be used to determine critical product and process parameters such as product temperature, vial heat transfer, product mass resistance, and primary drying endpoint (32).

Both MTM and TDLAS can also be used to determine the endpoint of primary drying. MTM uses a comparative pressure measurement tool which consists of a pirani gauge and a capacitance manometer. The pirani gauge works on the principle of measuring the thermal conductivity of the gas in the drying chamber and reads about 60% higher than the capacitance manometer. During primary drying, when all the gas in the chamber is essentially water vapor, the pirani gauge reads about 60% higher than the capacitance manometer, because the thermal conductivity of water vapor is ~1.6 times more than nitrogen gas. At the end of primary drying, when the gas composition in the chamber is essentially nitrogen, the pirani pressure decreases toward the capacitance manometer and that signals sublimation is essentially completed (33). For TDLAS, the end of primary drying is the point where the water vapor concentration shows a sharp decrease in the water vapor concentration profile, indicating that the gas composition is changing and hence sublimation is essentially complete (Fig. 4).

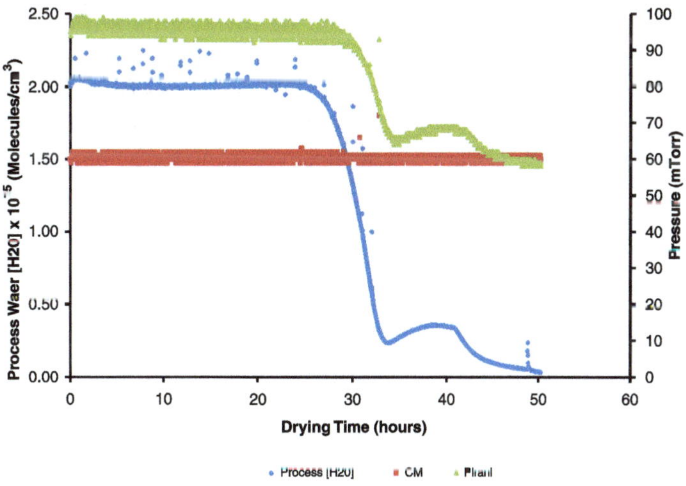

Fig. 4 Process water concentration from TDLAS and Pirani vs. Capacitance manometer can be used to determine the end-point of primary drying of biologics. In both instances, sharp decline in the curves depicts decrease in the concentration of water vapor, showing that sublimation is almost complete

4.4 Secondary Drying Step: Monitoring and Control of the Residual Moisture Content

For an optimized lyophilization cycle, it is imperative that the end-point of primary drying is accurately determined before progression into secondary drying, as premature progression could result in product collapse and ultimately batch rejection due to lack of cake elegance. Typically, primary drying is essentially over when the amount of unfrozen water in the amorphous matrix is less than 20% (34, 35).

The residual moisture in the final product at the end of secondary drying must also be accurately measured since product stability often correlates with residual moisture content. Both MTM and TDLAS have proved vital in characterizing the secondary drying stage of the freeze-drying process. TDLAS has been used for in situ monitoring of residual moisture content in real time during secondary drying on a laboratory scale (35).

4.5 Characterization of the Lyophilized Product

While there are not many tools for the real-time characterization of the lyophilized products, many off-line tools allow for both quantitative and qualitative characterization of the lyophilized cakes to ensure that product quality is consistent with the set target. For example, visual inspection for cake elegance, determination of reconstitution time, and offline determination of residual moisture content using Karl Fischer analyses are standard release tests that are required by the FDA. Other required information that are expected to be included in BLA or NDA include physico-chemical characterization information such as the glass transition temperature (T_g) of the dried cake by DSC, which is important in predicting optimum storage conditions, information about the crystallinity of the final product by Powder X-Ray diffraction (PXRD), the specific surface area of the lyophilized cake by nitrogen or krypton gas adsorption experiments, and secondary structure of the lyophilized biologic by Fourier Transform Infrared (FT-IR) Spectroscopy or Circular Dichroism (CD) Spectroscopy.

The desired improvements from the application of PAT are gains in quality and efficiency due to reduced production cycle time, increased automation of the process, and prevention of product rejection due to improved process consistency and understanding. Another major advantage is the possibility for real-time release, which means that the product quality can be ensured by data generated during production, and the batch can be released directly after completion of production without extensive additional final testing procedures.

5 Conclusion

The application of principles of QbD to the lyophilization of biologics would be mutually beneficial to both regulators and industry since it will ultimately lead to continuous process improvements. For regulators, it will improve the quality of information in regulatory submissions as well as the quality of review since decisions will be made on scientific information rather than on empirical information. For industry, this would ensure better design of products with fewer problems in manufacturing since decisions are made based on process understanding and risk mitigation. It would also allow for the implementation of new technology to improve manufacturing without regulatory scrutiny.

PAT is an enabling component of QbD which allows continuous real-time monitoring and control of a process, resulting in more consistent product quality and more efficient use of manufacturing capacity. This would likely facilitate technology or process transfer from laboratory to production and even from one site to another or one manufacturer to another since the process becomes less equipment and recipe-dependent and more a function of process outputs.

References

1. Kasper JC, Friess W (2011) The freezing step in lyophilization: physico-chemical fundamentals, freezing methods and consequences on process performance and quality attributes of biopharmaceuticals. Eur J Pharm Biopharm 78:248–263
2. Vasconcelos T, Sarmento B, Costa P (2007) Solid dispersions as strategy to improve oral bioavailability of poor water souluble drugs. Drug Discov Today 12:1068–1075
3. Reichert JM (2016) Antibodies to watch in 2016. MAbs 8(2):197–204. https://doi.org/10.1080/19420862.2015.1125583
4. Pikal MJ, Rambhatla S, Ramot R (2002) The impact of the freezing stage in lyophilization: effects of the ice nucleation temperature on process design and product quality. Am Pharm Rev 5:48–53
5. Tang X, Pikal M (2004) Design of freeze drying processes for pharmaceuticals: practical advice. Pharm Res 21:191–200
6. Chang BS, Kendrick BS, Carpenter JS (1996) Surface-induced denaturation of proteins during freezing and its inhibition by surfactants. J Pharm Sci 85(12):1325–1330
7. Bedu-Addo FK (2004) Understanding lyophilization formulation development. Pharmaceutical Technology – Lyophilization pp 10–18
8. Food and Drug Administration (2009) Q8 (R2) pharmaceutical development. https://www.fda.gov/downloads/drugs/guidances/ucm073507.pdf. Accessed on 23 May 2017
9. Jameel F, Khan MA (2009) Quality-by-design as applied to the development and manufacturing of a lyophilized protein product. Am Pharm Rev (November/December): 20–24
10. Guidance for industry: PAT — a framework for innovative pharmaceutical development, manufacturing and quality assurance (2004) https://www.fda.gov/downloads/drugs/guidances/ucm070305.pdf. Accessed on 23 May 2017
11. Woodcock J (2005) Pharmaceutical quality in the 21st century – an integrated systems approach. In: AAPS Workshop on Pharmaceutical Quality Assessment – A Science and Risk-Based CMC Approach in the 21st Century
12. Guidance for industry; Q9 quality risk management (2006) https://www.fda.gov/downloads/Drugs/Guidances/ucm073511.pdf. Accessed on 23 May 2017
13. Guidance for industry: Q10 pharmaceutical quality systems (2009) https://www.fda.gov/downloads/Drugs/.../Guidances/ucm073517.pdf. Accessed 23 May 2017
14. Nasr MM (2011) Implementation of Quality by Design (QbD) – current perspectives on opportunities and challenges topic introduction and ICH update. Presented at Advisory Committee for Pharmaceutical Science and Clinical Pharmacology, US Food and drug Administration, 27 July, 2011
15. Rathore SA, Winkle H (2009) Quality by Design for biopharmaceuticals. Nat Biotechnol 27(1):26–34
16. Kenett RS, Kenett DA (2008) Quality by Design applications in biosimilar pharmaceutical products. Accred Qual Assur 13:681–690

17. Awotwe-Otoo D, Agarabi C, Wu GK et al (2012) Quality by design: impact of formulation variables and their interactions on quality attributes of a lyophilized monoclonal antibody. Int J Pharm 438(1-2):167–175
18. Tang X, Nail SL, Pikal MJ (2006) Evaluation of manometric temperature measurement, a process analytical technology tool for freeze-drying: Part I, Product temperature measurement. AAPS PharmSciTech 7(1):E1–E9
19. Nail SL, Searles JA (2008) Elements of quality by design in development and scale-up of freezed-dried parenterals. Bio Pharm Int 21 (1):44–50
20. Kasper JC, Winter G, Freiss W (2013) Recent advances and further challenges in lyophilization. Eur J Pharm Biopharm 85:162–169
21. U.S. Food and Drug Administration. Guide to inspections of lyophilization of parenterals. http://www.fda.gov/ICECI/Inspections/Inspectionguides/UCM074909.htm. Accessed 3 Nov 2017
22. Skrabanja ATP, de Meere ALJ, Rien d R, van der Oetelaar PJM (1994) Lyophilization of biotechnology products. PDA. J Pharm Sci Technol 48(6):311–317
23. Meister E, Gieseler H (2009) Freeze-dry microscopy of protein/sugar mixtures: drying behavior, interpretation of collapse temperatures and a comparison to corresponding glass transition data. J Pharm Sci 98(9):3072–3087
24. Mujat M, Greco K, Galbally-Kinney KL, Hammer DX, Ferguson RD, Iftimia N et al (2012) Optical coherence tomography-based freeze-drying microscopy. Biomed Opt Express 3 (1):55–63
25. Greco K, Mujat M, Galbally-Kinney KL, Hammer DX, Ferguson RD, Iftimia N et al (2013) Accurate prediction of collapse temperature using optical coherence tomography-based freeze-drying microscopy. J Pharm Sci 102 (6):1773–1785
26. Awotwe-Otoo D, Agarabi C, Read EK et al (2013) Impact of controlled ice nucleation on process performance and quality attributes of a lyophilized monoclonal antibody. Int J Pharm 450(1-2):70–78
27. Konstantinidis AK, Luu W, Otten L, Nail SL, Sever RR (2011) Controlled nucleation in freeze-drying: effects on pore size in the dried product layer, mass transfer resistance and primary drying rate. J Pharm Sci 100:3453–3347
28. Searles JA, Carpenter T, Randolph TW (2001) The ice nucleation temperature determines the primary drying rate of lyophilization for samples frozen on a temperature controlled shelf. J Pharm Sci 90:860–871
29. Tang X, Nail SL, Pikal MJ (2005) Freeze-drying process design by manometric temperature measurement: design of a smart freeze dryer. Pharm Res 22:685–700
30. De Beer TRM, Vercruysse P, Burggraeve A, Quinten T, Ouyang J, Zhang X, Vervaet C, Remon JP, Baeyens WR (2009) In-line and real-time process monitoring of a freeze-drying process using Raman and NIR spectroscopy as complementary process analytical technology (PAT) tools. J Pharm Sci 98(9):3430–3446
31. Patel SM, Pikal MJ (2009) Process analytical technologies (PAT) in freeze-drying of parenteral products. Pharm Dev Technol 14 (6):567–587
32. Awotwe-Otoo D, Agarabi C, Khan MA (2014) An integrated process analytical technology (PAT) approach to monitoring the effect of supercooling on lyophilization product and process parameters of model monoclonal antibody formulations. J Pharm Sci 103:2042–2052
33. Patel SM, Doen T, Pikal MJ (2010) Determination of end-point of primary drying in freeze-drying process control. AAPS PharmSciTech 11(1):73–84
34. De Beer TR, Allesø M, Goethals F et al (2007) Implementation of a process analytical technology system in a freeze-drying process using Raman spectroscopy for in-line process monitoring. Anal Chem 79(21):7992–8003
35. Schneid SC, Gieseler H, Kessler WJ, Luthra SA, Pikal MJ (2011) Tunable diode laser absorption spectroscopy (TDLAS) as a residual moisture monitor for the secondary drying stage of freeze drying. AAPS PharmSciTech 12(1):379–387

Chapter 9

Container and Reconstitution Systems for Lyophilized Drug Products

T. Page McAndrew, Douglas Hostetler, and Frances L. DeGrazio

Abstract

Lyophilization is the process of dehydrating a material at low temperature and reduced pressure. It is used to extend the shelf life of many biologic drug products. This paper discusses two systems essential to these products: container systems and reconstitution (i.e., rehydrating) systems.

Key words Container systems, Closures, Container closure integrity, Extractables, Leachables, Reconstitution systems, Seals

1 Background

Lyophilization (also called freeze drying) is the process of dehydrating a material at low temperature and reduced pressure. It is used to extend the shelf life of many biologic drug products. This paper discusses two systems essential to these products—container systems and reconstitution (i.e., rehydrating) systems. Lyophilization was documented as early as 1908 at the Laboratory of Biophysics at the College of France [1]. Upon removal of a sufficient level of water, rates of metabolic processes are reduced substantially—so lyophilization can be used to extend the shelf life of a biologic product. A first pharmaceutical application was the preservation of live rabies viruses—which enabled vaccine development. During World War II, lyophilization played a crucial role in the transport of blood serum—refrigerated transport being unavailable [1]. Through to the end of 2014, the FDA had approved over 400 drug products in lyophilized form:

- infectious disease: 40%
- oncology: 23%
- cardiology: 12%
- other (e.g., immune, metabolic, neurology): 25%

Kevin R. Ward and Paul Matejtschuk (eds.), *Lyophilization of Pharmaceuticals and Biologicals: New Technologies and Approaches*, Methods in Pharmacology and Toxicology, https://doi.org/10.1007/978-1-4939-8928-7_9,

Over 90% are delivered in single-use vials. In 2014, over two billion doses were produced worldwide, up from 2010 at a combined annual growth rate >10%.

Crucial to understanding lyophilization is understanding sublimation. Sublimation is the transition of a material from the solid phase *directly* to the gas phase—without the intermediate liquid phase. Like melting and evaporation, it is an endothermic phase transition. For water, the enthalpy of sublimation (i.e., the amount of energy required to convert 1 mole of water to gas when solid and gas are in equilibrium) is 51×10^3 J. See Fig. 1—a schematic of the phase diagram of water [2]. As a function of pressure and temperature, the phase diagram shows the state of a substance—solid, liquid, or gas. Lines indicate where phases are in equilibrium. For water, liquid *cannot* exist at conditions of temperature below 0.01 °C *and* below 0.006 atm (i.e., conditions of the triple point). These conditions are shown by the yellow box in Fig. 1. Thus any phase transition occurring at these conditions necessarily involves solid to gas. At temperatures below 0 °C, vapor pressure of water is very low. See Table 1 [3]. However, at reduced pressure, the rate of vaporization is substantially increased. As such, lyophilization is performed at reduced pressure and can be accomplished in a cost-effective time period.

The lyophilization of a drug product has several stages. See Fig. 2—a schematic diagram depicting lyophilization parameters in terms of time, temperature, and water content [1]. Note the parameters of these phases will depend upon the drug product.

- *Freezing*. Product is frozen well below 0 °C. Actual freezing rate depends upon the drug product—emphasis is on preventing degradation. Large ice crystals generally are favored as: (a) easier to sublimate, and (b) promoting larger pores which promotes subsequent reconstitution.

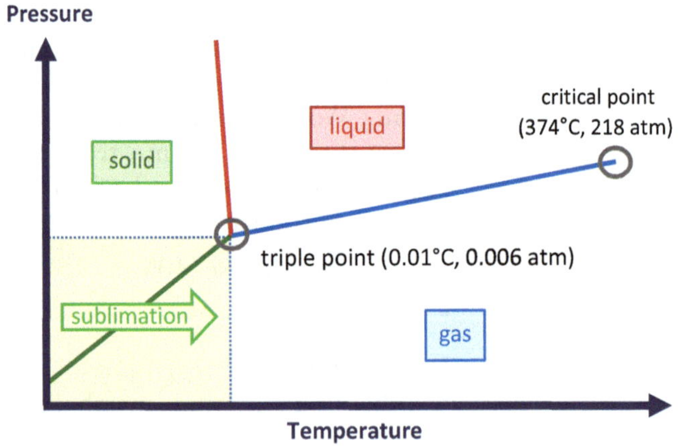

Fig. 1 Schematic Phase diagram of water. Not to scale. Yellow box indicates conditions in which only [solid ↔ gas] transition can occur

Table 1
Vapor pressure of water [3]

Temperature (°C)	−60	−50	−40	−30	−20	−10	0	10	20	30	40	50
Pressure (atm)	1.1×10^{-5}	4.0×10^{-5}	1.3×10^{-4}	3.8×10^{-4}	0.001	0.0024	0.006	0.012	0.023	0.042	0.073	0.12

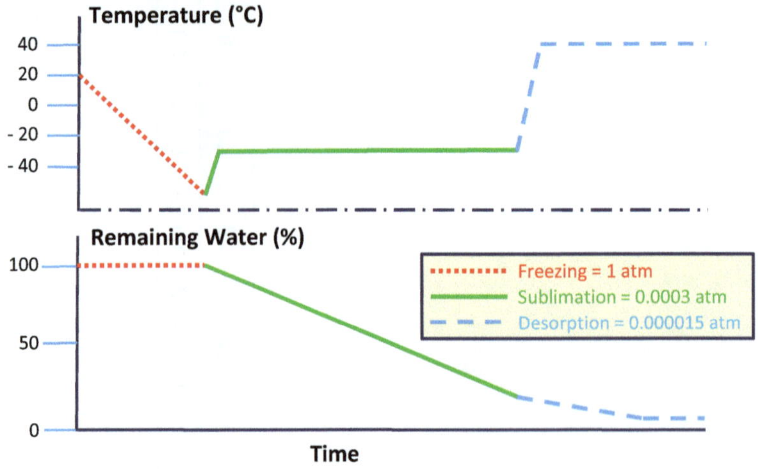

Fig. 2 Lyophilization parameters. Not to scale. Parameters vary depending upon drug product. Reproduced from data in [1]

- *Sublimation* (Primary Drying). Majority of water is removed—going directly from solid to gas phase at reduced pressure.
- *Desorption* (Secondary Drying). Water that was not in the form of crystalline ice, but adsorbed on drug product, is removed. Note temperature is elevated to increase vapor pressure of water, but the process is still performed at reduced pressure. Temperature is selected so as to prevent degradation.

Once the parameters are set for the lyophilization of a drug product, the challenge is execution—a key feature of which is the container closure system, i.e., vial, stopper, and seal.

2 Container Systems

The proper container system is essential to maintain the integrity of a lyophilized drug product through its shelf life, until it is reconstituted and subsequently administered. It must:

- maintain container closure integrity
- have no deleterious interaction with drug product
- minimize potential for water migration
- minimize potential for leachables migration
- have good durability during handling
- be suitable for sealing within the lyophilization chamber (under vacuum or inert atmosphere)

Defining the proper container system begins with component selection. Components are considered individually.

2.1 Components: Vials

Vials comprise either glass or polymer:

- *Glass.* Typically glass vials are made according to ISO specifications from Type 1 borosilicate glass tubing. Production from tubing is preferred over injection molding for better dimensional uniformity. Typical composition is ca. 80% SiO_2, ca. 13% B_2O_3, ca. 4% Na_2O, and other compounds [4]. Type 1 is preferred for pharmaceutical and fine chemical applications because of the low Na_2O content, and the reduced risk for Na^+ leaching. An interior coating of polysiloxane may be present to reduce risk of interaction with drug product.
- *Polymer.* Made by injection molding, polymer vials often comprise cyclic olefin polymer—a transparent polymer with very good resistance to water permeation (a combination of properties unique in a polyolefin). Examples are Daikyo Crystal Zenith® COP and Becton Dickinson and Company Crystal Clear Polymer. COP typically comprises either norborene (bicyclo[2.2.1]hept-2-ene derivative), or a copolymer of norborene with ethene. A copolymer example is Schott AG TopPac® product. See Fig. 3. Polymer vials have the advantage of being mechanically more durable, i.e., less likely to fracture during handling/use than glass vials. Typical composition is ca. 90% carbon, ca. 10% hydrogen. With essentially only carbon and hydrogen present, the possibility of interaction with drug product is reduced, as compared to glass.

Since lyophilization occurs under vacuum, most heat transfer to/from drug product occurs directly between vial bottom and chamber shelf. Some heat transfer can occur by liquid/vapor trapped between vial bottom and shelf, or by radiation. However, the dominant effect is by direct contact [5]. To facilitate this best, vial bottoms must be:

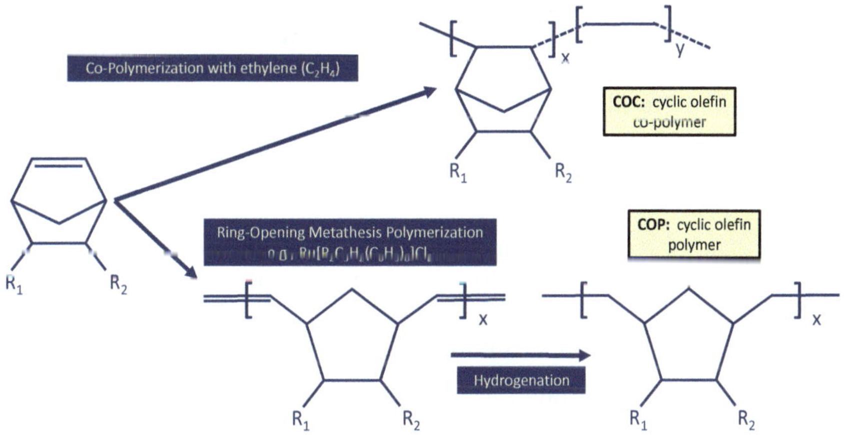

Fig. 3 Structures of cyclic olefin polymers

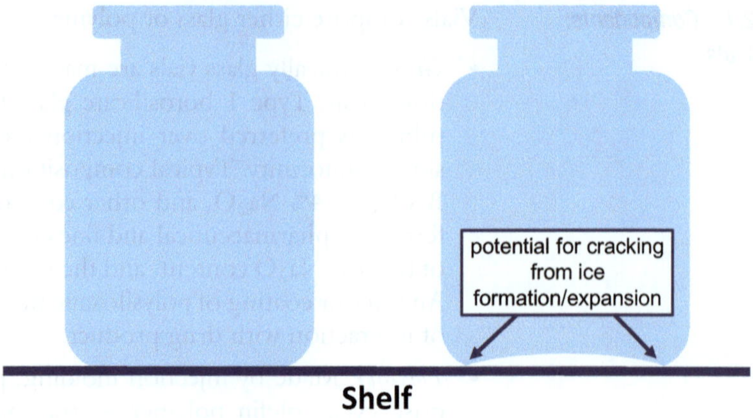

Fig. 4 Schematic drawings of vials

- *Flat.* See Fig. 4—schematic drawing comparing vials. A flat bottom maximizes contact and thus heat transfer. In contrast, a concave bottom has substantially reduced contact (air/liquid/vapor/vacuum exists between vial and shelf). Moreover, a concave bottom enables crevices where expansion from water to ice during freezing may occur and cause breakage.
- *Thin.* This minimizes thermal resistance between shelf and drug product.
- *Uniform.* Variations in thickness promote uneven heat transfer, and increase risk of breakage from residual stress (a common issue in glass articles with sections of uneven thickness).

For example, a Schott 2R glass vial (capacity to ca. 4 mL) has a bottom surface area of 2 cm^2, and a bottom thickness of 0.06–0.07 cm. Typically bottom thickness is ca. 70% of wall thickness (i.e., ca. 0.1 cm). A Daikyo Crystal Zenith® COP 2 mL vial has a bottom surface of 1.7 cm^2, and a bottom thickness of ca. 0.1–0.2 cm.

From a thermal conductivity perspective, glass is better than polymer because of a higher thermal conductivity coefficient, i.e., it conducts heat more efficiently:

- Glass ~1.05 $W\ m^{-1}\ K^{-1}$
- Polymer ~0.2 $W\ m^{-1}\ K^{-1}$

Lyophilization reduces, but does not eliminate, potential for interaction of drug product with vial, and subsequent drug product alteration. Before lyophilization, drug product is liquid or contains a substantial amount of water. Potential issues are:

- reaction of drug product with Si-OH groups on glass surface
- dissolution of silicates from glass and migration into drug product—especially at high or low pH

- ion exchange between drug product and glass (e.g., Na^+, K^+)
- migration of leachates from glass into drug product

However, once water is frozen, and through completion of lyophilization, risk of these issues is substantially reduced. In fact, some drug product manufacturers may offer lyophilized product for just this reason. In this regard, polymer vials have a much lower risk than glass vials. Comprising essentially only carbon and hydrogen, the risk of interaction, or migration of leachate, is reduced. Moreover, polymer vials do not have the issue of glass delamination [6]. So as a first consideration, polymer vials provide for less risk. Still, potential issues with polymer must be considered—if there are compounds (e.g., residual monomer) that will volatilize at reduced pressure in lyophilization chamber and be absorbed and interact with drug product.

2.2 Components: Stoppers

Stoppers are composed of elastomers because of the need to make a complete, durable, seal with the vial, and enable needle/spike insertion for reconstitution and withdrawal. They are formed by a compression molding process during which curing is performed. Most elastomers are thermoset (i.e., require a curing process), however thermoplastic elastomers also can be used. A particular formulation of an elastomer can be fabricated into any stopper design. Typically an elastomer formulation comprises:

- elastomer (usually bromo- or chloro-butyl—based on inherent resistance to permeation by water and oxygen)—ca. 50% by weight
- fillers
- pigments
- curing agents
- accelerators
- activators
- plasticizers
- pigments
- antioxidants and stabilizers

Development of a particular formulation (i.e., elastomer type and molecular weight, types and levels of ingredients, curing conditions) requires considerable research because of the many performance requirements that a stopper must meet. See Table 2.

Good stopper/vial seal integrity is essential for lyophilized products. The secondary seal (i.e., outer seal), comprising aluminum or plastic, that holds the stopper in place, may not be placed immediately after stopper insertion, but up to several hours later. Contact between stopper and vial is the primary seal.

Table 2
Stopper elastomer performance requirements

Parameter	Reason
Glass transition temperature <−55 °C	Maintains rubber characteristic at all temperatures of lyophilization
Hardness (Shore A) = 45–55 Low compression set Good sealing against glass/polymer Low level of coring and fragmentation	Enables easy stopper insertion, good seal integrity over time, good spike/needle penetration and reseal while minimizing formation of fragments
Low level of water absorption Low level of water permeability Low level of oxygen permeability	Maintains shelf life of drug product
Low level of potential extractables Low level of volatiles	Minimizes risk of interaction of drug product with a chemical compound from stopper
Low level of surface tackiness	Eases handling prior to insertion in vial
Ease of processing	Minimizes production costs

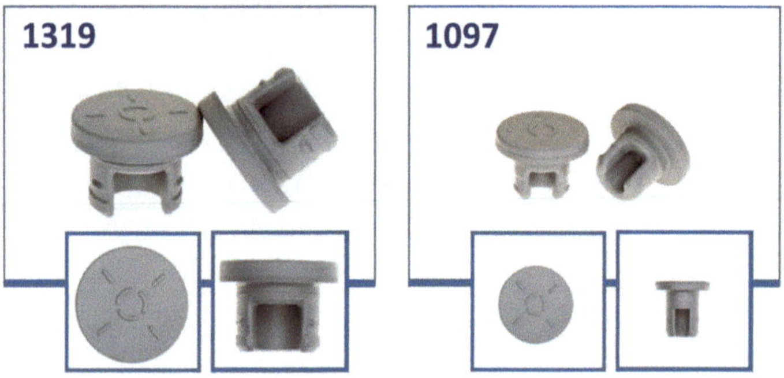

Fig. 5 Lyophilization stoppers—"Igloo" format. West Article 1319 (20 mm) and Article 1097 (13 mm). Both are in formulation 4023/50 gray

As noted above, a given formulation can be fabricated into any stopper design. Most lyophilization stoppers are "igloo" format—depicted in Fig. 5. Some lyophilization stoppers are "two-leg" format—depicted in Fig. 6.

Stoppers may be laminated with fluoropolymer films or coated with silicone-oil-based coatings or fluoropolymer coatings—see Fig. 7:

- *Fluoropolymer Laminate.* To minimize interaction of drug product with stopper (either directly with stopper surface, or migration of leachate from stopper), a fluoropolymer film is placed on areas that could contact drug product. To facilitate easy insertion of stopper into vial, a fluoropolymer film is likewise placed on outer surfaces. To prevent adherence of stopper to upper

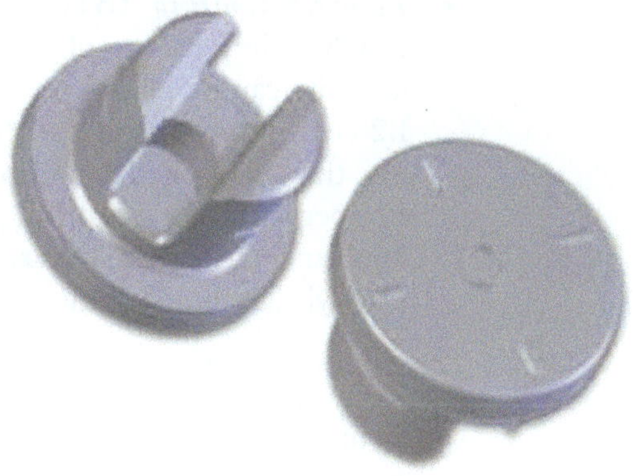

Fig. 6 Lyophilization stopper—"Two-Leg" format. West Article 1097 (20 mm). Formulation is 4023/50 gray

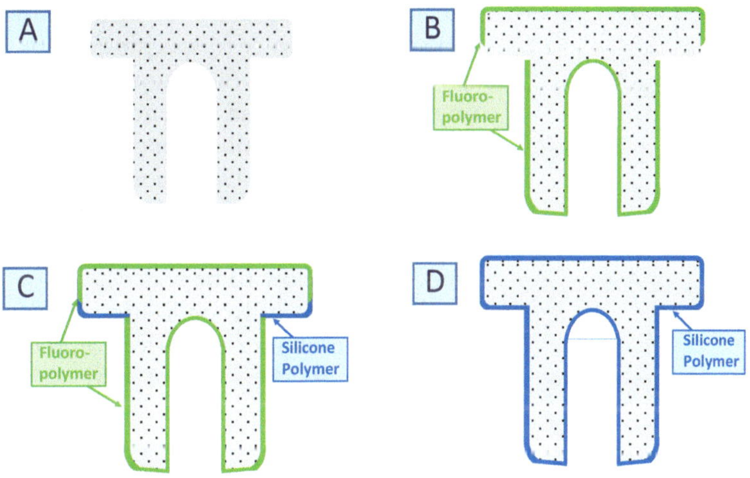

Fig. 7 Schematic of lyophilization stopper displaying positions of fluoropolymer film and silicone polymer coating. A two-leg stopper is used as an example. (**A**) neither film nor coating. (**B**) fluoropolymer film only. (**C**) fluoropolymer film and silicone polymer coating. (**D**) silicone polymer coating only

shelf during closure of container system at completion of lyophilization process, a fluoropolymer film may be placed on the top surface of stopper (West Lyotec® stoppers). West Pharmaceutical Services, Inc. FluroTec® film is based on ethylene tetrafluoroethylene copolymer (ETFE). No film is placed on areas of stopper that contact glass and serve as primary seal, i.e., land seal (contact of stopper flange to top horizontal plane of vial—see Fig. 12). This is because FluroTec® film is a thermoplastic and will not conform as well under pressure to make a good seal—especially important in areas of glass vial variability.

- *Lubricity Coating*. To facilitate insertion of stopper into vial and easy handling during fill/finish operation, a coating to enhance lubricity can be placed on stopper surfaces. An example is West B2 coating—a silicone polymer (also called polysiloxane) coating that is applied as a solution, and chemically bonded to stopper surface by a curing process. Fluoropolymer-based coatings can be used also, for example Omniflex® coatings offered by Datwyler Sealing Solutions.

In some cases, a thin layer of silicone oil is placed over the entire stopper. This is done by washing stoppers in a solution comprising emulsified silicone oil. This aids movement of stoppers during container system assembly and insertion into vials, and prevents stoppers from adhering to upper shelf during closure. However, it raises the risk of interaction of lyophilized drug product with silicone oil—a risk that is increased if the reconstitution liquid is partly organic. Given the complexity of biologic drug products, a safer option is the presence of chemically bonded fluoropolymer and silicone polymer to specific areas of the stopper.

Initial insertion of a lyophilization stopper into a vial is part way—resulting in the presence of a vent. See Fig. 8. Notice that design of lyophilization stopper is such to permit escape of water from drug product. Upon completion of lyophilization, while still in chamber, vials are sealed by complete insertion of stopper (done typically by lowering of upper shelf which forces systems on shelf immediately below to be sealed).

The process of lyophilization has been examined for the purpose of determining the effect of vent area on sublimation rate [7]. See Fig. 9.

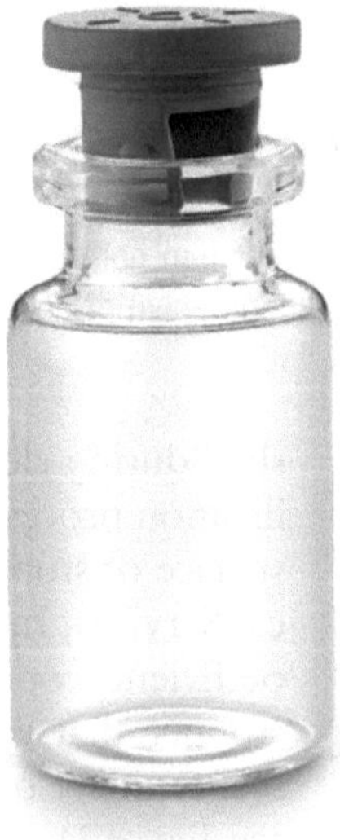

Fig. 8 Stopper/vial system. Stopper is partly inserted—this is the configuration during lyophilization process

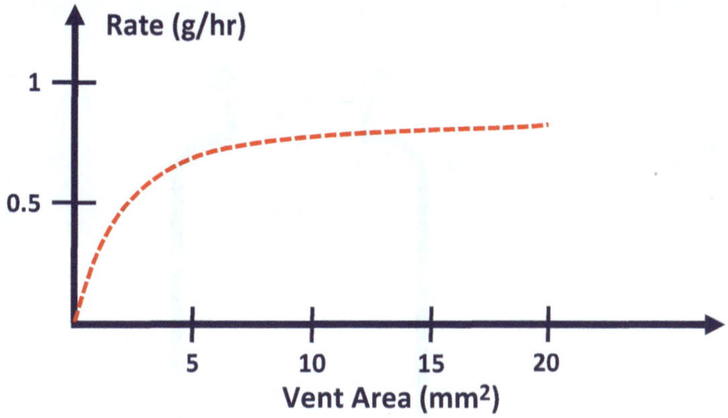

Fig. 9 Lyophilization—effect of vent area on sublimation rate. Depicted are results of experiments showing rate of water loss vs. vent area—20 mL samples of 4% mannitol ($C_6H_{14}O_6$) solutions lyophilized in 100 mL vials at 0 °C and 2.6×10^{-4} atm. Graph is reproduced from reference data [7]

Notice there is little benefit above a vent area of 5 mm^2. Evidently 5 mm^2 enables adequate water vapor transport—even for a large volume of solution, sublimation is the rate limiting step, not water escape. The practical impact is that a vent area of ca. 5 mm^2 should be well adequate for most cases.

It is important to match stoppers with vials properly to ensure a good seal. The first step is selecting a combination that has the right interference fit. Interference fit is defined in Eq. (1):

$$\text{Interference fit} = 100\{[(\text{stopper diameter}) - (\text{vial inner neck diameter})]/(\text{stopper diameter})\} \quad (1)$$

All suppliers furnish precise drawings and dimensions of components. For example, consider a Schott vial (6R) and a West stopper (Article 1319 "igloo"). See Fig. 10. Dimensions are:

- d4 (vial inner neck diameter) = 12.6 mm ± 0.2 mm
- D2 (stopper diameter) = 13.2 mm ± 0.1 mm

For this system the interference fit is 3%. The recommended interference fit historically is from ca. 3–5%. This is to ensure that the stopper diameter is slightly larger than the vial inner neck diameter, so the stopper is always under compression and applying a radially outward force against the inner wall of the vial. This ensures a good seal. Note that an interference fit that is too large would indicate difficulty in stopper insertion and a greater likelihood of stopper dislodging. Note however that the most important seal is the land seal (contact of stopper flange to top horizontal plane of vial—see Fig. 12).

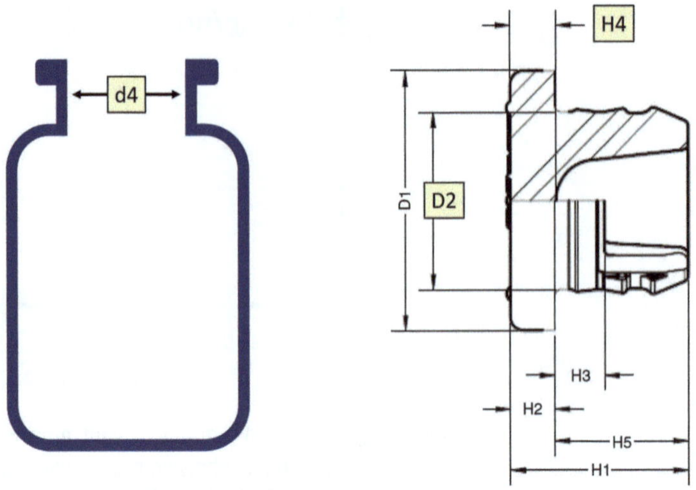

Fig. 10 Diagram of a typical vial (e.g., Schott) and a West stopper

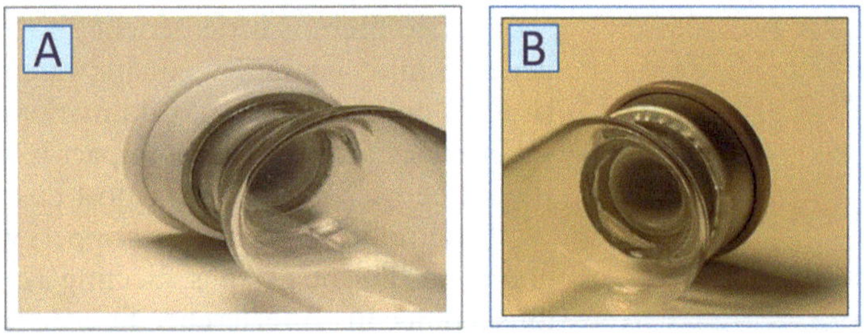

Fig. 11 Seals. (**A**) acceptable. (**B**) unacceptable (wrinkling due to skirt length being too long)

2.3 Components: Metal Seals

Seals are fixtures, typically comprising aluminum, applied to closed vial/stopper systems by crimping, to maintain contact between the stopper and vial, and hold stopper in place over the shelf life of drug product. See Fig. 11—photographs of sealed vials showing seals of different quality. Application of a seal ordinarily involves some compression of flange of rubber stopper (between 5% and 30% of stopper flange thickness—H4 in Fig. 10). Figure 12 shows a schematic of a lyophilization stopper in a vial. There are three areas of contact that are maintained by the seal:

- land seal—contact of stopper flange to top horizontal plane of vial
- transition seal—contact of stopper flange to mouth of vial
- valve seal—contact of vertical side of stopper to vial interior wall—sometimes called the "plug seal"

Selection of the proper seal is critical—it is made based on what is called a "stack up" calculation to obtain the proper excess skirt length. See Eq. (2).

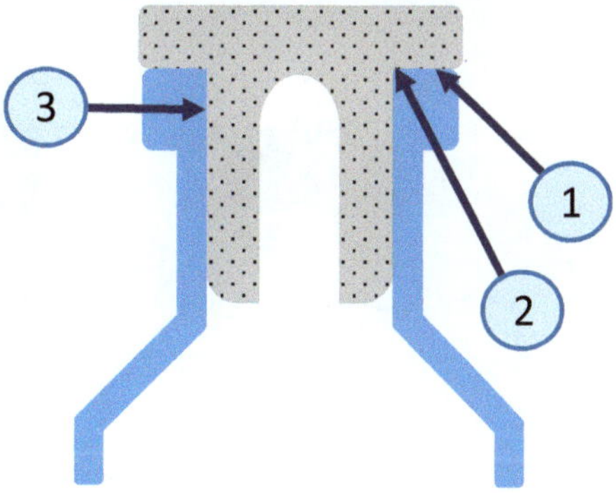

Fig. 12 Schematic diagram of lyophilization stopper in a vial. *1.* land seal. *2.* transition seal. *3.* valve seal [8]

$$\begin{aligned}\text{Excess skirt length} = {} & [\text{mean skirt length} - \text{aluminum thickness}] \\ & -[\text{vial crown height} + ((\text{flange thickness}) \\ & \times[(100 - \%\text{compression})/100])]\end{aligned} \quad (2)$$

Target for excess skirt length typically is 0.76 mm, or slightly greater. To select the proper mean skirt length, Eq. (2) is rearranged as Eq. (3).

$$\begin{aligned}\text{Mean skirt length} = {} & \text{excess skirt length} \\ & + \text{aluminum thickness} \\ & + [\text{vial crown height} + ((\text{flange thickness}) \\ & \times [(100 - \%\text{compression})/100])]\end{aligned} \quad (3)$$

Consider the example—West ART 1319 4023/50 gray stopper and Schott 6R vial

- excess skirt length = 0.76 mm
- aluminum thickness = 0.20 mm
- vial crown height = 3.6 ± 0.2 mm
- flange thickness = 3.3 ± 0.25 mm
- compression = 20%

The proper skirt length for this system is ≥7.20 mm.

Typically seals have a removable plastic (usually polypropylene-based) button on top to protect rubber stopper from damage during storage/handling. This button is removed before reconstitution. If lyophilized product is to be stored at low temperature, it must be considered whether said button can withstand said low temperature. An alternative is an all-aluminum seal.

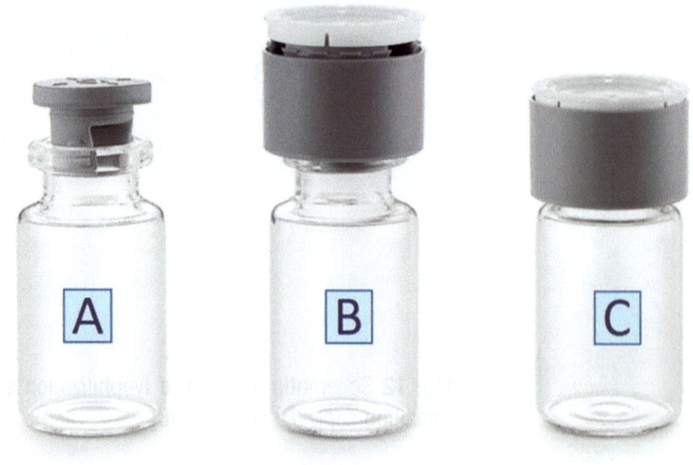

Fig. 13 Vial/stopper system with plastic seal. (**A**) with stopper inserted. (**B**) after application of cap. (**C**) after closure

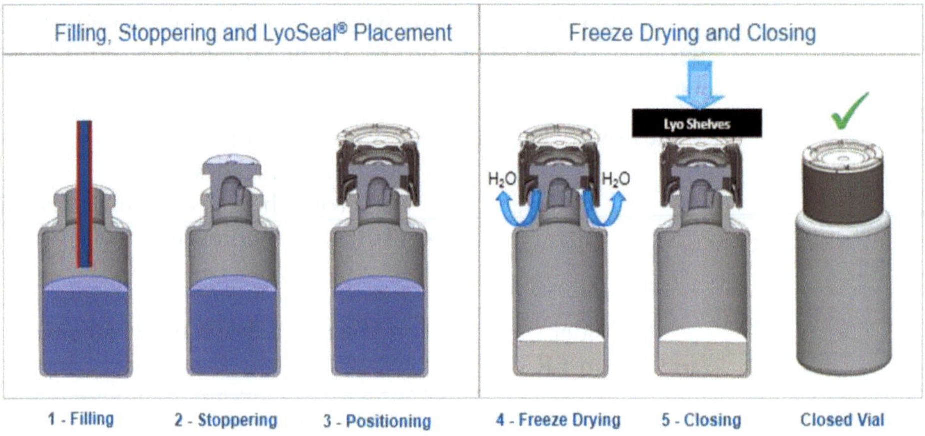

Fig. 14 Application/use of plastic seal. Shown is a schematic of process from filling vial through closure

2.4 Components: Plastic Seals

An alternative to metal seals is plastic seals (e.g., West LyoSeal® caps or Daikyo Plascap® caps). Metal seals are applied to closed vial/ stopper systems after removal from lyophilization chamber. This introduces the risk that vial/stopper seal can be compromised before seal application. Plastic seals reduce this risk. See Figs. 13 and 14. Applied to stopper before introduction of vial/stopper system to lyophilization chamber, the seal is affixed at completion of process when chamber shelf is lowered. Since plastic seals are applied in situ, systems are sealed before exit from lyophilization chamber. Plastic caps comprise polypropylene (a polymer with low surface energy) in the case of LyoSeal® product. This eliminates risk of adherence to chamber shelf after closure. Moreover, use of plastic caps removes a unit operation from the entire lyophilization process—since the separate step to apply metal seal is not required.

3 Container System Performance

The purpose of any container system is to protect drug product from the time it is introduced in liquid form before the lyophilization process begins, through the process of lyophilization, and through storage (i.e., shelf life) in lyophilized form until reconstitution. Two aspects of this are considered:

- *Container Closure Integrity.* This is ability of a container system to exclude external materials over drug product shelf life. It is related intrinsically to performance and fit of components.
- *Extractables and Leachables.* This is the consideration of chemical compounds that can move from, or through, system components over shelf life of drug product and potentially affect drug product performance.

3.1 Container Closure Integrity (CCI)

CCI is a container system's ability to prevent bacterial or chemical ingress from exceeding the maximum allowable leak limit (MALL)—the limit above which drug product performance can be affected. MALL will vary depending upon the drug product. In essence, confirmation of CCI is verification that system components fit together well, and have minimal leak. United States Pharmacopeia has recently issued Chapter <1207> *Package Integrity Evaluation—Sterile Products* (www.usp.org). This Chapter discusses methods to evaluate CCI—it strongly recommends use of deterministic methods, as opposed to probabilistic methods:

- *Deterministic*: Leakage event detected/measured is based on phenomena that follow a predictable chain of events—measurement is based on technologies that are readily controlled/monitored, and yield quantitative data.
- *Probabilistic*: Leakage event measurement relies on a series of sequential and/or simultaneous events, each associated with random outcomes described by probability distributions. Findings are associated with uncertainties and require large sample sizes and rigorous test controls.

Methods presented in Chapter <1207> are:

- laser-based headspace analysis (typically oxygen)
- high-voltage leak detection

- tracer gas leak detection (typically helium)
- mass extraction
- vacuum decay
- tracer liquids (*probabilistic*)

For any drug product, container system CCI must be demonstrated experimentally to be acceptable over shelf life. A recent publication describes an overall strategy of how CCI evaluation should be approached [9].

Before consideration of extractables and leachables, or movement of water from or through system components, it must be verified that the CCI of the container system meets requirements. If a system cannot meet CCI requirements, there is no point in considering it further.

3.2 Extractables and Leachables

Chemicals that can move from, or through, container components, and contact drug product may pose a risk. These chemicals are considered under the category of extractables and leachables. Definitions are:

- *Extractables.* Chemical entities (organic or inorganic, including metal ions) that are released from container system components (either by vaporization, or dissolution in an extraction solvent) under laboratory conditions (which may be very vigorous). Extractables, or derivatives thereof, *have the potential* to leach into drug product.
- *Leachables.* Chemical entities (organic or inorganic, including metal ions) that can migrate from container system components into drug product under ordinary conditions.

For any drug product and container system, extractables and leachables must be considered. Usually container system component manufacturers make available listings of potential extractables (e.g., West Verisure® data packages). In view of the composition of the drug product, and the list of potential extractables, a risk-based analysis can be made to determine what chemicals should be considered potential leachables. Studies then are conducted with container systems and drug product, *under actual conditions of use and length of shelf life* (i.e., not accelerated) to determine presence of said potential leachables, and determine whether level of release (if any) presents a risk to drug product or patient. It is emphasized that for lyophilized products, consideration must be given to volatile extractables and leachables, which could migrate from components during reduced pressure phases of lyophilization, and subsequent storage at reduced pressure.

3.3 Water

For a lyophilized product, the leachable of greatest concern is water. There are four potential sources:

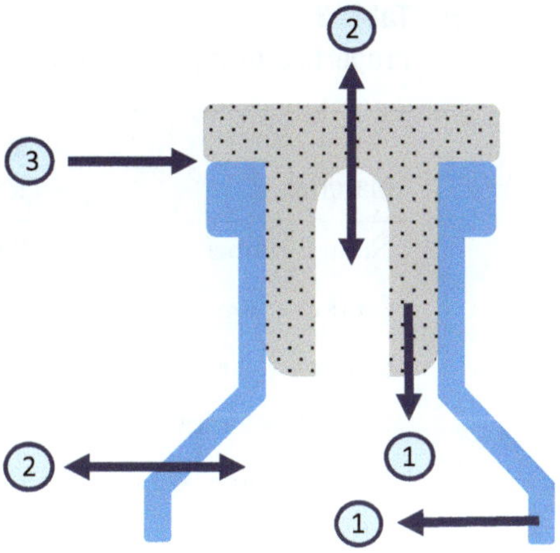

Fig. 15 Sources of water ingress into sealed container system. (1) water in container components. (2) water transmitted through container components. (3) water transmitted through seal

- *Residual Water after Lyophilization.* This is the source of lowest concern, since the lyophilization process is designed to reduce water level to an acceptable value.
- *Water in Container Components.* This is illustrated in Fig. 15. Water can be present either in, or absorbed on the surface of, a component. Consideration must be given to the fact that components are often sterilized by autoclave (e.g., ca. 120 °C steam for ca. 1 h), followed by drying at elevated temperature (e.g., ca. 105 °C for several hours). The level of water contained in/on components after these processes must be quantified in order to verify the quantity is below a level such that a theoretical complete release into lyophilized drug product would not result in alteration. This type of analysis must be done for every drug product and container system. Note that in the case of glass vials, as a practical matter, only water adsorbed on the surface is an issue.
- *Water Transmitted through Container Components.* This is illustrated in Fig. 15. Once a container system is assembled, it can reside in an uncontrolled atmosphere. The concern is movement of water through components to drug product. Even though this process is slow, over the span of drug product shelf life (e.g., several years) there may be enough transmission for alteration. Table 3 lists the moisture vapor transmission rates (MVTR) and oxygen permeability values (added only as reference) for container system materials of construction. Stoppers typically comprise chlorobutyl rubber or bromobutyl rubber (e.g., West formulations 4432 and 4023), because of their very good resistance to water and oxygen transmission—especially as compared to natural rubber or isoprene. Glass, as expected, is essentially impervious to water (and oxygen) transmission. A Poly(norborene) polymer (e.g., Daikyo Crystal Zenith® COP) does not have

Table 3
Properties of materials of container system components

Material	Moisture vapor transmission rate[a]	O_2 Permeability[b]
Natural rubber	9.0	23
Synthetic isoprene	14	–
Chlorobutyl rubber	0.1	~1–4
Bromobutyl rubber	0.3	~1–4
Poly(norborene)[c]	<10	1.2
Glass	-0-	-0-

[a]$(g - mm)/(m^2 - day)$
[b]Barrer = $[10^{-11} \times (cm^3\ (STP)) \times cm]/[(cm^2) \times (s) \times (Torr)]$
[c]Daikyo Crystal Zenith® cyclic olefin polymer

Table 4
Comparison of moisture vapor transmission rate to water uptake for selected rubber stopper formulations

Stopper formulation	Moisture vapor transmission rate[a]	Water uptake (weight %)[b]
Ethylene propylene diene monomer	2.15	0.48
Butyl-1	0.35	0.27
Butyl-2	0.40	1.39
Butyl-3	0.10	1.31
Butyl-4	0.65	0.87
Butyl-5	0.50	1.95

Water uptake is relative increase at equilibrium after drying
Data reproduced from reference [10]
[a]$(g - mm)/(m^2 - day)$
[b]Measured by Karl-Fisher titration

resistance as good as glass—however as noted above, glass vials present a higher risk of breakage and a higher potential for interaction with drug product. Choice of glass versus polymer must be made on a case-by-case basis.

- *Water Transmitted through Seal.* This will result if the container system does not maintain a good seal. This is illustrated in Fig. 15.

A very important point to consider is that, counterintuitively, MVTR is not always related to the level of water absorbed at equilibrium (see Table 4). Formulations that have a low MVTR in

Table 5
Water uptake of lyophilized sucrose

Stopper formulation	Water content immediately post lyophilization (weight %)[a]	Water content after storage for 3 months (weight %)[a]
Butyl-W	1.95	2.65
Butyl-X	2.34	3.12
Butyl-Y	2.25	3.91
Butyl-Z	2.45	3.62

Data reproduced from reference [10]
[a]Measured by Karl-Fisher titration

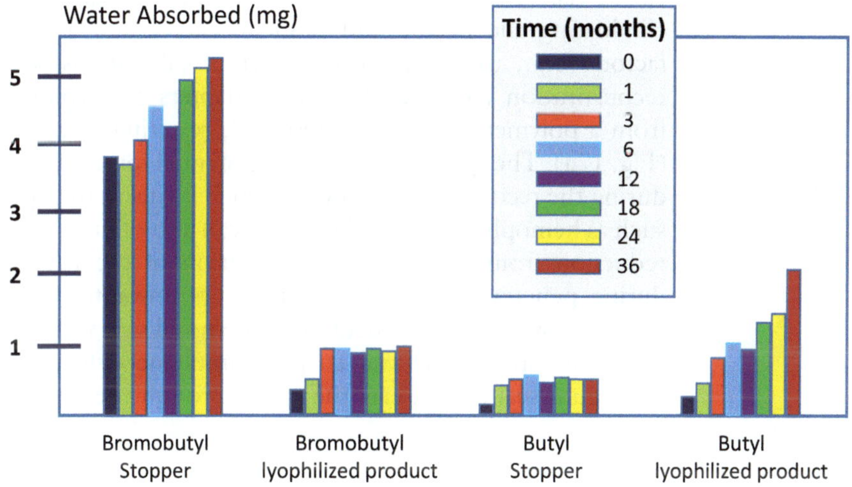

Fig. 16 Water absorption by stoppers and lyophilized products. Reproduced from data in reference [11]

stopper form can absorb a relatively high level of water, and vice versa. This is important because water absorbed in a stopper can be transferred to a lyophilized drug product, as shown in Table 5. Upon consideration, this makes sense. Referring to Table 1, at room temperature, the vapor pressure of water is approximately 0.03 atm. Considering the lyophilized drug product is stored under reduced pressure the vaporization rate is thus much higher, and as seen in Table 5, a significant amount of water can be transferred [10].

This is further illustrated in Fig. 16 [11]. While a bromobutyl stopper absorbs more water than a butyl stopper, it transmits less water as evidenced by a lower water adsorption value of the lyophilized product.

The key point is that in selection of a stopper, or a vial, consideration must be given to both water absorption and water transmission—such that considering shelf life of drug product, and amount of drug product contained in system, the total amount of water potentially available or absorbed does not pose a risk. Practically, this means considering each system case-by-case.

4 Reconstitution Systems

Reconstitution of a lyophilized drug product must be performed before it can be administered. In simple terms this involves mixing with a fixed amount of water-based liquid (i.e., diluent) and agitating the resultant mixture until the drug product is dissolved or dispersed. The logistics of this can be complex.

Reconstitution necessarily involves needle insertion into the closed vial. A vial adapter can make this process safer and easier by eliminating the needle and reducing steps, and addressing risk factors (e.g., use of incorrect level of diluent) associated with reconstitution (see Fig. 17). Vial adapters are typically molded from a polymer (e.g., polycarbonate), resulting in a spike design (Fig. 17a). The spike eliminates the potential for needle stick injury during the reconstitution process, which is vital in therapeutic areas such as hemophilia. The spike design can also offer a significant risk reduction from coring or fragmentation of the rubber stopper during penetration. Further, it prevents unwanted foaming and agitation by directing diluent flow down vial side wall via windows along the spike. The vial adapter simultaneously affixes to the aluminum seal and inserts the spike through the rubber stopper.

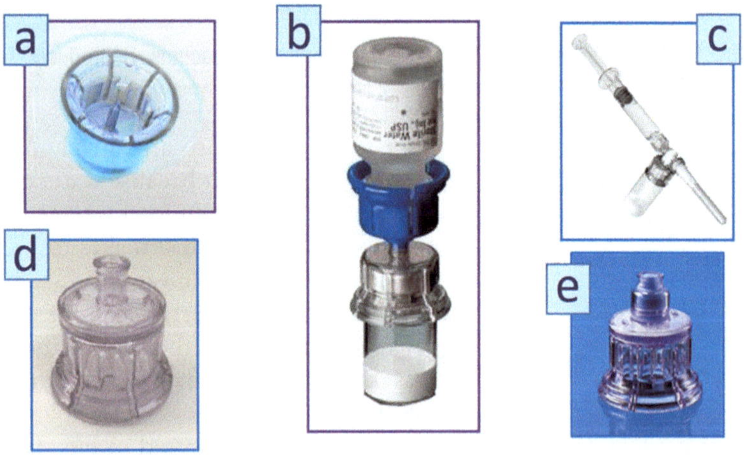

Fig. 17 Components of reconstitution systems. (**a**) vial adapter displaying polymer spike. (**b**) Mix2Vial® paired vial adapters for a 1:1 transfer from diluent filled vial. (**c**) MixJect® vial adapter system with attached needle for prepackaged diluent-filled PFS. (**d**) vial adapter with air filter/vent. (**e**) vial adapter with swabable port and air filter/vent

The opposite end of the vial adapter, which typically is a female Luer Lock connection, is then connected to a Luer Lock syringe filled with diluent for reconstitution. To eliminate steps, vial adapters can be paired (Fig. 17b). Such a configuration is designed to utilize the vacuum already present in a vial of lyophilized product and where the diluent is supplied in a vial format. Vial adapter systems also exist in support of processes where the diluent is pre-packaged in a pre-filled syringe (PFS). These systems typically have a pre-attached needle (Fig. 17c). Other benefits associated with using a vial adapter system include:

- *Consistent control in withdrawing drug product.* Unlike a needle, the vial adapter spike is rigid and fixed in place. Once reconstituted, the drug product flows into the spike through a series of windows positioned around the side of the spike. Thus, use of a vial adapter reduces the dependence on effectiveness of withdrawing the drug product, and ensures a consistent withdrawal and deliverable volume, as compared to using a needle where the position is not fixed.
- *Reduced concerns with undissolved particulates.* Using a vial adapter with an inline filter can capture undissolved particulates—preventing entry into the syringe barrel and eliminating concerns with potential injection.
- *Elimination of vacuum build-up.* Vial adapters that contain a vent allow for air to pass through a filter (e.g., 0.2 μm)—eliminating the need to manually pressurize the vial prior to withdrawal, and eliminating the risk of over-pressurizing sensitive drug products (Fig. 17d).
- *Maintenance of sterility in multi-dose, multi-access formats.* Using a vial adapter that contains a swabable port connection (Fig. 17e) allows for a closed and sterile system between activations. In addition, using a vial adapter of this nature results in only one spike penetration—as opposed to multiple penetrations when using a needle. This greatly reduces any risk of coring and fragmentation

Clearly, the vial adapter approach enables a much safer and more efficient reconstitution process and outcome.

5 Summary

Lyophilization is an essential process to the safe delivery of a very large number of drug products. In order to enable this, selection of proper package and reconstitution systems is critical. In this selection, several factors must be very well understood:

- component materials properties—compatibility with drug product and ability to prevent ingress of water and deleterious compounds
- component fit—ability to maintain CCI over shelf life
- component performance—compatibility with lyophilization process
- reconstitution system—ability to safely and conveniently use lyophilized drug product

Understanding these factors, the right systems can be selected.

Acknowledgments

Mix2Vial® and MixJect® are registered trademarks of West Pharma. Services IL, Ltd., a subsidiary of West Pharmaceutical Services, Inc. FluroTec®, LyoTec®, LyoSeal®, Verisure®, are trademarks or registered trademarks of West Pharmaceutical Services, Inc. FlurоTec® and Daikyo Crystal Zenith® technology are licensed from Daikyo Seiko, Ltd. Daikyo Crystal Zenith® and Plascap® are trademarks or registered trademarks of Daikyo Seiko, Ltd. TopPac® is a registered trademark of Schott AG.

References

1. Rey L (2004) Glimpses into the realm of freeze-drying: fundamental issues. In: Rey L, May J (eds) Freeze drying/lyophilization of pharmaceutical and biological products, 2nd edn. Marcel Dekker, Inc., New York, NY. (ISBN: 0-8247-4868-9, pp 1–32
2. Castellan GW (ed) (1971) Physical chemistry, 2nd edn. Addison-Wesley, Reading, MA, p 272
3. Linde D (ed) (1995) Handbook of chemistry and physics, 76th edn. CRC Press, Inc., New York, NY, pp 6–14 15
4. http://glassproperties.com/glasses/
5. Scutella XB, Passot S, Bourles E, Fonseca F, Trelea IC (2017) How vial geometry variability influences heat transfer and product temperature during freeze-drying. J Pharm Sci 106:770–778
6. https://www.fda.gov/Drugs/DrugSafety/ucm248490.htm
7. Mungikar A, Ludzinski M, Kamat M (2010) Effect of the design of the stopper including dimension, type, and vent area on lyophilization process. PDA J Pharm Sci Technol 64:507–516
8. Parenteral Drug Association Technical Report No. 76: Identification and classification of visible nonconformities in elastomeric components and aluminum seals for parenteral packaging. https://store.pda.org/TableOfContents/TR76_TOC.pdf
9. DeGrazio F (2018) A holistic strategy for container closure integrity: selecting and evaluating an integral packaging system. PDA J Pharm Sci Technol 72(1):15–34
10. DeGrazio F (2010) Closure and container considerations in lyophilization. In: Rey L, May J (eds) Freeze drying/lyophilization of pharmaceutical and biological products, 3rd edn. CRC Press, Inc., New York, NY. (ISBN: 9781439825754, pp 396–412
11. Kofler H (2015) Selecting stoppers for use in the lyophilisation of moisture-sensitive drugs. Manufacturing Chemist p 47–49

Chapter 10

Scale-Up of Freeze-Drying Cycles, the Use of Process Analytical Technology (PAT), and Statistical Analysis

Erwan Bourlès, Gael de Lannoy, Bernadette Scutellà, Fernanda Fonseca, Ioan Cristian Trelea, and Stephanie Passot

Abstract

Traditionally, the quality of pharmaceutical drugs is tested on the final freeze-dried product following a regulatory framework known as Quality-by-Testing (QbT) (Yu, Pharm Res 25: 781–91, 2008). In this system, product quality and performance are ensured by performing extensive tests on the final product, and by using a fixed formulation and manufacturing process. In contrast, the US Food and Drug Administration (FDA) proposed the Quality by Design (QbD) initiative with the idea that quality cannot be "tested into" the product, but it should be built into it (FDA, Guidance for industry, Q8 (R2) pharmaceutical development. Dept. of Health and Human Services, Center for Drug Evaluation and Research. Rockville, MD, 2009). Quality by Design consists of a systematic approach to pharmaceutical product development that begins with predefined objectives and emphasizes product and process understanding and process control, based on sound science and quality risk management (FDA, Guidance for industry, Q8(R2) pharmaceutical development. Dept. of Health and Human Services, Center for Drug Evaluation and Research. Rockville, MD, 2009; Mockus et al, Pharm Dev Technol 16: 549–76, 2011; Yu, Pharm Res 25: 781–91, 2008). In this chapter, a statistical model for the sublimation step in freeze-drying was used to construct the design space for the cycle development and to select adequate parameters for scaling up from pilot to commercial scale. Three critical operating variables of the process were tested: freezing rate, shelf temperature, and chamber pressure in primary drying. The model was used to predict the sublimation rate and the product temperature, since their selection is of paramount importance to obtain a product of high quality. The obtained results were then used to define the design space of the product at pilot scale.

Key words Quality by design (QbD), Statistical model, Scale-up, Edge effects, Heat transfer coefficient, Process analytical technology (PAT)

Nomenclature

A	Cross sectional area (m^2)
b	Model parameters
ΔH	Latent heat of sublimation ($J\ kg^{-1}$)
K_v	Vial heat transfer coefficient ($W\ m^{-2}\ K^{-1}$)
L	Product layer thickness (m)

Kevin R. Ward and Paul Matejtschuk (eds.), *Lyophilization of Pharmaceuticals and Biologicals: New Technologies and Approaches*, Methods in Pharmacology and Toxicology, https://doi.org/10.1007/978-1-4939-8928-7_10,

m	Mass (kg)
$\dot{m}$	Sublimation rate (kg s^{-1})
P	Pressure (Pa)
$\dot{Q}$	Heat flow rate (W)
R_p	Mass transfer resistance (kPa s m^2 kg^{-1})
T	Temperature (K)
T_g'	Glass transition temperature (K)
T_{coll}	Collapse temperature (K)
T_{eu}	Eutectic melt temperature (K)
y	Critical process parameters
x	Operating variable

Greek

ε	Random error assumed to follow a Gaussian distribution
λ	Thermal conductivity (W m^{-1} K^{-1})

Subscripts

b	Vial bottom
c	Chamber
ice	Ice
i	Interface
max	Maximum
s	Shelf

1 Introduction

Freeze-drying is a water or solvent removal process typically used to preserve perishable materials, to extend shelf life or make the product more convenient for transportation. This process is often used for vaccine production since it allows removal of water from the product at low temperature and then avoids or decelerates the degradative pathways of labile materials such as antigens or live attenuated viruses that can occur in aqueous media [1, 2]. Moreover, the low residual water content (and low water activity) allows extending shelf life of the product for several years [2]. The process typically works in three main phases: freezing, primary drying (sublimation), and secondary drying (desorption). Firstly, the liquid drug product is filled into glass vials. These vials are partially stoppered to allow water vapor to escape during the process. Vials are then loaded on the shelves of the freeze-dryer. After the loading step, shelves are cooled down to temperatures generally below −45 °C in order to maintain the product, in the case of amorphous formulations, below its glass transition temperature. During the freezing step, free water completely solidifies and converts to ice crystals. A part of the water remains unfrozen in the cryoconcentrated matrix (around 10–20%) [3]. Following freezing, primary drying is started by reducing the pressure in the drying chamber of the freeze-dryer and raising the temperature of the shelves. When pressure reaches a value below the saturated vapor pressure of ice at the frozen product temperature, sublimation begins. After complete sublimation of ice crystals, shelf temperature is raised and secondary drying starts. This process allows desorption of water molecules from the cryoconcentrated matrix until desired residual moisture content is achieved. At the end of the freeze-drying cycle, the chamber is backfilled with dry nitrogen to a pressure slightly lower than atmospheric pressure and the stoppers are fully inserted into the vials by collapsing the shelves to insert the stoppers. Once stoppering is completed, the chamber pressure is equilibrated to atmospheric pressure for unloading. The vials are then unloaded and oversealed with aluminum flip off caps [4].

A successful freeze-drying cycle is achieved when the final formulation meets the following criteria [5]:

- A low residual water content (generally below 3%) [2, 6];
- An elegant pharmaceutical appearance (no collapse or meltback visible);
- A fast reconstitution time;
- A target protein activity retained;
- An extended shelf life of the product when stored below its glass transition temperature.

To achieve this goal, process parameters of the freeze-drying cycle have to be adapted to take into account not only the formulation physical properties but also the equipment performance. The three steps of the process may affect the final product quality. It is well known that some proteins are sensitive to the freezing rate applied at the beginning of the freeze-drying process. A schematic illustration of the state diagram of a sucrose solution (Fig. 1) describes the different regions of the physical state of materials and shows the relationships between temperatures (equilibrium crystallization/melting T_m, glass transition temperature T_g) and the sucrose content. At the slow cooling rates generally applied when freeze-drying aqueous solutions, progressive conversion of water into ice concomitantly induces the increase of solute concentration of the matrix surrounding the ice crystals until the maximal solute cryoconcentration and the concentrated matrix reaches the glassy state (point X in Fig. 1). In these conditions a significant increase of solute concentration upon freezing, up to 16 times its initial concentration, can occur [3]. Proteins can thus be unfolded when exposed to such highly concentrated solutions.

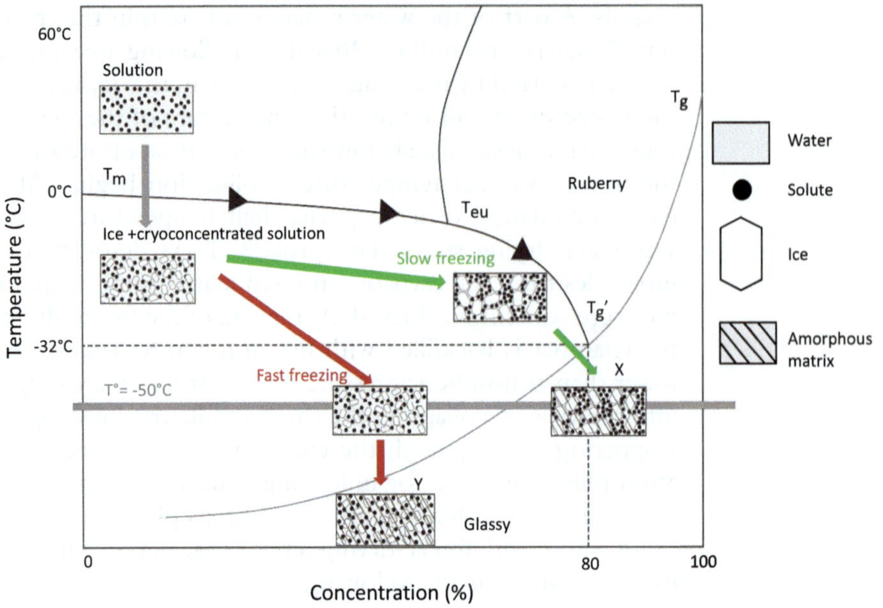

Fig. 1 Schematic illustration of the impact of the freezing step on a sucrose matrix in a freeze-dryer

On the other hand, when fast freezing is applied to a product, growth of ice crystals will be limited and hence cryoconcentration occurs to a lesser extent (point Y in Fig. 1) resulting in a lower value of T_g. However, fast cooling rates have been shown to result in small ice crystals thus providing high surface areas. Some studies [7, 8] reported denaturation of proteins during freezing as closely related to surface-induced denaturation phenomenon. This denaturation could be reduced or stopped by adding some surfactants to the formulation or adapting the freezing rate applied to the product.

Primary drying is usually considered the most critical and time-consuming step of the freeze-drying process, affecting several characteristics of the product such as the visual aspect and the reconstitution time. Prediction and monitoring of the product temperature during this part of the process is a fundamental step for cycle development. If during primary drying the product temperature becomes higher than a critical value, the material will undergo viscous flow, resulting in the loss of the pore structure obtained by freezing. This phenomenon, known as collapse [9], will result in a higher and non-homogeneous moisture content within the batch, an inelegant cake appearance, longer reconstitution times, and often poor stability upon storage [10, 11]. The maximum allowable product temperature (T_{max}) achievable during primary drying, associated with the collapse temperature (T_{coll}), depends on the physical state of the frozen product. For crystalline formulations, the limit temperature T_{max} is defined by the eutectic melting temperature of the crystallizing solute, whereas for an amorphous material, T_{max} is usually associated with the glass transition temperature of the maximally freeze-concentrated phase (T_g') (Fig. 1). Moreover, collapse temperatures of simple aqueous solutions of disaccharides are low and usually 1–3 °C higher than their T_g' value [9, 12]. The product temperature is strictly related to the operating variables (shelf temperature and chamber pressure) and thus, their selection is of paramount importance in designing an appropriate freeze-drying cycle. If cycle conditions are designed far from optimum, unnecessarily long primary drying times can result. Conversely, if overly aggressive conditions are selected, the product can experience an excursion above its collapse temperature during sublimation. However, product temperature depends also on other several factors during primary drying, such as the container design [13–15], the thermal characteristics of the equipment (e.g., emissivity of the shelf), and the position of the vial on the shelf [16]. Vials located at the periphery of the shelf show a higher product temperature because they receive the radiation from the walls and door of the freeze-dryer. This phenomenon, known as "*edge vial effect*," may cause the collapse of the edge vials if the product is processed at a temperature close to the critical temperature [17].

Sublimation rate cannot be increased beyond a maximum value corresponding to the capability of the freeze-dryer. If the process is run above the equipment capability, choked flow may occur. This phenomenon was described in detail by Searles [18] and corresponds to the velocity at which water vapor reaches the speed of sound between the drying chamber and the condenser. The consequences in a freeze-dryer can be dramatic for the process because when the choked flow phenomenon appears, pressure control is lost and rises above its set point, thus increasing product temperature due to additional heat transfer.

Since different freeze-dryers can show different thermal properties and capabilities, the application of the same cycle between pilot and commercial scale can lead to an unacceptable or heterogeneous batch product quality. This generally happens when the conditions selected at pilot scale are not robust enough to fit in different freeze-dryers. The development of an accurate methodology for the cycle transfer and adaptation between different freeze-dryers is of paramount importance for successful scale-up [19, 20].

In the present work, two approaches based on mathematical modeling (statistical or mechanistic) are proposed and compared, to calculate the design space for cycle design and scale-up in agreement with the quality by design paradigm. Both approaches make it possible to identify optimal freeze-drying cycle parameters for freezing and primary drying in order to preserve product from collapse while driving sublimation as fast as possible.

2 The Quality by Design Paradigm

Traditionally, the quality of pharmaceutical drugs is tested on the final freeze-dried product following a regulatory framework known as Quality-by-Testing (QbT) [21]. In this system, product quality and performance are ensured by performing extensive tests on the final product, and by using a fixed formulation and manufacturing process. However, this framework has several drawbacks, e.g., no attention on how the design of the product formulation and of the manufacturing process can ensure product quality and no investigation on the causes responsible for product quality variability and/or failure [21]. In contrast with this quality-by-testing approach, the US Food and Drug Administration (FDA) proposed the Quality by Design (QbD) initiative with the following idea: "*the quality cannot be tested into the product, but it should be built into it*" [22]. Quality by Design consists of a systematic approach to pharmaceutical product development that begins with predefined objectives and emphasizes product and process understanding and process control, based on sound science and quality risk management [21–23].

Figure 2 shows a schematic overview of the implementation of the Quality by Design initiative in a pharmaceutical process. A preliminary step for a successful implementation of QbD in pharmaceutical freeze-drying is the definition of the *quality target product profile* (QTPP), which describes the design criteria of the product for quality, safety and efficacy and forms the basis for its development [22]. The QTPP could include for example the dosage, the container system, the drug quality criteria (e.g., potency). Once the QTPP has been defined, the next step is to identify the relevant *critical quality attributes* (CQAs). The CQAs are the physical, chemical, and biological properties of a product that should remain within an appropriate limit, range or distribution to assure the desired product quality [22]. Example of CQAs for freeze-dried vaccines are the visual aspect, the final moisture content, and the potency of the product [24]. The CQAs (and thus the quality of the product) are related to the manufacturing process through the *critical process parameters* (CPPs). The CPPs are the process parameters whose variability has an impact on one or more CQAs of the product and therefore should be monitored or controlled to ensure that the process produces the desired quality [22]. In order to avoid the loss of the product structure (collapse) and thus to guarantee an elegant visual aspect, product temperature should be maintained below a critical value (T_{coll}) during the primary drying step of the freeze-drying process [9, 24]. Furthermore, in order to assure homogeneous product quality, the same thermal history of the product should be reproduced between vials and in cycles performed in different equipment. Hence, the product temperature

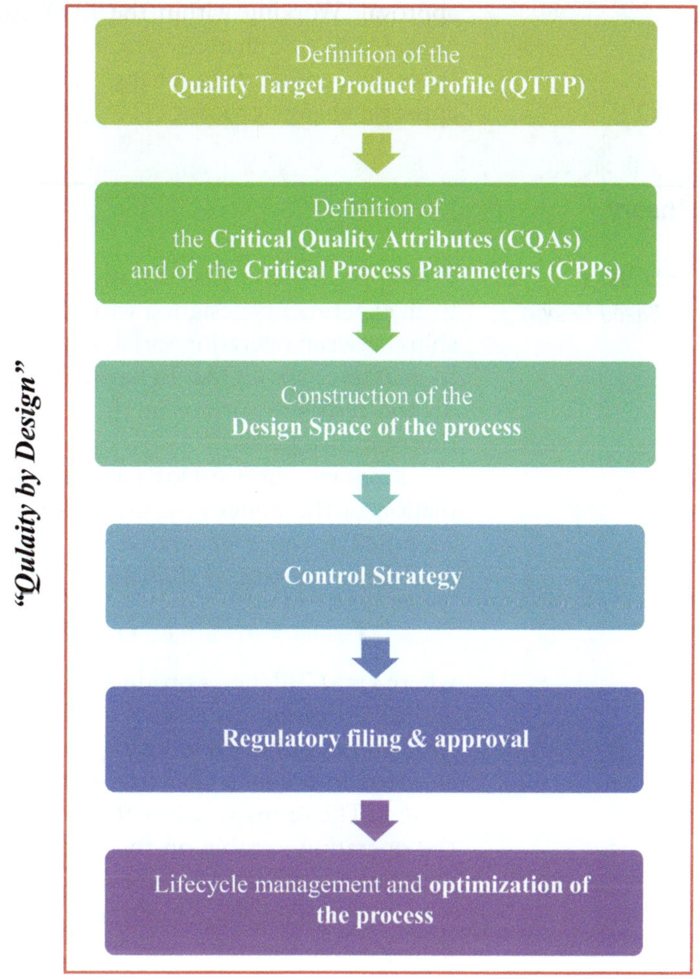

Fig. 2 Schematic overview for the implementation of the Quality by Design approach in pharmaceutical processes

T_b and the sublimation rate $\dot{m}$ can be defined as the CPPs of the primary drying step and their values should be reproducible during the cycle transfer or scale-up.

Based on the acceptable range of CQAs, the risk assessment of the process can be performed by constructing the *design space* of CPPs. The design space is defined as "*the multidimensional combination of input variables and process parameters that have been demonstrated to provide assurance of product quality*" [22]. With regard to the primary drying step of freeze-drying process, the input variables are the chamber pressure and shelf temperature, whereas the process parameters are the product temperature and sublimation rate. The design space is strongly dependent on the product and the equipment considered. It is usually proposed by the applicant and it is subject to regulatory assessment and approval. Working within the FDA approved design space is not considered as a change, whereas a movement out of the design space is considered a change and requires a regulatory post-approval change process.

3 Theory

3.1 Statistical Model-Based Design Space

This approach consists of statistically modeling the data obtained from experiments designed with the purpose of detecting relationships between operating variables and CPPs of the process, in order to guarantee the CQAs. In particular, a DoE (for Design of Experiments) response surface methodology (RSM) was considered for this objective [25].

Response surface DoEs are empirical models for the approximation of the underlying unknown physical mechanisms that are supposed to have generated the experimental data. A statistical model fits the data, as shown in Eq. (1):

$$y = b_0 + b_1 x_1 + b_2\, x_2 + b_3 x_1^2 + b_4\, x_2^2 + b_5 x_1 x_2 + \varepsilon \qquad (1)$$

where y is a CPP (i.e., a product temperature or sublimation rate), x_i are the operating variables (i.e., shelf freezing rate, shelf temperature, and chamber pressure in primary drying), ε is a random error assumed to follow a Gaussian distribution, and b_i are model parameters. The terms x_i^2 allow the evaluation of a quadratic impact of the operating variable on the CPPs, and the term x_1x_2 allows the test for an interaction between operating variables. The objective is then to estimate the b_i parameters from experimental data which best predict the CPP values from observed operating variable values.

Experiments can be a priori designed in order to optimize the statistical quality of the model parameters and to minimize the variance of the error. Response surface designs are experimental designs having this objective and were therefore considered in the current case study [25].

3.2 Mechanistic Model-Based Design Space

Classical equations describing heat and mass transfer phenomena during freeze-drying [15, 26] were used to construct the mechanistic design space. Two main model parameters need to be determined in order to calculate the design space: the vial heat transfer coefficient and the product resistance.

3.2.1 Vial Heat Transfer Coefficient K_v

The vial heat transfer coefficient (K_v) characterizes the heat transfer between the freeze-dryer shelf and the vial. It can be defined as [14, 15]:

$$K_v = \frac{\Delta H \dot{m}}{A_b\,(T_s - T_b)} \qquad (2)$$

where A_b is the outer vial bottom area, ΔH is the latent heat of sublimation, T_s is the temperature of the shelf, T_b is the bottom product temperature, and $\dot{m}$ is the sublimation rate.

The bottom product temperature was evaluated from the heat balance in the ice layer [15]:

$$\dot{Q} = \frac{\lambda_{ice}}{L_{ice}} A_i (T_b - T_i) \tag{3}$$

where λ_{ice} is the ice thermal conductivity, A_i is the inner base area of the vial, L_{ice} is the ice thickness, and T_i is the ice-vapor interface temperature.

The temperature at the ice-vapor interface T_i was calculated using the Clausius-Clapeyron relation as reported in Scutellà et al. [15]:

$$P_{vi} = e^{-\frac{6139.6}{T_i}+28.8912} \tag{4}$$

where P_{vi} is the partial pressure of the vapor at the ice-vapor interface in the product. The sublimation rate $\dot{m}$ was measured gravimetrically. Selected vials were filled with 1.8 mL of distilled water and weighed before and after the run on a precision scale balance (±0.001 g; Mettler Toledo, Zaventem, Belgium). The sublimation rate was calculated as [15]:

$$\dot{m} = \frac{m_1 - m_2}{t_{sub}} \tag{5}$$

where m_1 and m_2 are the initial and final mass of the vials, respectively, and t_{sub} is the sublimation time. Sublimation time was measured from the moment when shelf fluid inlet temperature exceeded product temperature, meaning that there was a net heat flux from the shelf toward the vials.

3.2.2 Product Resistance R_p

The product resistance R_p represents the resistance imposed by the dried product layer to the sublimation rate during the primary drying step. It can be calculated as:

$$R_p = A_i(P_{vi} - P_{vC})m \tag{6}$$

where A_i is the sublimation interface area, P_{vC} is the partial pressure of the vapor in the drying chamber, usually assumed equal to the total chamber pressure during primary drying, and P_{vi} is the partial pressure of the vapor at the ice-vapor interface in the product, calculated using the Clausius-Clapeyron relation (Eq. 4). T_i is the product temperature at the sublimation interface theoretically determined from the heat balance at the vial scale (Eq. 3), with the product temperature T_b measured by the signal of the Tempris probes. The sublimation rate $\dot{m}$ was calculated from Eq. (2) knowing the previously determined vial heat transfer coefficient K_v and the measured product temperature profile T_b.

The product resistance R_p can be described as a function of the dried layer l_d [27, 28]. The evolution of dried layer thickness in time $\left(\frac{dl_d}{dt}\right)$ can be calculated as:

$$\frac{dl_d}{dt} = \frac{1}{\rho A_i} \dot{m} \tag{7}$$

where ρ is the density of the ice. Depending on the product, the product resistance can evolve differently with the dried layer thickness (linearly or nonlinearly). In order to construct the mechanistic design space, it will be considered in this work a constant value of product resistance at a specific l_d (i.e., 0.001 m).

4 Case Study

In this section, the previously described methodologies including an empirical approach based on statistical modeling of experimental data and a mechanistic modeling of the freeze-drying process are applied to the development of a design space for primary drying and scale-up of a vaccine product.

4.1 Materials

4.1.1 Vials

For the whole set of experiments described in the case study, siliconized glass tubing vials (3 mL) provided by Müller + Müller (Holzminden, Germany) were used. These vials are routinely used in commercial manufacturing.

4.1.2 Freeze-Dryer

The pilot scale freeze-dryer used was a LyoVac GT6 (Finn-Aqua Santasalo-Sohlberg SPRL, Brussels, Belgium). The drying chamber had a volume of 0.061 m^3 and was equipped with five shelves with an area of 0.14 m^2 each. Double stage high-performance compressors were connected specifically to the cooling system of the shelves in order to achieve high-speed freezing capacity. A butterfly valve was installed between the chamber and the condenser. The pressure in the freeze-dryer chamber was monitored with a capacitance manometer.

4.1.3 Process Analytical Tools Used in the Study at Pilot Scale

Wireless Temperature Remote Interrogation System (TEMPRIS®)

The equipment used in this study (Fig. 3) was described in detail by Schneid and Gieseler [29] and more recently by Nail et al. [30]. It consisted of a wireless and battery-free temperature monitoring system (IQ Mobil Solutions GmbH, Wolfratshausen, Germany) that is composed of 16 individual sensors, an interrogation unit (IRU) (including transmitter), and a compact PC system with the software installed to record the data. The sensing element consists of a quartz crystal that vibrates at a frequency that is a function of its temperature. The sensors are powered by excitation of the passive transponder by means of an amplitude-modulated electromagnetic signal in the internationally usable 2.4 GHz ISM band [31]. The signal is demodulated in the transponder by means of a diode

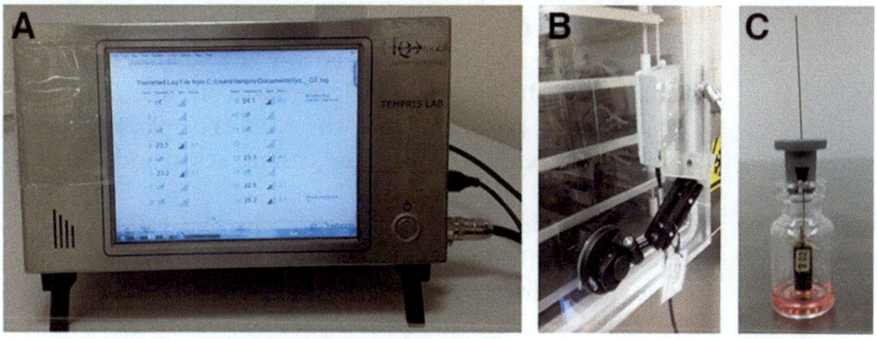

Fig. 3 Picture of the TEMPRIS wireless sensor experimental setup (**A**: compact computer to monitor product temperature from the sensors; **B**: transmitter antenna fixed to the laboratory freeze-dryer front door; **C**: temperature sensor placed at the bottom-center of vials which was filled with a model vaccine formulation for the study)

detector and used to stimulate the quartz-based resonance circuit. In the second step, the amplitude modulation is deactivated and only the continuous wave (CW) carrier is radiated. The stimulated resonance circuit continues to oscillate at its characteristic frequency which depends on its temperature. This free oscillation frequency is mixed with the CW carrier and re-transmitted to the interrogation unit. The IRU measures the frequency of the response modulation and the exponential drop in amplitude. In combination with statistical parameters of several consecutive responses the key variable "temperature" is derived [29, 30]. These sensors were placed in the bottom center of selected vials (Fig. 3C) to record product temperature during the experiments.

Cold Plasma Ionization Sensor (Lyotrack Adixen, France)

This system measures the humidity in the drying chamber based on Inductively Coupled Plasma/Optical Emission Spectrometry. The device consists of a plasma generator and an optical spectrometer which is normally used in chemical and gas analysis [32]. The plasma generator is plugged into the drying chamber of the freeze-dryer via a tri-clamp flange. The system ionizes the gas present in the chamber, and the spectrometer identifies the gas species based on the wavelengths of the emitted photons [31]. In a freeze-dryer, this equipment measures the ratio of water vapor to nitrogen in vacuum conditions (from 3 to 0.005 mbar). This ratio is labeled as humidity in the software. The signal ranges from 0 to 1 with 0 indicating that there is no water vapor and 1 that the freeze-dryer is saturated with water vapor. Based on the curve profile, it is possible to easily detect the endpoint of primary drying [32].

As stated by Patel and Pikal [31], as this technique involves ionization of the gas species in the drying chamber, there could be potential in-process drug product degradation via free radical oxidation. Therefore, a placebo formulation (same formulation without antigen) was preferred for the validation experiments at full load in the pilot freeze-dryer, to avoid free radical occurrence on the active product during the cycle. The placebo model formulation was composed of lactose, amino acids, and sorbitol.

4.2 Glass Transition and Collapse Temperatures

For developing a freeze-drying cycle, the first step involves the identification of the maximal temperature of the formulation allowable during freezing and primary drying. The target product temperature during the primary drying stage of an optimized lyophilization process is several degrees below a critical threshold value corresponding to the glass transition temperature of the freeze-concentrated phase (T_g') or to the collapse temperature (T_{coll}) [33].

The glass transition temperature of the maximally freeze-concentrated phase formed during freezing (T_g') and the collapse temperature of the product during sublimation (T_{coll}) are the two main properties of amorphous formulations to be determined [9, 34]. For this purpose, two methods are usually employed: differential scanning calorimetry (DSC) and freeze-drying microscopy for determining T_g' and T_{coll} respectively.

For identifying T_g' of vaccine formulations described in this chapter, differential scanning calorimetry (DSC) measurements were performed on a power compensation DSC instrument (Pyris Diamond, Perkin Elmer LLC, Norwalk, CT, USA) equipped with a mechanical cooling system. Samples were frozen from ambient temperature to -55 °C at 10 °C min^{-1} and warmed to ambient at the same rate. Glass transition temperatures were measured during the heating ramp (data not shown).

The collapse temperature (T_{coll}) of the frozen product (vaccine formulation) was measured using a freeze-drying cryo-stage (BTL Lyostat 3, Biopharma Process Systems, Winchester, UK). Samples were frozen to -50 °C at 10 °C min^{-1}, heated at 3 °C min^{-1} to -40 °C and 0.5 °C min^{-1} from -40 °C until the appearance of collapse became evident on the microscope. T_{coll} values obtained are summarized in Fig. 4. The model vaccine formulation is characterized by a glass transition temperature close to -38.2 °C and a collapse temperature of -37.4 °C.

4.3 Experimental Design

The response surface DoE used in the experiments was a cubic face centered composite design where three operating variables (freezing rate, shelf temperature, chamber pressure in primary drying) were varied as shown in Table 1 for a total of 15 DoE conditions (14 DoE conditions and one center point). Furthermore, the position of the vials in the freeze-dryer was also considered an additional model parameter in order to take into account the variability due to the position of the vials on the shelves (edge versus center).

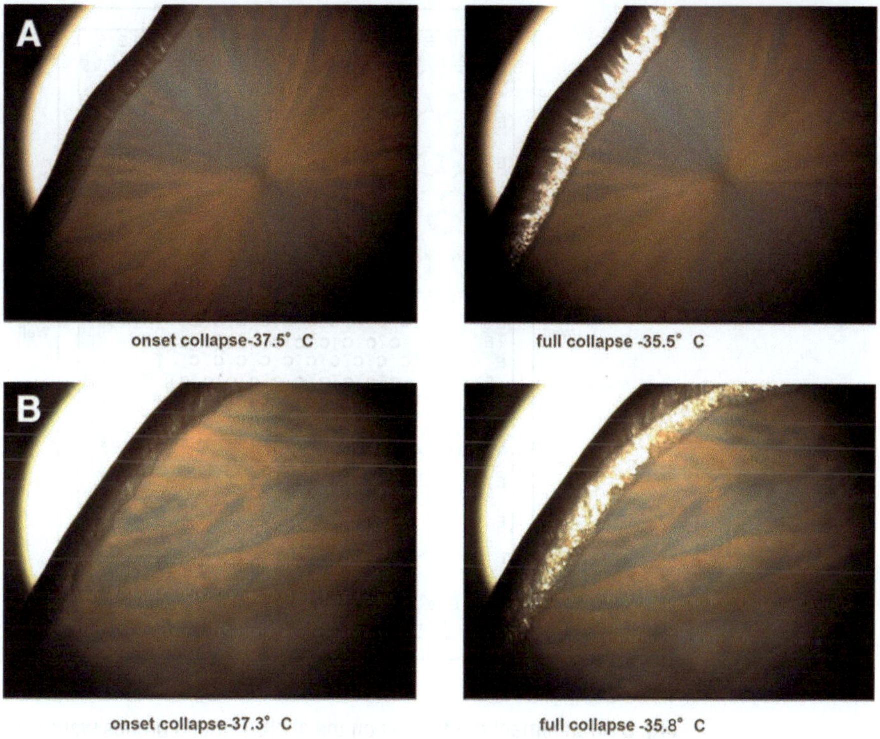

Fig. 4 Pictures taken from the cryomicroscope instrument of the formulation collapse temperature (**A**: run 1; **B**: run 2)

Table 1
Operating variable (freezing rate, pressure, shelf temperature) evaluated for design of experiment purpose

Operating variables	Unit	Low range	Medium range	High range
Freezing rate target	°C min^{-1}	0.5	3.75	7
Pressure	Pa	3	5	9
Shelf temperature	°C	−35	−32	−29

The following experimental procedure was applied throughout the experiments. First, 580 vials were arranged in hexagonal clusters in a bottomless tray, as shown in Fig. 5. A stainless steel frame was used to fully shield the vials from the chamber walls. The vials were filled with 0.4 + 0.02 mL of vaccine model formulation solution, and bromobutyl stoppers were partially inserted in the neck of all vials. The vials were then loaded onto the middle shelf of the freeze-dryer by using a stainless steel tray, which was removed immediately after to allow direct contact between the vials and the shelf during the cycle. Depending on the process parameters

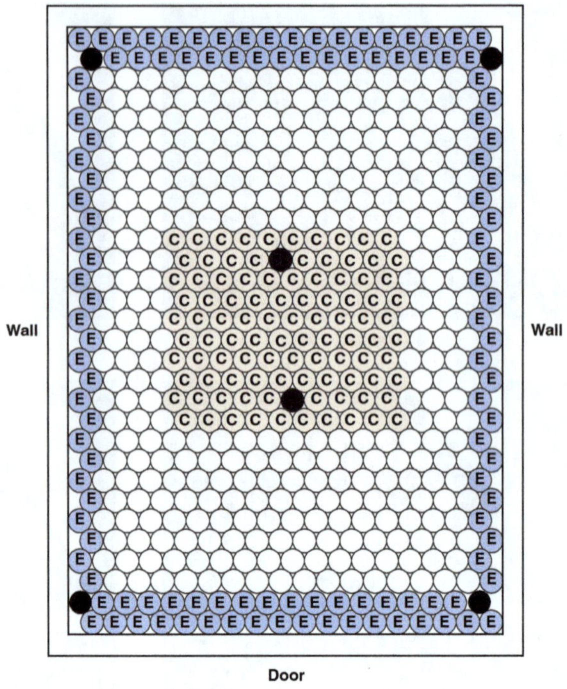

Fig. 5 Arrangement of the vials on the shelf. Tempris probes were placed in four edge vials (marked with letter E) and in two central vials (marked with letter C). All edge and center vials were gravimetrically analyzed

applicable to each run, the freezing step was performed by decreasing the shelf temperature from 4 to −50 °C at about 0.5 °C min^{-1}; 3.75 or 7 °C min^{-1} (the latter of which corresponds to loading the vials onto precooled shelves and was estimated from the evolution of product temperature after ice nucleation). The vials were then held at constant temperature for 1 h. After the freezing step, the chamber pressure was decreased and shelf temperature was raised to the target primary drying temperature in 30 min. Three different values of chamber pressure, i.e., 3, 5, and 9 Pa, and of shelf inlet temperature, i.e., −29, −32 or −35 °C, were tested. The cycles were run long enough to dry up to 20–30% of the initial mass. A total of 124 edge vials (marked with E in Fig. 5) and 100 central vials (marked with C in Fig. 5) were individually weighed before and after the experiment using a precision scale balance (±0.001 g; Mettler Toledo, Zaventem, Belgium). The arrangement of the weighed vials within the shelves is shown in Fig. 5. The product temperature data used to construct the statistical response surface were collected at the end of each freeze-drying cycle.

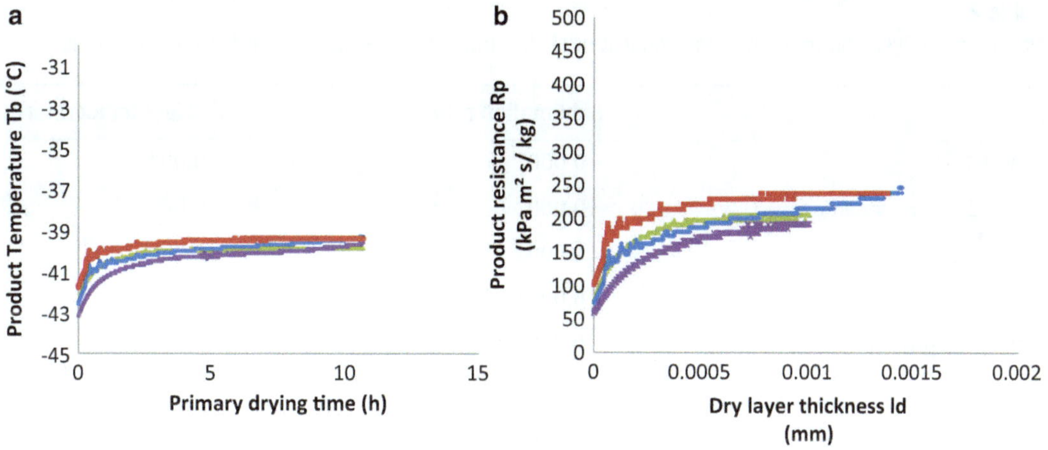

Fig. 6 Measured signal of the wireless temperature probes in time (**a**), which was used for the calculation of the product resistance R_p in function of the dried layer thickness l_d (**b**)

4.4 Evaluation of K_v and R_p for the Construction of the Mechanistic Design Space

The vial heat transfer coefficient K_v was determined for 100 central vials (Fig. 5) by using the gravimetric method, as previously described [15].

The product resistance was estimated from the product temperature measured by using the signals of two temperature sensors placed in central vials during a freeze-drying cycle performed in the GT6 pilot scale freeze-dryer at 6 Pa and −32 °C, as reported in Sect. 3.2.2. The evolution of the product resistance as a function of the dried layer thickness for the considered product is shown in Fig. 6 for two central vials and two repetitions of the cycle. An average product resistance of 213 kPa s m^2 kg^{-1} (for $l_d = 0.001$ m) was considered for the construction of the design space.

4.5 Statistical Model Optimization

ANOVA results are shown in Table 2 for the two CPPs (sublimation rate $\dot{m}$ and bottom product temperature T_b). As can be seen, the full quadratic model (i.e., including all simple effects, quadratic effects, and two-way interactions) is highly significant (p-value < 0.001) and can be considered for response surface analysis. Model prediction reliability is also confirmed by the plot of predictions against measured values in Fig. 7. The adjusted R^2 and the R^2 of predictions for both models are shown in Fig. 7. The adjusted R^2 measures the quality of fit of the model, adjusted with respect to the number of parameters included in the model. The prediction R^2 measures how close the predictions are from their observed values. In our case, prediction and adjusted R^2 for the T_b and $\dot{m}$ parameters are equal to 0.86 and 0.72, respectively. These values were considered sufficiently high for the studied purpose. There is a higher variability between vials for the $\dot{m}$ measurements, which explains the lower R^2 values and the higher dispersion of points around the trending regression line.

Table 2
Variance analysis table of the statistical model, the operating variables and their interactions

	Sublimation rate	Product temperature
Model	<0.0001	<0.0001
A—Chamber pressure	<0.0001	<0.0001
B—Shelf temperature	<0.0001	<0.0001
C—Freezing rate	<0.0001	<0.0001
D—Vials position	<0.0001	<0.0001
AB	0.002929	<0.0001
AC	<0.0001	<0.0001
AD	<0.0001	<0.0001
BC	0.001769	<0.0001
BD	<0.0001	<0.0001
CD	<0.0001	0.844245[a]
A^2	<0.0001	<0.0001
B^2	0.05691	<0.0001
C^2	<0.0001	<0.0001

[a]Interaction CD for product temperature is not significant and was not considered in the model development

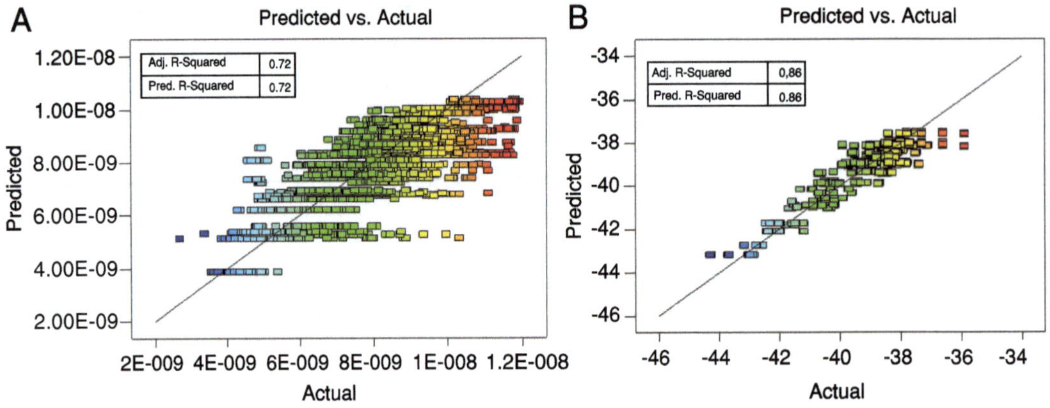

Fig. 7 Predictions against observed values of the sublimation rate (**A**) and product temperature (**B**)

4.6 Response Surface Analysis for Product Temperature and Sublimation Rate

The response surface generated by the statistical model described in the previous section is shown in Fig. 8 for the product temperature (T_b) and in Fig. 9 for the sublimation rate ($\dot{m}$), considering edge and central vials at freezing rates of 0.5 and 7 °C min^{-1}. Increasing freezing rate from 0.5 to 7 °C min^{-1} would generally cause product temperature to rise (sublimation cooling effect decreased for samples with high freezing rate), probably because smaller ice crystals

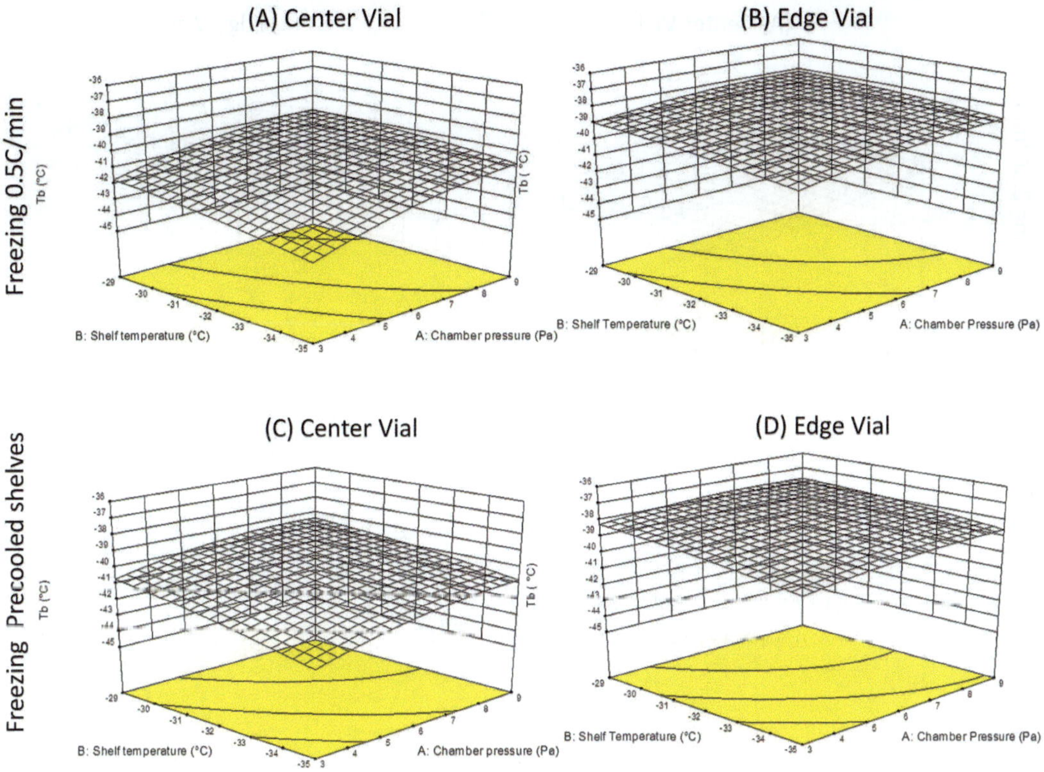

Fig. 8 Response surface generated by the statistical model for product temperature for low (**A**, **B**) and high freezing rate (**C**, **D**) and for one central (**A**, **C**) and one edge vial (**B**, **D**)

are formed and dry layer resistance R_p increases. This hypothesis can be confirmed by the observation of the sublimation rate (Fig. 9) that tends to decrease under the same conditions. Increasing shelf temperature and pressure results in an increase of the product temperature and sublimation rate (higher heat transfer due to additional conduction between shelf and vial bottom and additional gas conduction in the chamber).

The same information is also shown for front edge vials in Figs. 8 and 9. Furthermore, edge vials are warmer than center vials (radiation and additional gas conduction effect) and sublimate faster [16, 17].

4.7 Design Space

Figure 10 shows an example of a two-dimensional design space of primary drying for a pilot freeze-dryer obtained by using (Fig. 10A) the statistical model and (Fig. 10B) the mechanistic model for center vials at the highest freezing rate (7 °C min^{-1} obtained by precooled shelves), thus representing the conditions associated with high risk of product collapse.

The statistical design space was constructed by superimposing the two response surfaces taken from product temperature and sublimation rate for a high freezing rate and center vials, whereas

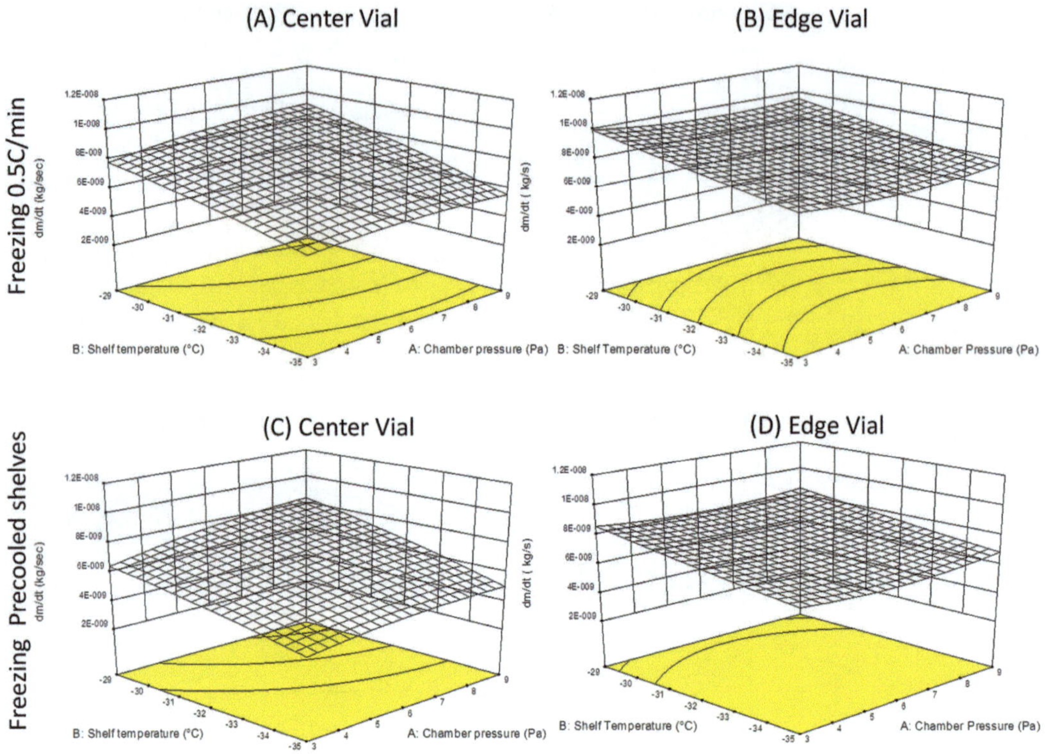

Fig. 9 Response surface generated by the statistical model for sublimation rate for low (**A**, **B**) and high freezing rate (**C**, **D**) and for one central (**A**, **C**) and one edge vial (**B**, **D**)

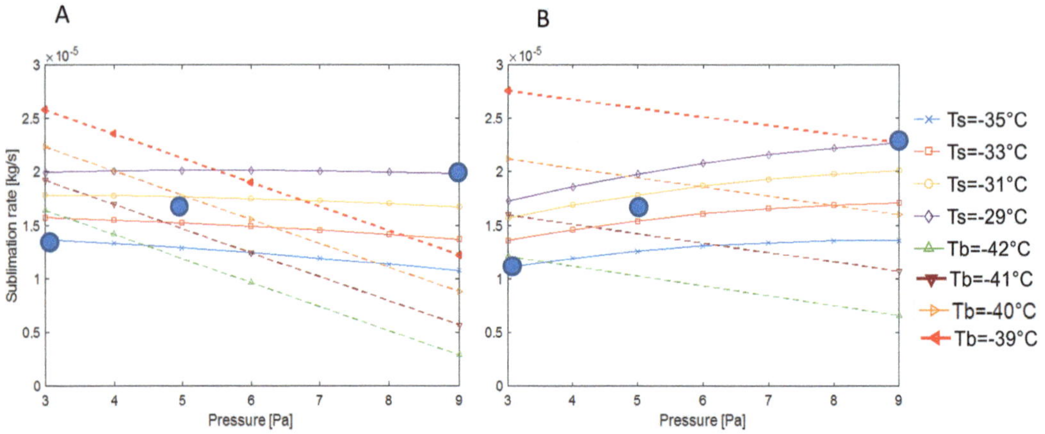

Fig. 10 (**A**) mechanistic design space. (**B**) statistical design space, for the considered product at a high freezing rate. T_B is the product temperature, T_s is the shelf temperature

the mechanistic design space was calculated from the model proposed by Pikal [26]. In agreement with previous works [8, 35], both design spaces show that the sublimation rate and the product temperature tend to decrease as the shelf temperature and chamber pressure decrease. As a consequence, the use of a very low shelf temperature (e.g., −40 °C, Fig. 10B) results in a very low product temperature and low vapor pressure at the sublimation interface. However, if the vapor pressure becomes lower than the chamber pressure, the sublimation cannot take place. For this reason, the sublimation rate tends to decrease at very low shelf temperature as the chamber pressure increases. This observation, confirmed by a previous work of Bhatnagar et al. [36], is visible in the mechanistic design space in Fig. 10B. In contrast, the same trend is not observed with the statistical design space where experimental data show that sublimation rate reaches a plateau in the same conditions (Fig. 10a).

At defined shelf temperature and pressure, the sublimation rate calculated by using the statistical and mechanistic model (Fig. 10A, B) is quite similar. However, differences can be observed for the estimated product temperature, which is lower with the statistical design space. This discrepancy can be explained by the different methods used for the estimation of T_b. In the mechanistic design space, the product temperature was calculated from a local value of the sublimation rate determined from the R_p value at l_d equal to 0.001 m (Fig. 6). This value corresponds to the highest estimated T_b in primary drying before losing the accuracy of the R_p calculation. In contrast, in the statistical design space, product temperature measured at 20–30% of the cycle time was considered.

A product temperature of −37.5 °C was considered for the definition of the safe area in the design space, since the collapse temperature of the considered formulation was −37.4 °C. In this case study, the maximum allowed product temperature was the main critical boundary considered for the design space given that the pilot equipment capability was found to be very high (Fig. 11A, B).

4.8 Robustness Study at Pilot Scale

Based on the statistical and mechanistic design space (Fig. 10 A, B) obtained for this formulation, the parameters reported in Table 3 were selected for the robustness study at pilot scale. Moreover, a fast freezing rate was selected for the design space, since better potency and stability of the vaccine, formulated with model formulation components, was achieved post-lyophilization using such process parameters.

The pilot scale freeze-dryer was fully loaded with 2700 vials and sublimation was monitored with the Lyotrack instrument (Fig. 12) [32].

The results are presented in Tables 4 and 5, and show that consistent residual moisture was obtained using the selected process parameters. Elegant pharmaceutical appearance was observed for standard and low worst case cycle whereas samples of the high

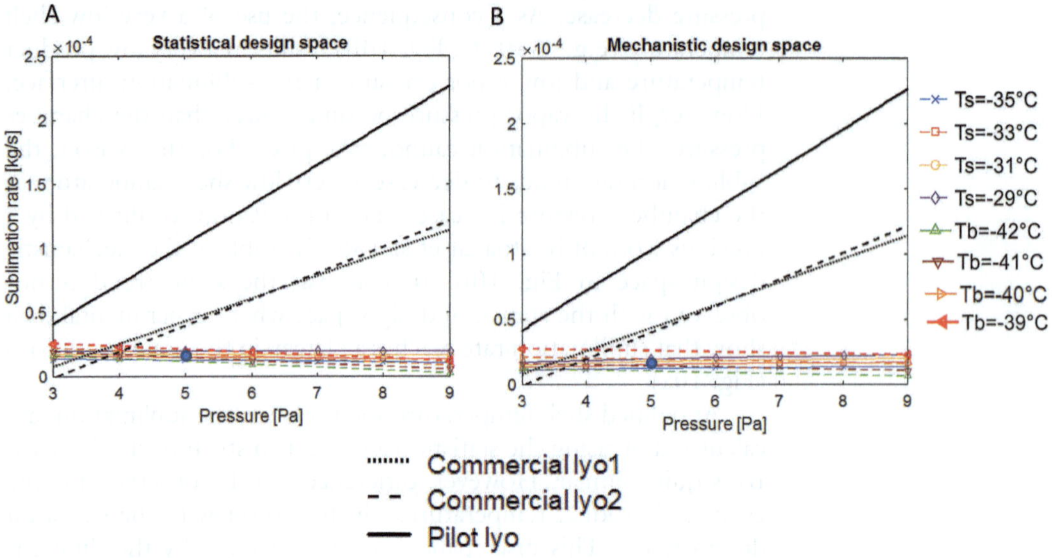

Fig. 11 (**A**) Statistical design space. (**B**) mechanistic design space, for the considered product at a high freezing rate plotted with the equipment capability curve. T_b is the product temperature, T_s is the shelf temperature. The equipment capability refers to the commercial and pilot scale freeze-dryers used in the study (lyo 1 and 2, respectively). The spot at 5 Pa corresponds to the process parameters selected for the cycle to be transferred to the commercial scale equipment

Table 3
Selection of operating variables to establish the process acceptable range of the primary drying phase of the freeze-drying cycle based on the estimations of the design spaces

	Freezing rate (°C min^{-1})	Shelf temperature (°C)	Pressure (Pa)	Estimated product temperature with mechanistic design space (°C)	Estimated product temperature with statistical design space (°C)
Low temperature low pressure	7	−35	3	−43	−42
Standard cycle (mid temperature mid pressure)	7	−32	5	−40.5	−40.5
High temperature high pressure	7	−29	9	−37.5	−39

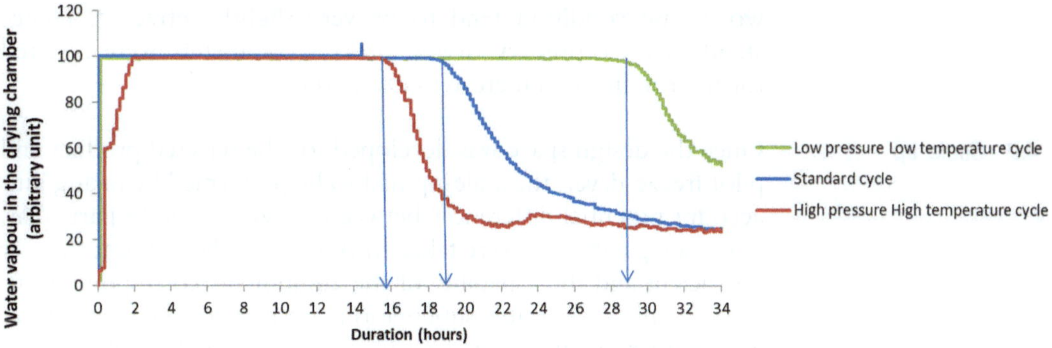

Fig. 12 Lyotrack curves obtained during the robustness study at pilot scale

Table 4
Duration of the sublimation step and final moisture content obtained at pilot scale

	Sublimation time (full saturation of the chamber) (h)	Moisture content (%) Edge front vials ($n = 10$)	Moisture content (%) Central vials ($n = 10$)
Low temperature low pressure	29	1.74 (±0.58)	1.46 (±0.05)
Standard cycle (mid temperature mid pressure)	19	1.33 (±0.05)	0.95 (±0.05)
High temperature high pressure	15	1.58 (±0.18)	1.15 (±0.10)

Sublimation was carried at full saturation of the chamber

Table 5
Visual aspect of the freeze-dried cakes (edge and central vials) obtained from the robustness study at pilot scale for different cycles

	Visual appearance edge front vials	Visual appearance center vials
Low temperature/low pressure	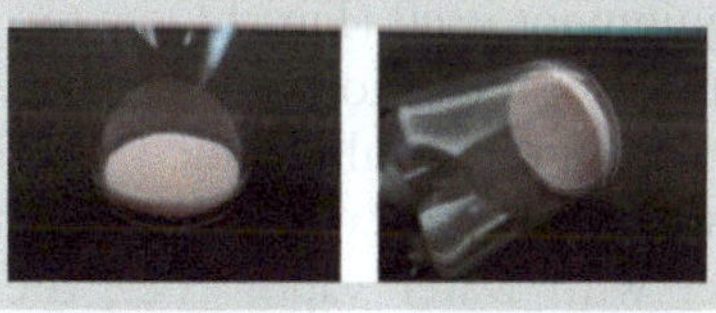	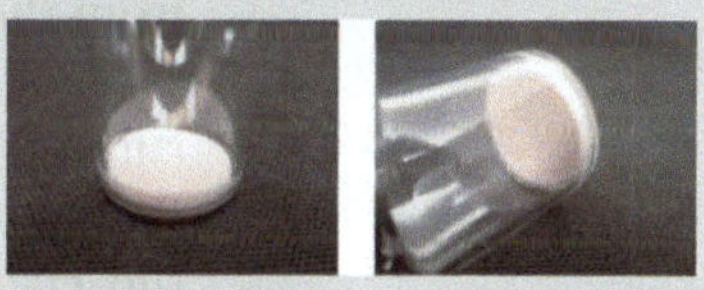
Mid temperature/mid pressure	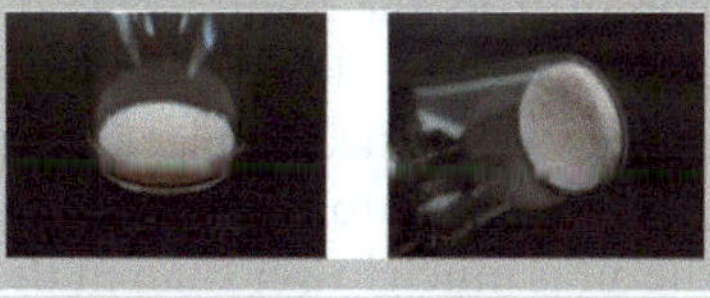	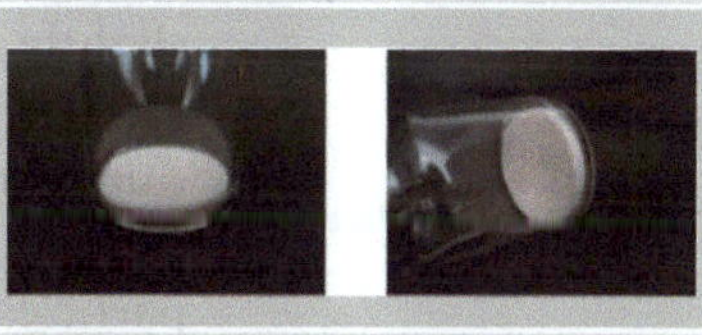
High temperature/high pressure	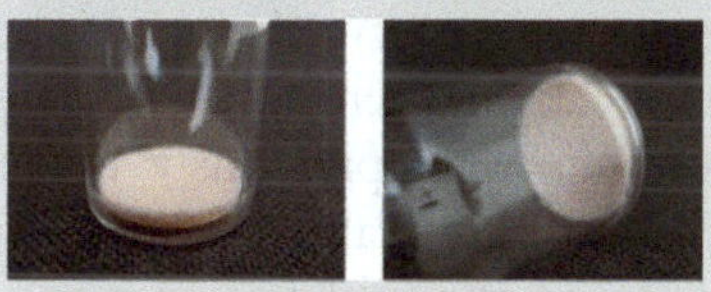	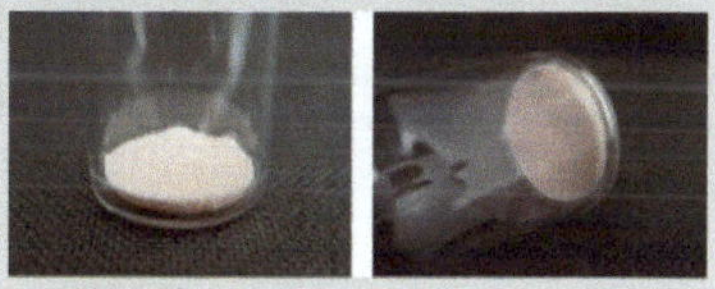

worst case condition tend to be very slightly retracted. Hence standard cycle primary drying process parameters were selected for the run in a commercial freeze-dryer.

4.9 Scale-Up

Once the design space was developed for the selected product and pilot freeze-dryer, the scale-up had to be performed by taking into account potential differences between freeze-dryers. In particular, two main parameters were taken into account: the vial heat transfer coefficient and the capability of the equipment (corresponding to the maximum achievable sublimation rate at which the freeze-dryer is able to run fully loaded with water, without loss of pressure control).

Firstly, differences in the heat transfer characteristics among freeze-dryers were assessed by determining the vial heat transfer coefficient in different freeze-dryers for edge and central vials. The heat transfer coefficients evaluated at 4 Pa for central vials were found to be similar in both pilot and commercial freeze-dryers, as shown in Fig. 13A. The vial heat transfer coefficient determined in edge vials (vials marked with letters E in Fig. 5) at pilot scale is shown in Fig. 13B and appears to be higher than central vials due to the additional radiation received from the walls of the equipment. However, similar K_v values were found at commercial scale for edge and central vials, evidencing that the edge vial effect is less important at commercial scale than at pilot scale.

In a second trial, the equipment capability was determined in the pilot and two commercial freeze-dryers using the protocol described in Searles et al. [18]. The results are shown in Fig. 14 for three different chamber pressures. The maximum allowable sublimation rate increased at higher pressure, as expected [18, 37]. Furthermore, commercial freeze-dryers showed a lower capability than the pilot dryer. In the present case study, the parameters of the cycle to be transferred to the manufacturing scale were selected below the capability to guarantee a low risk of failure from the equipment itself (Fig. 11).

Following K_v evaluation and capability testing, an industrial run was carried out in a fully loaded freeze-dryer equipped with a Pirani probe. Results indicated that the period of full saturation of the chamber with water vapor (i.e., the sublimation time) was slightly longer than in the pilot freeze-dryer (23 h vs. 19 h) for primary drying (data not shown). This difference may be mainly due to the supercooling taking place during freezing being more pronounced in a production environment where the number of particles in the air is much lower than in the development area. This can lead to smaller ice crystal size, higher product resistance to sublimation rate, and thereby to a longer sublimation process. Such observations were previously made by Searles et al. [38] who showed experimentally that the higher the supercooling degree is, the lower the sublimation rate would be.

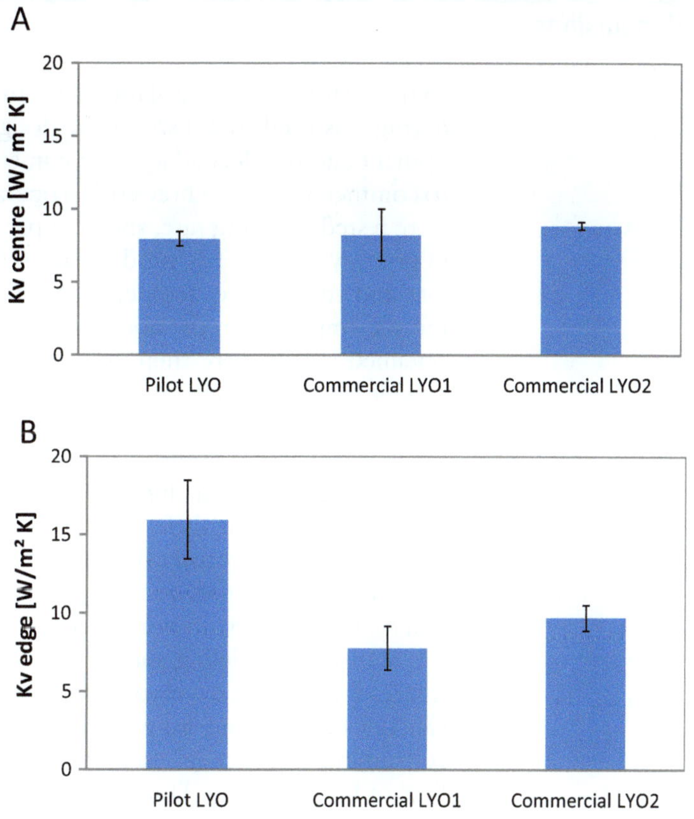

Fig. 13 Kv for central (**A**) and edge (**B**) vials. Note that Kv edge was evaluated from data at −40 °C at pilot scale, and at −25 °C at commercial scale

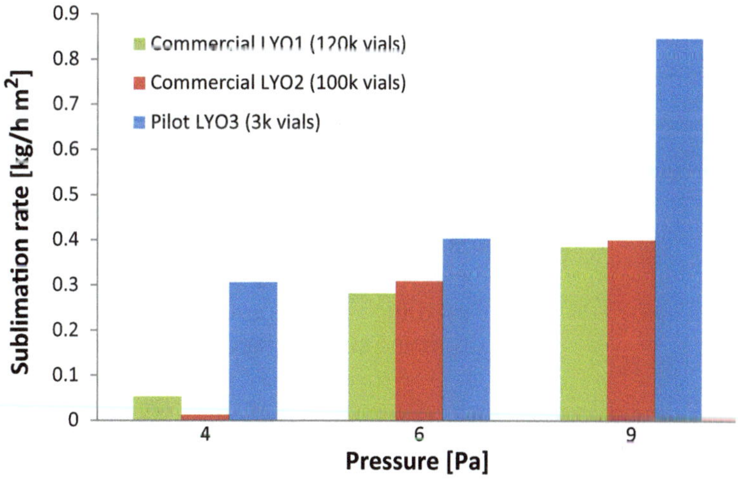

Fig. 14 Equipment capabilities in two commercial scales and one pilot scale freeze-dryer (lyo 1, 2 and 3, respectively)

5 Conclusions

In this chapter, a statistical model for the sublimation step in freeze-drying was used to construct the design space for the cycle development and to select adequate parameters for scaling up from pilot to commercial scale. Three critical operating variables of the process were tested: freezing rate, shelf temperature, and chamber pressure in primary drying. The model was used to predict the sublimation rate and the product temperature, since their selection is of paramount importance to obtain a product of high quality. The obtained results were then used to define the design space of the product at pilot scale. In order to validate this approach, a design space was calculated by using the mechanistic model classically proposed in the literature [26]. The two design spaces showed a good agreement with slightly higher estimated product temperature with the mechanistic method. The design space calculated for vials located in the center of the shelf was then used to perform the scale-up from pilot to commercial scale, as the "edge vial effect" was found to be less important at commercial scale.

Statistical modeling should be used with accurate PAT for the freeze-drying cycle development. This methodology has the disadvantage of requiring numerous experiments which can be time-consuming but can be easily performed by a non-expert in the field of freeze-drying. During the validation of the selected process parameters for process scale-up, vial heat transfer estimation both at pilot and commercial scale is essential. In our study, close values of heat transfer for center vials were indeed observed between the different pilot and manufacturing freeze-dryers. Some adaptations of the design space would be needed if higher or lower values of heat transfer coefficient were observed. In that case, the statistical design space would represent a less efficient process, since all characterization would have been done in the pilot freeze-dryer. Mechanistic design space appears to be more attractive since fewer experiments are required (for the estimation vial heat transfer and product resistance) and changes of scale are taken into account. However, the method used to measure the product resistance experimentally has to be selected with care, since the value of R_p used for calculation can greatly affect the sublimation rate estimation and the product temperature.

Acknowledgments

The authors would like to thank Yves Mayeresse and Benoît Moreau (Manufacturing Science and Technology Belgium, GSK) for reviewing this work and Vincent Ronsse, Olivier Despas and Alain Philippart (Technical Research and Development, Belgium) for all the experimental work performed for this project.

Conflict of Interest: Erwan Bourlès, Gael De Lannoy and Bernadette Scutella are employees of the GSK group of companies. Stephanie Passot, Fernanda Fonseca, and Ioan Cristian Trelea report no financial conflicts of interest.

Funding: This work was funded by GlaxoSmithKline Biologicals S. A., under a Cooperative Research and Development Agreement with INRA (Institut National de la Recherche Agronomique) via the intermediary of the UMR (Unité Mixte de Recherche) GMPA (Génie et Microbiologie des Procédés Alimentaires) at the INRA Versailles-Grignon research centre.

Author Contributions: All authors were involved in the conception of the model and design of the study. Erwan Bourlès acquired the data. Erwan Bourlès Bernadette Scutellà, Stephanie Passot, Fernanda Fonseca, and Ioan Cristian Trelea analyzed and interpreted the experimental results. Erwan Bourles, Gael de Lannoy, Bernadette Scutellà, Stephanie Passot, Fernanda Fonseca, and Ioan Cristian Trelea were involved in the model development. All authors were involved in drafting the manuscript or revising it critically for important intellectual content. All authors had full access to the data and approved the manuscript before it was submitted by the corresponding author.

References

1. Carpenter JF, Chang BS, Garzon-Rodriguez W, Randolph TW (2002) Rational design of stable lyophilized protein formulations: theory and practice. In: Carpenter JF, Manning MC (eds) Rational design of stable protein formulations: theory and practice. Springer, Boston, MA
2. Hansen LJJ, Daoussi R, Vervaet C, Remon JP, De Beer TRM (2015) Freeze-drying of live virus vaccines: a review. Vaccine 33:5507–5519
3. Franks F (1998) Freeze-drying of bioproducts: putting principles into practice. Eur J Pharm Biopharm 45:221–229
4. Jennings TA (1999) Lyophilization: Introduction and Basic Principles. Interpharm Press, Denver, CO
5. Passot S, Trelea IC, Marin M, Fonseca F (2010) The relevance of thermal properties for improving formulation and cycle development: application to freeze-drying of proteins. In: Rey L, May JC (eds) Freeze drying/lyophilization of pharmaceutical and biological products. Informa Healthcare, New York, NY
6. Rexroad J, Wiethoff CM, Jones LS, Middaugh CR (2002) Lyophilization and the thermostability of vaccines. Cell Preserv Technol 1:91–104
7. Cao E, Chen Y, Cui Z, Foster PR (2003) Effect of freezing and thawing rates on denaturation of proteins in aqueous solutions. Biotechnol Bioeng 82:684–690
8. Chang BS, Kendrick BS, Carpenter JF (1996) Surface-induced denaturation of proteins during freezing and its inhibition by surfactants. J Pharm Sci 85:1325–1330
9. Pikal MJ, Shah S (1990) The collapse temperature in freeze drying: dependence on measurement methodology and rate of water removal from the glassy phase. Int J Pharm 62:165–186
10. Johnson R, Lewis L (2011) Freeze-drying protein formulations above their collapse temperatures: possible issues and concerns. Am Pharm Rev 14:50–54
11. Rambhatla S, Obert JP, Luthra S, Bhugra C, Pikal MJ (2005) Cake shrinkage during freeze drying: a combined experimental and theoretical study. Pharm Dev Technol 10:33–40
12. Fonseca F, Passot S, Cunin O, Marin M (2004) Collapse temperature of freeze-dried Lactobacillus bulgaricus suspensions and protective media. Biotechnol Prog 20:229–238
13. Hibler S, Gieseler H (2012) Heat transfer characteristics of current primary packaging systems for pharmaceutical freeze-drying. J Pharm Sci 101:4025–4031
14. Pikal MJ, Roy ML, Shah S (1984) Mass and heat transfer in vial freeze-drying of pharmaceuticals: role of the vial. J Pharm Sci 73:1224
15. Scutellà B, Passot S, Bourlès E, Fonseca F, Trelea IC (2017a) How vial geometry variability influences heat transfer and product

temperature during freeze-drying. J Pharm Sci 106:770–778

16. Scutellà B, Plana-Fattori A, Passot S, Bourlès E, Fonseca F, Flick D, Tréléa IC (2017b) 3D mathematical modelling to understand atypical heat transfer observed in vial freeze-drying. Appl Therm Eng 126:226–236
17. Rambhatla S, Pikal MJ (2003) Heat and mass transfer scale-up issues during freeze-drying, I: atypical radiation and the edge vial effect. AAPS PharmSciTech 4:E14
18. Searles JA (2010) Optimizing the throughput of freeze-dryers within a constrained design space. In: Rey L, May JC (eds) Freeze-drying/lyophilization of pharmaceutical and biological products. 3rd edition. Informa Healthcare, New York, NY
19. Pisano R, Fissore D, Barresi AA, Rastelli M (2013) Quality by design: scale-up of freeze-drying cycles in pharmaceutical industry. AAPS PharmSciTech 14:1137–1149
20. Tchessalov S, Dixon D, Warne NW (2007) Principles of lyophilization cycle scale-up. Am Pharm Rev 10:88–92
21. Yu LX (2008) Pharmaceutical quality by design: product and process development, understanding, and control. Pharm Res 25:781–791
22. FDA (2009) Guidance for industry, Q8 (R2) pharmaceutical development. Food and Drug Administration U.S. Dept. of Health and Human Services, Center for Drug Evaluation and Research, Rockville, MD
23. Mockus LN, Paul TW, Pease NA, Harper NJ, Basu PK, Oslos EA, Sacha GA, Kuu WY, Hardwick LM, Karty JJ, Pikal MJ, Hee E, Khan MA, Nail SL (2011) Quality by design in formulation and process development for a freeze-dried, small molecule parenteral product: a case study. Pharm Dev Technol 16:549–576
24. Van Bockstal PJ, Mortier S, Corver J, Nopens I, Gernaey KV, De Beer T (2017) Quantitative risk assessment via uncertainty analysis in combination with error propagation for the determination of the dynamic Design Space of the primary drying step during freeze-drying. Eur J Pharm Biopharm 121:32–41
25. Box GEP, Hunter WG, Hunter JS (2005) Statistics for experimenters: design, innovation, and discovery, 2nd edn. Wiley-Blackwell, New York, NY
26. Pikal MJ (1985) Use of laboratory data in freeze drying process design: heat and mass transfer coefficients and the computer simulation of freeze drying. PDA J Pharm Sci Technol 39:115–139
27. Pikal MJ (2000) Heat and mass transfer in low pressure gases: applications to freeze drying. In: Lee PI, Amidon GL, Topp EM (eds) Transport processes in pharmaceutical systems. CRC Press, New York, NY
28. Scutellà B, Cristian Trelea I, Bourlès E, Fonseca F, Passot S (2018) Determination of the dried product resistance variability and its influence on the product temperature in pharmaceutical freeze-drying. Eur J Pharm Biopharm 128:379
29. Schneid S, Gieseler H (2008) Evaluation of a new wireless temperature remote interrogation system (TEMPRIS) to measure product temperature during freeze drying. AAPS PharmSciTech 9:729–739
30. Nail S, Tchessalov S, Shalaev E, Ganguly A, Renzi E, Dimarco F, Wegiel L, Ferris S, Kessler W, Pikal M, Sacha G, Alexeenko A, Thompson TN, Reiter C, Searles J, Coiteux P (2017) Recommended best practices for process monitoring instrumentation in pharmaceutical freeze drying-2017. AAPS PharmSciTech 18:2379–2393
31. Patel SM, Pikal M (2009) Process analytical technologies (PAT) in freeze-drying of parenteral products. Pharm Dev Technol 14:567–587
32. Mayeresse Y, Veillon R, Sibille P, Nomine C (2007) Freeze-drying process monitoring using a cold plasma ionization device. PDA J Pharm Sci Technol 61:160–174
33. Passot S, Fonseca F, Barbouche N, Marin M, Alarcon-Lorca M, Rolland D, Rapaud M (2007) Effect of product temperature during primary drying on the long-term stability of lyophilized proteins. Pharm Dev Technol 12:543–553
34. Chang BS, Randall CS (1992) Use of subambient thermal analysis to optimize protein lyophilization. Cryobiology 29:632–656
35. Patel SM, Pikal MJ (2013) Lyophilization process design space. J Pharm Sci 102:3883–3887
36. Bhatnagar BS, Bogner RH, Pikal MJ (2007) Protein stability during freezing: separation of stresses and mechanisms of protein stabilization. Pharm Dev Technol 12:505–523
37. Patel SM, Chaudhuri S, Pikal MJ (2010) Choked flow and importance of Mach I in freeze-drying process design. Chem Eng Sci 65:5716–5727
38. Searles JA, Carpenter JF, Randolph TW (2001) The ice nucleation temperature determines the primary drying rate of lyophilization for samples frozen on a temperature-controlled shelf. J Pharm Sci 90:860–871

Chapter 11

Through Vial Impedance Spectroscopy (TVIS): A Novel Approach to Process Understanding for Freeze-Drying Cycle Development

Geoff Smith and Evgeny Polygalov

Abstract

Through vial impedance spectroscopy (TVIS) provides a new process analytical technology for monitoring a development scale lyophilization process, which exploits the changes in the bulk electrical properties that occur on freezing and subsequent drying of a drug solution. Unlike the majority of uses of impedance spectroscopy, for freeze-drying process development, the electrodes do not contact the product but are attached to the outside of the glass vial which is used to contain the product to provide a non-sample-invasive monitoring technology. Impedance spectra (in frequency range 10 Hz to 1 MHz) are generated throughout the drying cycle by a specially designed impedance spectrometer based on a 1 GΩ trans-impedance amplifier and then displayed in terms of complex capacitance. Typical capacitance spectra have one or two peaks in the imaginary capacitance (i.e., the dielectric loss) and the same number of steps in the real part capacitance (i.e., the dielectric permittivity). This chapter explores the underlying mechanisms that are responsible for these dielectric processes, i.e., the Maxwell-Wagner (space charge) polarization of the glass wall of the vial through the contents of the vial when in the liquid state, and the dielectric relaxation of ice when in the frozen state. In future work, it will be demonstrated how to measure product temperature and drying rates within single vials and multiple (clusters) of vials, from which other critical process parameters, such as heat transfer coefficient and dry layer resistance, may be determined.

Key words Impedance spectroscopy, Process-analytical-technology, PAT, Freeze-drying, Lyophilization, Maxwell-Wagner, Polarization, Dielectric relaxation, Ice

Abbreviations

ADC Analog digital converter
AWG American wire gauge
BDS Broadband dielectric spectroscopy
DAQ Data acquisition card
DSC Differential scanning calorimetry
DTA Differential thermal analysis
ER Electrical resistivity measurements

Kevin R. Ward and Paul Matejtschuk (eds.), *Lyophilization of Pharmaceuticals and Biologicals: New Technologies and Approaches*, Methods in Pharmacology and Toxicology, https://doi.org/10.1007/978-1-4939-8928-7_11,

ETA	Electrical thermal analysis
FDM	Freeze drying microscope
IS	Impedance spectroscopy
IVC	Current to voltage converter
MW	Maxwell-Wagner polarization process
OUT	Object under test
TSC	Thermally stimulated current spectroscopy
TVIS	Through vial impedance spectroscopy

Symbols

–	Series arrangement of two elements in an electrical circuit
C'	Real part capacitance or dielectric storage of complex capacitance
C''	Imaginary part capacitance or dielectric loss of complex capacitance
$C'(\infty)$	Real part capacitance at high frequency
C''_{PEAK}	Peak amplitude of the imaginary capacitance
C'_{fit}	Real part capacitance from equivalent circuit modelling
C''_{fit}	Imaginary part capacitance from equivalent circuit modelling
C_{a}	Capacitance of adhesive layer
$C_{\mathrm{a-g}}$	Capacitance of the composite glass wall and adhesive layer in series
$C_{\mathrm{a-G}}$	Total capacitance of the composite glass wall and adhesive layer in series
C_{g}	Capacitance of glass-sample interface
C_{G}	Total glass-sample interface capacitance
C_{i}	Capacitance of the interfacial layer between glass and sample
C_{o}	Capacitance of empty cell
C_{s}	Capacitance of sample
$C_{\mathrm{s}}(\infty)$	Capacitance of sample in the limit of high frequency
$C_{\mathrm{s}}(0)$	Capacitance of sample in the limit of low frequency
$C_{\mathrm{s}}(f)$	Capacitance of sample as a function of frequency
$\mathrm{CPE_G}$	Constant phase element of glass wall
$C'_{\mathrm{fit}}(\infty)$	Real part capacitance from modelling at high frequency
$C'_{\mathrm{fit}}(f)$	Real part capacitance from modelling as the function of frequency
$C'_{\mathrm{fit}}(o)$	Real part capacitance from modelling at low frequency
$\mathrm{DE_s}$	Distribution element of sample
F_{PEAK}	Peak frequency of the imaginary capacitance
I_{o}	Current amplitude
Q_{o}	Admittance of a constant phase element at an angular frequency of $\omega = 1$ rad s^{-1}
R_{s}	Resistance of sample
T_{c}	Collapse temperature
T_{eu}	Eutectic temperature
T_{g}	Glass transition temperature
T'_{g}	Glass transition of the maximally freeze concentrated solution
T_{m}	Melting temperature
T_{b}	Ice temperature at the base of a vial
T_{i}	Ice temperature at the sublimation interface
V_{o}	Voltage amplitude
$\lvert\Upsilon\rvert$	Admittance magnitude

Υ_{C}	Admittance of a capacitor
Υ_{CPE}	Admittance of a constant phase element
Υ_{R}	Admittance of a resistor
Z'	Real part impedance
Z''	Imaginary part impedance
Z^*	Complex impedance
Z_{C}	Impedance of capacitance
Z_{CPE}	Impedance of constant phase element
Z_{R}	Impedance of resistance
d_{g}	Glass wall thickness
k_{g}	Cell constant of glass
k_{s}	Cell constant of sample
ε_{∞}	Permittivity in the limit of high frequency
ε_{a}	Permittivity of adhesive
ε_{g}	Permittivity of glass
ε_{o}	Permittivity of free space
ε_{r}	Relative permittivity
ε_{s}	Static permittivity
ρ_{s}	Sample resistivity
ω_{c}	Angular frequency at cross over between the dominance of two circuit elements
$\|Z\| \sin\varphi$	Imaginary part of the complex impedance or reactance
$\|Z\|$	Impedance magnitude
$=$	Parallel arrangement of two elements in an electrical circuit
$\Delta C'$	Increment in the real part capacitance
C	Capacitance
h	Electrode height
I/O	Input/output
N	A number of sine wave periods
Ø	Fill factor in relation to the electrode height
R	Resistance
α	Exponent parameter describing the broadening of a dispersion process
ρ	Density
A	Electrode area
CPE	Constant phase element
I	Current
V	Voltage
Υ	Admittance
Z	Impedance
d	Separation of two electrodes
f	Frequency
i	Notation for an imaginary number
k	Cell constant
p	Frequency independent parameter (CPE exponent) which corresponds to the phase angle
t	Time
w	Electrode width
τ	Time constant or relaxation time
φ	Phase difference between the voltage and current
ω	Angular frequency
ϑ	Phase angle

Units

°	Degree
°C	Degree Celsius
dB	Decibel
$F\ m^{-1}$	Farad per meter
fF	Femtofarad
g	Gram
$g\ cm^{-3}$	Gram per cubic centimeters
GΩ	Gigaohm or 10^9 ohm
Hz	Hertz
K	Kelvin
$kg\ m^{-3}$	Kilogram per cubic meters
kHz	Kilohertz or 10^3 hertz
MHz	Megahertz or 10^6 Hertz
min	Minute
mL	Milliliter
mm	Millimeter
mm^2	Square millimeter
ms	Millisecond
pF	picoFarad
$rad\ s^{-1}$	radians per second
s	Second
V	Volt
μs	Microsecond
Ω	Ohm

1 Introduction

A study of the electrical impedance of materials has been used for many years for the investigation of various processes associated with freeze drying. However, in the main, these studies have been restricted to the determination of critical temperatures. In one of the earliest reports, Greaves [1] monitored the crystallization process through the measurement of changes in electrical conductivity at a single excitation frequency of an applied AC voltage. The basis for this assessment is that the formation of ice, within a solution, increases the viscosity while reducing the volume of the unfrozen (i.e., non-ice) fraction; and as a consequence the mobility of the ionic species within the unfrozen fraction decreases which in turn is reflected in a reduction of the measured electrical conductivity. Some years later, similar measurements were used to determine the eutectic temperature of a solution by measuring the electric resistance as a function of the temperature of a frozen material on reheating [2–4]. A number of other authors have followed suit by using electrical thermal analysis techniques to measure the eutectic

Table 1
Eutectic temperature (T_{eu}) of various materials

	T_{eu} (°C)		
Test samples	**ETA**	**DTA/DSC**	**References**
$CaCl_2$	−54.0		[5]
KBr	−12.9		[3]
KCl	−11.1		[3]
Lactose	−5.4		[3]
Mannitol	−24.0 −5.0 −2.24	−22.0 −2.0	[6] [7] [3]
Methylphenidate HCl	−11.7		[3]
Methylphenidate HCl with Lactose	−11.9		[3]
Methylphenidate HCl with mannitol	−11.7		[3]
Methylphenidate methanesulfonate	−10.1		[3]
Methylphenidate phosphate	−4.29		[3]
NaCl	−21.0 −21.6 −21.6 −21.5	−20.9 −21.6	[7] [3] [8] [4]
Phentolamine HCl	−1.3		[3]
Phentolamine methanesulfonate	−11.0		[3]
Phentolamine phosphate	−0.75		[3]

ETA (electrical thermal analysis) is a generic term for a number of techniques that measure the electrical properties of a material as a function of temperature, including electrical resistivity measurements (ER), broadband dielectric spectroscopy (BDS), thermally stimulated current spectroscopy (TSC), and impedance spectroscopy (IS)
DTA (differential thermal analysis) and DSC (differential scanning calorimetry) are thermal analysis techniques typically used for the determination of phase transitions

temperatures (T_{eu}) of salts, sugars, and the occasional drug substance (Table 1). The basis for the assessment is that the resistance of a solidified frozen mass suddenly decreases when the temperature is heated through the eutectic temperature, but this time as a consequence of the increased mobility of ions which results from a combination of reduced viscosity and increased volume of the non-crystalline (liquid) fraction. Single frequency measurements have also been widely employed for off-line characterization of the glass transition temperature (T_g) and/or collapse temperature (T_c) of a number of pharmaceutical relevant excipients such as sugars, polymers salt solutions, and proteins (Table 2).

Table 2
Critical temperatures T_g' and T_c of various materials

	T_g' (°C)		T_c (°C)		
Test samples	**ETA**	**DTA/DSC**	**ETA**	**FDM**	**References**
Azactam™			−17.7	−17.0	[9]
Dextran 8.8K	−14.2	−16.5			[10]
Dextran 39.1K	−13.2	−15.4			[10]
Dextran 70K	−13.6	−15.4			[10]
Dextran 503K	−13.0	−15.0			[10]
Dextrose (D-glucose)	−40.6	−49.5			[10]
Ficoll 70K	−22.6	−23.9			[10]
Ficoll 400K	−23.4	−23.9			[10]
Gelatin	−12.8	−14.2			[10]
Lactose	−29.5	−30.3			[5]
		−33.4			[10]
Maltodextrin	−16.0	−17.0			[11]
Mannitol	−33.7	−33.9			[10]
PVP 10K	−28.3	−32.3			[10]
PVP 30K	−22.0	−22.8		−23.0	[12]
PVP 40K	−23.5	−26.6			[10]
Sorbitol			−47.2	−45.0	[9]
	−41.6	−52.1			[10]
Sucrose		−34.0			[13]
	−32.0				[5]
			−35.0	−32.0	[9]
	−33.5	−38.7			[10]
Trehalose			−33.4	−32.0	[9]
	−31.2	−34.4			[10]

ETA (electrical thermal analysis) is a generic term for a number of techniques that measure the electrical properties of a material as a function of temperature, including electrical resistivity measurements (ER), broadband dielectric spectroscopy (BDS), thermally stimulated current spectroscopy (TSC), and impedance spectroscopy (IS)
DTA (differential thermal analysis) and DSC (differential scanning calorimetry) are thermal analysis techniques typically used for the determination of phase transitions
FDM (freeze drying microscope) is a technique for determining critical collapse temperature of freeze drying formulations

Various experimental approaches have been used for characterizing the temperature dependence of the passive electrical properties of frozen solutions, which combine an electrode system with a temperature sensor and a reheating regime from temperatures as low as −100 °C. The electrode designs range from a pair of rods to a pair of flat plates or a set of multiple inter-digitated "comb-like" electrodes mounted on a flat surface [7, 9]. In each system the temperature sensor (usually a platinum resistance thermometer) is mounted in close proximity to the electrodes. In the vast majority of these studies a single frequency voltage is applied (usually 1 kHz) and the ratio of the voltage amplitude (V_o) to the current amplitude (I_o) is used to determine the impedance magnitude ($|Z| = V_o/I_o$) and the phase difference between the two vector quantities of voltage and current is used to define the phase angle (theta, ϑ). In some studies [10] the sensor is calibrated against a known solution resistivity (or conductivity) so that the measured electrical resistance of the frozen solution may also be expressed in terms their dimensionless property (i.e., resistivity). In other studies, attempting to measure the dielectric properties of the frozen solution [9] a range of discrete frequencies are employed to construct a dielectric spectrum of the real and imaginary permittivity against the log of the frequency of the applied field.

Only a few commercial systems are available for off-line and in-line applications. Lyotherm, from Biopharma Process Systems Ltd., is an integrated electrical impedance ($|Z| \sin \varphi$) and differential thermal analyzer (DTA) designed to measure the critical temperatures associated with: (1) the glass transition of the maximally concentrated solutes (T'_g), (2) the melting of any eutectic mixture that has crystallized from solution on freezing (T_{eu}), and (3) the melting of the ice fraction (T_m). $|Z| \sin \varphi$ is the imaginary part of the complex impedance (Z^*) otherwise known as the reactance. While it is restricted to the analysis of certain critical temperatures it nevertheless highlights the unique sensitivity of impedance measurements over thermal methods for characterizing phase behavior in frozen aqueous solutions. For example, the glass transition (T'_g) of 10% w/v sucrose formulation that was determined by this technology agrees with the published value ($T'_g = -32$ °C) [5]. To the best of our knowledge, the LyoRx system (from Martin Christ GmbH) is currently the only commercially available process analytical technology, based on electrical impedance that is used for in process measurements. This system monitors the temperature of the product and its electrical resistance (at a fixed frequency of 1 kHz) to deliver the freezing/eutectic points while enabling process optimization by automatically controlling the energy supply to the individual shelves during the main drying phase, which then reduces the risk of product collapse and thawing [14]. The main drawback of LyoRx is the invasive measurement principle involving immersion of the electrodes into the sample. More recently, a new non-contact has been proposed by Alkeev et al. [15] which uses a capacitive sensor connected to a self-oscillating circuit for the purpose of monitoring the lyophilization of biological products.

2 TVIS Method

2.1 TVIS Measurement System

TVIS is a process analytical technology, for development scale application, which measures the electrical impedance spectrum of a conventional freeze-drying vial and its contents, using electrodes which are located outside the vial, hence the term "through-vial impedance spectroscopy." The technique is therefore noninvasive in the sense that the electrodes do not contact the sample.

The technology has been developed, in the first instance, with electrodes attached to the external surface of a conventional glass freeze-drying vial. To date, the majority of the published work has been undertaken on Type I glass vials (nominal capacity 10 mL) with a single pair of electrodes, 5 mm in height, and with each surrounded by a guard electrode [6, 11, 13, 16–19].

In contrast, the majority of the data presented in this chapter has been generated using Type I glass vials (nominal capacity 10 mL) with a single pair of electrodes, 10 mm in height, but without the guard electrodes that were used in previous studies (Fig. 1a). The absence of the guard electrode makes it more straightforward to attach electrodes to form the TVIS measurement vials, whereas the increased electrode height from 5 to 10 mm has the additional benefit of being able to use TVIS to measure drying rates for typical fill volumes between 2 and 3 mL.

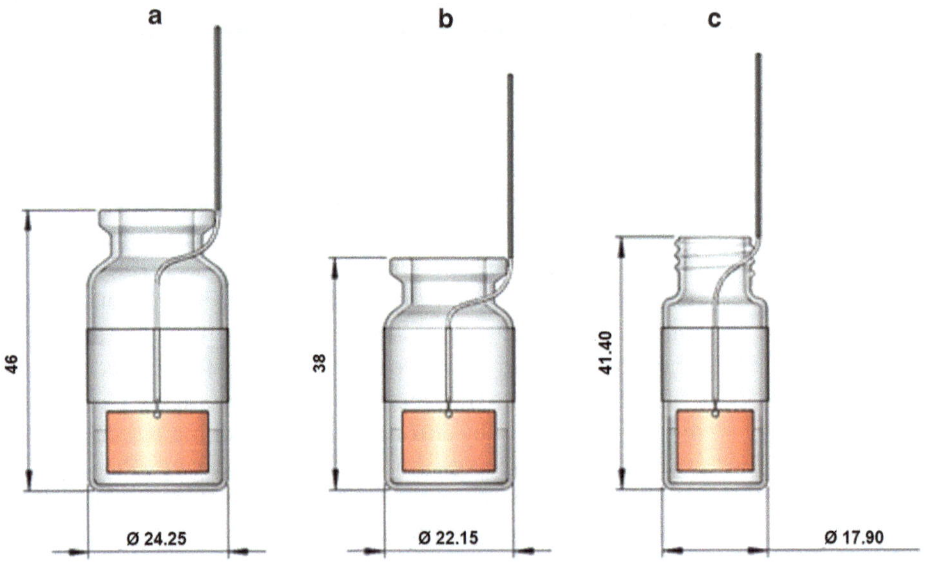

Fig. 1 Illustrations of the designs of various vials that have been modified with copper foil electrodes (10 mm in height and 3 mm from the base of each container). From left to right are non-ISO standard uncoated Type I borosilicate Fiolax® glass vials: (**a**) Adelphi VC010-20C (20 mm crimp-neck vial with 10 mL nominal capacity); (**b**) Adelphi VC005-20C (20 mm crimp-neck vial with 5 mL nominal capacity); (**c**) Adelphi VCD005 (screw-neck vial with 5 mL nominal capacity). Images have been provided courtesy of BlueFrog Design Ltd., Leicester, UK

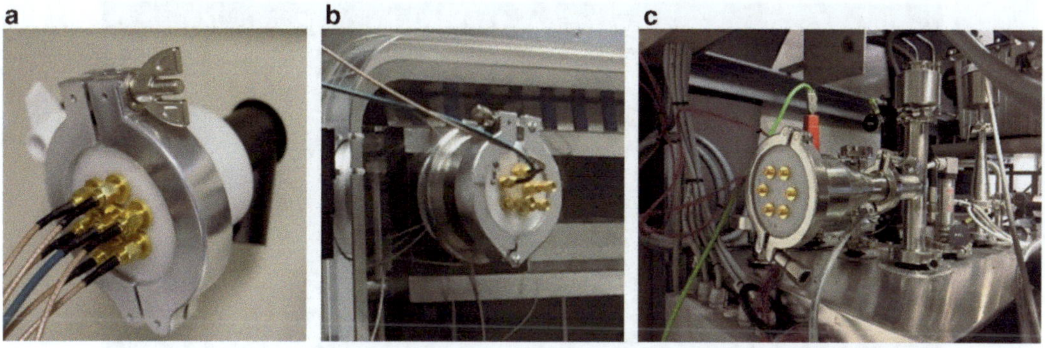

Fig. 2 Example pass-throughs for the TVIS instrument that have been deployed on a range of freeze-dryers at various institutions and companies: (**a**) Virtis Advantage Plus XL freeze-dryer (De Montfort University) in which the pass-through is connected via the manifold hose on the outside of the dryer; (**b**) Telstar LyoBeta freeze-dryer (Image courtesy of the National Institute of Biological Standards and Control) in which the pass-through is connected via the port on top left side of the door on the dryer; (**c**) GEA LYOVAC™ FCM2 LN2 pilot scale dryer (Image courtesy of GEA Lyophil GmbH) where the pass-through is connected to a port on the top of the drying chamber; Each pass-through has a minimum of six TE-connectivity-AMP SMA-jack to SMA jack bulk-head adapters (1054874-1): One adapter is used for the stimulating signal and the other five for the receiving signal. All pass-throughs were manufactured by GEA Pharma Systems (Eastleigh, UK)

Other vial types are possible (Fig. 1) with the only rule of thumb being that the combined width of the electrode pair does not occupy more than 50% of the vial circumference. The height of the electrode system, however, is variable, with the possibility for using tall electrodes which span the length of the vial. With the multichannel capability it is also possible to have multiple pairs of electrodes for predicting temperatures at the base of the ice (T_b) and at the sublimation interface (T_i).

When fitted to a commercial freeze-dryer, there is a requirement for a bespoke pass-through (Fig. 2) which carries the co-axial cabling from the impedance spectrometer, located outside the dryer, to the vial located inside the dryer.

The cabling and connections for the multichannel system, used to acquire the exemplar data for this book chapter, can be described as follows:

50 Ω 26 AWG RG316 double-shielded co-axial cables take the stimulating voltage from the analogue output (AO1) of a National Instruments PCI6110 Multi-function I/O device (inside the tower of a desk-top PC) via a National Instruments BNC 2120 connector block, to one of the TE-connectivity-AMP SMA-SMA jack adapters on the pass-through. On the inside of the dryer (i.e., on the other side of the pass-through) a 50 Ω 30 AWG RG178 co-axial cable takes the stimulating signal to a 5 way multiplexer inside the junction box (which is placed somewhere convenient within the dryer, Fig. 3). The splitter feeds the voltage, simultaneously, to five MCX coaxial stimulating ports on the top row of the junction box.

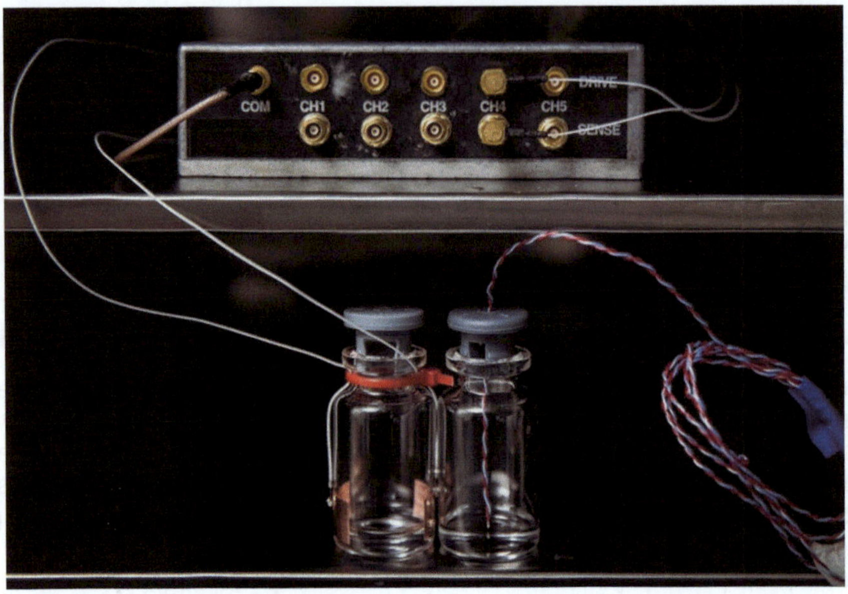

Fig. 3 *Top shelf* sits the five channel multiplexer. The COM channel receives the excitation signal from the NI DAQ PCI 6110 and distributes it to the stimulating ports on the top row of the multiplexer. The current passing through the vials (up to five in this particular system) flows through the individual receiving ports on the bottom row and then to the five channels IVC outside the freeze-dryer where the current from each vial is converted to a voltage and then passed via five channels reed relay multiplexer to the ADC input of NI DAQ PCI6110 in the computer and digitized. *Bottom shelf* (*left*) is the TVIS measurement vial. *Bottom shelf* (*right*) is a standard vial with a thermocouple inserted in the liquid such that the thermocouple bead is at a height which is equivalent to the mid-point of the volume of liquid in the region bounded by the electrodes in the TVIS vial (see Fig. 4 for an illustration)

Any one of the two fine coaxial cables from the measurement vial is then connected to one of the MCX co-axial stimulating ports on the multiplexer and the other connected to the corresponding MCX coaxial sensing port on the bottom row of the junction box via the right-angle MCX 50 Ω connector plugs (JOHNSON 133-3402-101) which terminate these cables. The coaxial cables attached to the measurement vial have an outer diameter of 0.533 mm, with a 36 AWG tinned copper inner-conductor, a 90% spiral tinned copper braid screening, and PFA polymer for both the external coating and insulation core. The cables are sufficiently flexible such that they do not apply any appreciable torsion to the vial that might otherwise cause the vial to tip or make it difficult to position on the shelf.

The signals from the five sensing ports on the bottom row of the multiplexer are then passed to the five individual trans-impedance amplifiers inside the current to voltage (IVC) converter unit (located outside the dryer), again via pairs of 50 Ω 30 AWG RG178 and 26 AWG RG316 co-axial cables (with the RG178 cable inside the dryer and the RG316 on the outside of the dryer).

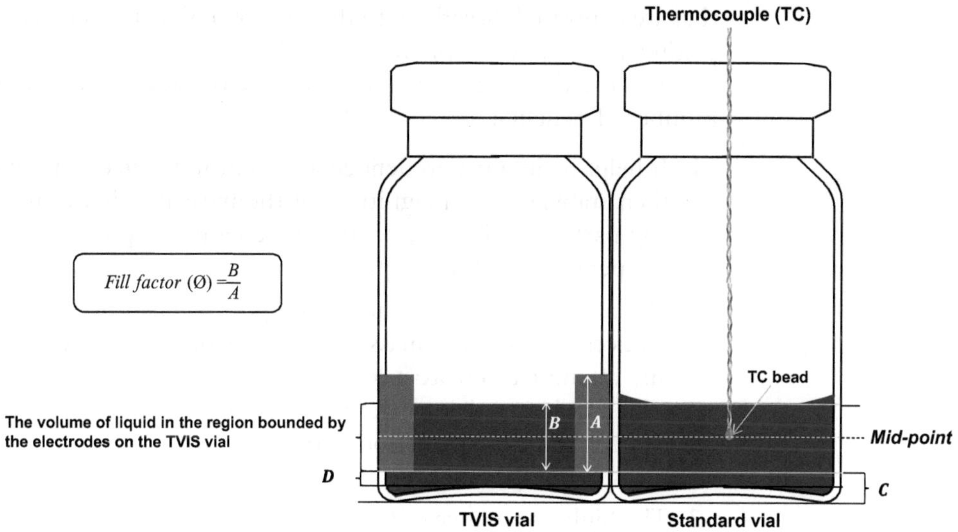

Fig. 4 Sketch of an Adelphi VC010-20C vial (20 mm crimp-neck vial with 10 mL nominal capacity and external diameter and internal diameters of 24.25 and 22.05 mm); *Right:* Unmodified "nearest neighbor" vial. *Left:* TVIS-modified vial showing the electrode pair of height 10 mm and width 19 mm, with a 3 mm separation between the bottom of the electrode and the external base of the vial (Dimension *C*). The Dimension *D* is the approximate height of the liquid on circumference of the volume space below the lower edge of the electrode. Its magnitude is given by dimension *C* minus the thickness of the base at the contact point with the external surface on which the vial is placed. The fill factor Ø shown here is 0.7 (which for a 10 mm high electrode means that the height of the liquid within the region bounded by the electrodes is 7 mm). The fill volume of water is approximately 3.4 mL. The position of the thermocouple, inserted in a nearest neighbor vial to the TVIS vial, is at a height which is equivalent to the mid-point of the volume of the liquid that is bounded by the electrodes on either side of the glass wall of the TVIS vial

The stimulating signal is fed to the ADC0 input of the 4 channel NI DAQ PCI6110 Multi-function I/O device whereas the five outputs from the IVC channels are fed to the ADC1 input, via a programmatically controlled reed relay multiplexer.

All connections inside the dryer are made with Belden 30 AWG RG178 coaxial cables which are terminated by SMA plug connectors (HUBER & SUHNER 11 SMA-50-1-4/111NE) on the pass through side and by MCX bulkhead Jack connectors (MULTICOMP 27-10M TGG) on junction box side. All outside connections are made with Belden coaxial cable 26 AWG RG316 terminated by SMA straight plug connectors (MULTICOMP MC23554).

The electrodes are formed from 19 mm wide copper adhesive tape (1181 3M™) consisting of a soft copper foil backing (0.04 mm) and an electrically conductive pressure-sensitive acrylic adhesive (0.026 mm) attached to the outer wall of the vial. This approach is only one of a number of possible design options. Others include foil electrodes with an adhesive "wrap-over" layer to avoid having glue between the electrode and the glass wall, and electrodes that are deposited directly onto the surface of the vial using electroplating and electroless-plating technologies.

The location of the electrodes on the outside of the vial has a number of benefits:

1. It helps maintain a predefined and immovable geometry which then stabilizes the magnitude of the measured impedance for any particular fill volume and/or condition (phase state and temperature) of the sample.
2. The electrodes do not require a support mechanism which then reduces the thermal mass of the electrode assembly, whereas any attempt to create a low thermal mass electrode assembly which is inserted into the vial will necessarily be fragile and susceptible to deformation with consequent alterations in the measured impedance.
3. The high impedance of the glass wall, in series with the sample, means that any variation in the layout of the cabling has negligible impact on the measured impedance response.
4. The electrode assembly does not provide additional (non-representative) nucleation sites for ice growth that would otherwise alter the ice crystal structure that develops during the freezing stage.
5. The thin electrode on the measurement vial means that the vials can be arranged in the conventional hexagonal array, thereby maintaining the inherent heat transfer between vials, shelf, and the gaseous environment.

The principle disadvantage is that, in its current manifestation, the method depends on cables to connect the electrodes on the vials to the measurement system which renders the system incompatible with an automatic vial-loading system.

The main challenge in making precise (low noise) measurements of the TVIS spectrum is the large dynamic impedance range encountered across individual spectra (from 10 Hz to 10 MHz) and across the entire freeze-drying cycle (Fig. 5) where the impedance magnitude can be as high as 10–100 GΩ (10^{10}–10^{11} Ω) at the low frequency end of the spectrum (10 Hz) for the vial at the end of drying (when the vial is effectively empty from an impedance point of view) to as low as 100 kΩ (10^5 Ω) at the high frequency end of the spectrum when the vial is full with a liquid, coupled to the requirements for a short spectrum acquisition/scan time of the order of 10 s so that spectra from multiple vials may be acquired sequentially in less than 1 min. This functionality is not provided by the current state-of-the-art broad band dielectric spectrometers, which can take as long as one minute to acquire a single spectrum from 1 MHz down to 10 Hz, and so the implementation of the TVIS method has required the design and development of a bespoke instrument for this purpose.

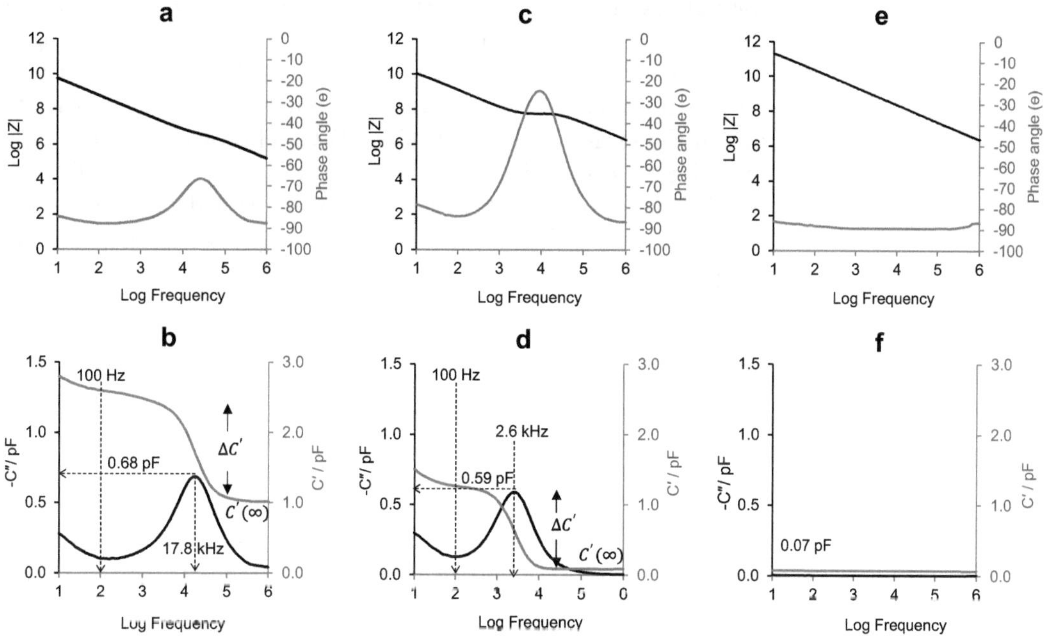

Fig. 5 (**a**) Impedance spectrum and (**b**) equivalent complex capacitance spectrum of 3.5 mL double distilled water in an Adelphi VC010-20C Type I glass tubing vial with a pair of 10 × 19 mm electrodes ($h \times w$) attached to the outside of the vial at a distance of 3 mm from the external base (Ø = 0.7), (**c**) impedance spectrum and (**d**) equivalent complex capacitance spectrum of the same vial containing water but frozen to −20 °C (**e**) impedance spectrum and (**f**) equivalent complex capacitance spectrum of the same vial but without the sample. $|Z|$ is the magnitude of the impedance and ϑ is the phase angle between the real and imaginary parts of the complex impedance, Z^*. C' is the dielectric storage and C'' is the dielectric loss components of the complex capacitance, respectively. The vertical dotted line at 100 Hz illustrates the frequency below which both the real and imaginary capacitances increase as a consequence of charge percolation through the porous nature of the glass

2.2 TVIS Measurement Instrumentation

The instrument used to generate the data for this book chapter has been developed by Evgeny Polygalov at De Montfort University (Innovate UK project grant LyoDEA 100527). It is based on an NI PCI 6110 data acquisition (DAQ) card with a 4 MHz sampling rate, five 1 GΩ trans impedance amplifiers (i.e., a current to voltage convertor, IVC) each with a trans-impedance gain of 180 dB, and five sequentially measuring impedance channels which share a common excitation signal. The instrument features an automatic adjustment of the excitation signal, whereby the output level from the instrument, i.e., the amplitude of output signal from the IVC, is maintained at 2 V, which is half of the maximum output level of 4 V so that the operational amplifier output does not experience any significant nonlinear distortion. This is achieved by adjustment of the stimulation voltage between 0.2 and 8 V and then fixing it at 8 V when the maintenance of this level is no longer achievable: In the sequence for the measurement of the first data point of each spectrum, the stimulating voltage is first set to 0.2 V; the system then checks for an overflow/underflow of the ADC and changes the gain of the data acquisition card until the ADC is functioning in its optimal regime. Then the system checks the amplitude of IVC output and adjusts the amplitude of simulating signal in order to obtain the target 2 V output of the IVC. This procedure can have several iterations until the optimal regime is achieved and only then the first data point is taken. For the subsequent data points in the spectrum, the optimal excitation signal amplitude and ADC gain are predicted on the basis of previous point measurement parameters. The same applies to the measurement of data points for subsequent spectra.

Another feature of the instrument is the methodology for improving the signal to noise ratio: The instrument integrates (i.e., averages) a number of sine wave periods (N); When the duration of that number of periods is longer than 0.05 s then N is fixed at a preset number (4 is recommended), otherwise N is calculated as $N = 0.05$ s $\times$ f Hz. It follows that $N = 4$ for a frequency of 80 Hz and below; while at 100 Hz, $N = 5$ (i.e., 0.05 s $\times$ 100 Hz); at 1 kHz, $N = 50$ (i.e., 0.05 s $\times$ 1000 Hz); at 10 kHz $N = 500$ (i.e., 0.05 s $\times$ 10,000 Hz); and so on. One or more first periods (which can be preset in the "Delay" box in "Experiment setup" window) are excluded from averaging to avoid any dynamic distortions that result from the essentially reactive impedance of the object under test (OUT). The integration and delay times for each frequency point of the spectrum then define the total scan time to acquire each individual spectrum during the freeze-drying cycle. For a spectrum recorded from 1 MHz to 10 Hz, with ten data points per decade, the instrument takes ~4 s to scan from 1 MHz to 100 Hz and then a further ~3–4 s to scan from 100 to 10 Hz. So, the total time taken to scan across the whole range frequency range of 10 Hz to 1 MHz is 7–8 s per channel. With the five channel instrument it is possible to measure five vials in sequence in less than 1 min.

2.3 TVIS Measurement Principles

The electrical impedance of an object (in our case a freeze-drying vial and its contents) defines the total opposition to the flow of charge (current) when a sinusoidal alternating voltage is applied. Given that the glass vial and its contents conduct electricity somewhat like a capacitor (rather than a conductor) then it can be more intuitive to present the electrical impedance of this object in terms of an electrical capacitance. By varying the frequency of the applied voltage, typically between 10 Hz and 1 MHz, the TVIS system generates an electrical impedance spectrum which when displayed in terms of the equivalent electrical capacitance spectrum is characterized by a peak in the imaginary capacitance (i.e., dielectric loss) spectrum and a step in the real part capacitance (i.e., dielectric permittivity) spectrum. This basic response is seen routinely when measuring pure water where the peak in the imaginary capacitance is located within the mid-range of the experimental frequency window of 10 Hz to 1 MHz. However, the exact position and amplitude of the loss peak depends on the physical state of sample (whether liquid or frozen), the temperature of whichever phase the sample is in, at any point in time during freezing, annealing and or primary drying, and the height of the frozen layer within the region bounded by the electrodes on the outside of the vial. In effect, any changes in the capacitance spectrum will mirror the condition of the solution throughout the lyophilization process and therefore TVIS may be used to monitor the physical state, composition, and temperature of the material throughout the lyophilization process.

Figure 5 shows example spectra for the TVIS vial (Adelphi VC010-20C of nominal volume 10 mL) containing 3.5 g water (at 20 °C), 3.5 g frozen water (ice at −20 °C) and empty. The impedance spectra on the left (displayed as Bode plots, i.e., log impedance magnitude and phase angle against log frequency) illustrate the extremely wide range of impedance values associated with the various transitions that occur on freeze-drying; from the initial liquid state to the frozen state, and then to the end state, once all the ice has been removed, to leave behind the empty cell. The capacitance spectra on the right illustrate how the amplitude (C''_{PEAK}) and frequency position (F_{PEAK}) of the main dielectric loss peak, in the imaginary capacitance spectrum, and the increment in capacitance ($\Delta C'$) and high-frequency capacitance ($C'(\infty)$) in the real part capacitance spectrum, change with those same transitions. For the TVIS vial containing liquid water there is a single peak located at the high-frequency end of the dielectric loss spectrum (~18 kHz), whereas for the TVIS vial containing frozen water (ice at −20 °C) the peak has now shifted to lower frequencies of the dielectric loss spectrum (~3 kHz). There is also a dramatic decrease in the high-frequency capacitance ($C'(\infty)$) in the real part spectrum.

2.3.1 Liquids and the Maxwell-Wagner Polarization of the Glass

In the case of simple, unfrozen liquids of relevance to pharmaceutical freeze-drying, such as water, ethanol, and tert-butanol, the peak in the imaginary capacitance (i.e., the dielectric loss) and the step in the real part capacitance (i.e., the dielectric storage) are due to a Maxwell-Wagner (MW) polarization process, otherwise known as space charge polarization or interfacial polarization. The MW process originates from the fact that the object under test is a composite of a relatively conductive material (i.e., the cylinder of liquid within the vial) in intimate contact with the poorly conductive material (i.e., the glass wall of the container). This particular type of MW process is manifest at the macroscopic scale of the glass-sample interface (i.e., ions migrate through the solution and accumulate at the interface between the solution and the glass). It should be stressed that the observation of the frequency-dependent response of the composite object does not mean that the dielectric properties of the liquid have any frequency dependence of its own. The dielectric permittivity of water, for example, is constant within the frequency range of the TVIS instrument (10 Hz to 10 MHz) and its conductivity can be described by a simple dc conductivity.

When a MW process occurs at the intermediate (meso-) scale (i.e., within the sample) because of inner dielectric and/or conductive boundaries which trap charge carriers within the material, then the object may display dielectric and conductive properties which are frequency dependent. This is a feature of many composite and microstructured materials, including:

1. Multilayered polycrystalline composites [20] owing to the juxtaposition of thin films of alternating dielectric and conductive properties.
2. Ceramics [21] (e.g., as a result of grains and grain boundaries within the bulk material).
3. Biological cells and tissues [22, 23] as a consequence of the relatively non-conductive (dielectric) property of the cytoplasmic membrane and the high conductivity of the intra- and extracellular fluid.

The physical origin and characteristics of the MW process (observed for the TVIS vial containing liquid water) can be considered follows: When a voltage (V) is applied to the composite object of the freeze-drying vial and its contents, via the electrodes attached to the outside of the vial, then current will start to flow and the electrical capacitance of the glass wall begins to accumulate charge at a rate which is dependent largely on the electrical resistance of the solution inside the vial.[1]

The charges accumulating at the glass boundary layer with the solution are neutralized to some degree by the accumulation of ionic charges that have diffused through the solution contained within the vial to the solution boundary layer with the glass. The net result is that a proportion of the applied voltage is dropped across the glass wall and the remaining voltage is dropped across the material within the vial.

According to the classical electric circuit theory, the time constant (τ) for the rate of charging of the glass wall capacitance, through the solution resistance, is defined as the time it takes to reach 63.2% of its maximum charge holding capacity. This time

[1] Note that the impact on the flow of charge, from the cabling from the measurement instrument and the vial, is negligible given that the cables are made from conductive metal of significant lower resistance than that of the sample within the vial (i.e., the liquid/frozen solution or pure water/ice). This is one of the intrinsic benefits of the TVIS approach over instruments which place the electrodes in contact with the sample.

constant may be approximated by the product of the sample resistance (R_s) and the glass-sample capacitance (C_g),

$$\tau \approx R_s C_g \tag{1}$$

One can rationalize the dependency of the time constant on both parameters, R_s and C_g, by considering that it is the sample resistance that regulates the flow of charges to the capacitance of the glass wall (hence restricting the rate of charging) whereas it is the capacitance of the glass wall-sample interface which defines the amount of charge that the glass can accommodate (hence defining the total magnitude of charges that must first pass through the solution resistance for the capacitor to become fully charged). It follows that, if either the resistance or the capacitance increases then it will take longer for the charging process to complete which would then be reflected in the value of the time constant (τ).

One should also recognize that the solution is not simply behaving as an electrical resistor, it also has an electrical capacitance owing to the fact that the space between the two glass walls has a dielectric (charge storage) property which is due to the polarization of permanent dipoles (e.g., the molecular dipole of water and other small molecules). The actual time constant for the process is impacted by the additional time required for the solution capacitance to charge, such that

$$\tau = R_s(C_g + C_s) \tag{2}$$

where C_s is the approximate value for the electrical capacitance of the liquid contained primarily within the volume of the vial that is bounded by the electrodes but with a lesser contribution coming from the volume of liquid that is within the fringing fields extending beyond the boundaries of the electrodes.

2.3.2 Impedance Spectroscopy

The above treatment of the composite object of the glass wall and the liquid contents of a freeze-drying vial considers the response of the object to a static (i.e., time invariant) voltage. However, when studying the charging of the glass wall through the solution resistance, using impedance spectroscopy, an oscillating sinusoidal voltage, $V = V_o \sin(\omega t)$, is applied and the resultant current $I = I_o \sin(\omega t + \varphi)$ is measured, where ω is the frequency of the applied field in radians and φ is the phase difference between the voltage and current [24]. The phase difference for a pure resistor is zero and that for a pure capacitor is $-90°$ or $-\pi/2$ radians (The negative sign means that the voltage lags behind the current by 90°). The ratio of the voltage amplitude (V_o) to the current amplitude (I_o) is known as the impedance magnitude, $|Z| = V_o/I_o$ whereas the inverse ratio (I_o/V_o) is known as the admittance, $|Y| = 1/|Z|$.

2.3.3 Basic Model for the TVIS Spectrum of the Liquid State

The interpretation of impedance spectra is facilitated by using an equivalent circuit comprising individual elements that have characteristics which collectively reflect the physicality of the object while modeling the impedance of the object as a function of the applied frequency. For example, an object that is a good conductor is represented by a resistor whereas an object that does not conduct well (i.e., an insulator) is represented by a capacitor. The basic characteristics of the TVIS vial, comprising a non-conductive glass wall and a relatively conductive sample, have already been discussed in the previous section, and so now it is only a question of arranging these elements in an appropriate circuit layout which reflects the pathways for the flow of charge (i.e., current) (Fig. 6).

In the model for the liquid filled vial the electrical impedance of the solution is represented by a resistor (R_s) and capacitor (C_s) in parallel with each other, which reflects the fact that the solution has a measureable conductivity associated with delocalized charges, i.e., ions (which can diffuse through the solution) as well as a dielectric constant, which is associated with the polarization of charges that are more localized (i.e., molecular dipoles). The arrangement of R_s and C_s in parallel reflects the fact that current can flow

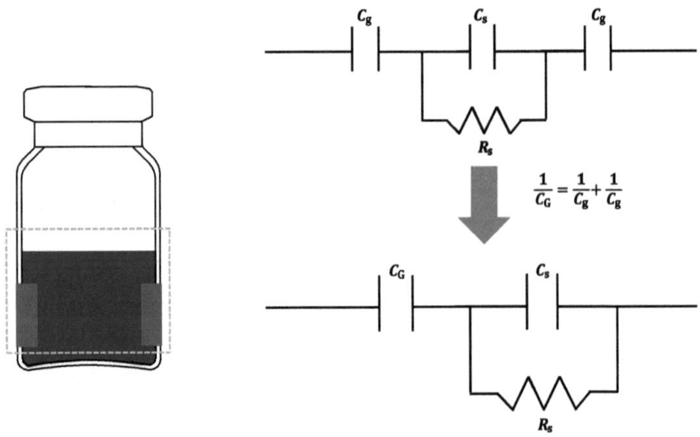

Fig. 6 Basic equivalent circuit model that approximately fits the experimental data for simple systems such as a water filled vial with copper foil electrodes attached to the outside of the glass. C_g is an approximation for the capacitance of the glass wall-sample interface and C_S and R_S are the capacitance and resistance of the sample respectively. The interface capacitances of the two segments of glass juxtaposed with the electrodes can be combined into a single capacitance using the inverse sum rule for capacitances in series, where the reciprocal of the total capacitance equals the sum of the reciprocal values of the two individual capacitances $1/C_G = 1/C_g + 1/C_g$; $C_G = C_g^2/(C_g + C_g)$. Note the use of capital subscript G for the combined capacitance from two glass segments in contact with the external electrodes

independently as a result of the admittance of each component.[2] The final element in the model is a capacitor in series with the sample impedance, which accounts for the dielectric behavior of the glass wall of the vial. Each of these impedance elements (C_s, R_s, C_g) will be considered in turn.

The *sample capacitance* (C_s) is largely defined by the static permittivity (ε_s) of the liquid (e.g., water) and the height of the liquid according to Eq. 3:

$$C_{\mathrm{s}} = \varepsilon_{\mathrm{o}} \varepsilon_{\mathrm{s}} k_{\mathrm{s}} \tag{3}$$

where ε_o is the permittivity of free space (8.854×10^{-12} F m^{-1}) and k_s is the geometric cell constant. The value of k_s is dominated by the volume of liquid in the region of the vial bounded by the electrodes but with a smaller contribution from the liquid in the fringing fields of the electrodes. In the case of a parallel plate capacitor (with two planar electrodes of equal size and in close proximity to one another relative to their surface area) the cell constant k_s would be defined by A/d, where A is the area of an electrode and d is the separation between the electrode pair. In the case of two curved electrodes, on opposite sides of a cylindrical object, then it is more difficult to define the cell constant in these simple geometric terms, owing to the fact that the fringing field effect is more significant the further apart the electrodes are. The characteristics of these fringing fields are illustrated later in Fig. 9.

The *sample resistance* (R_s) is largely defined by the concentration and valency (charge carrying capacity) of ions in the solution, according to Eq. 4:

$$R_{\mathrm{s}} = \rho_{\mathrm{s}} / k_{\mathrm{s}} \tag{4}$$

where ρ_s is the resistivity of the solution and k_s is the same geometric cell constant as for the capacitance.

The high-frequency contribution to the *glass wall capacitance* (C_g) is associated with the instantaneous atomic and electronic polarizations that create a macroscopic dipole moment which largely defines the instantaneous (i.e., frequency independent) relative permittivity of the glass (ε_g) and hence its electrical capacitance. An analogous equation to that for the static sample capacitance of the sample may be applied to the instantaneous capacitance of the glass wall (C_g).

$$C_{\mathrm{g}} = \varepsilon_{\mathrm{o}} \varepsilon_{\mathrm{g}} k_{\mathrm{g}} \tag{5}$$

[2] While it does not matter which element is placed above the other in a parallel circuit, we have adopted a rule that the element which dominates the impedance of the $R = C$ circuit at high frequency is placed above the element which dominates the impedance of the $R = C$ circuit at low frequency. Note that the use of the symbol "=" signifies a parallel arrangement of two elements, whereas the same elements in series will be indicated by the use of the symbol "–."

The relative permittivity of the Fiolax® glass used for the Adelphi VC010-20C vial (which comprises 75% SiO_2, 10.5% B_2O_3, 5% Al_2O_3, 7% Na_2O and 1.5% CaO) is reported by the manufacturer (Schott) to be 5.7 at 1 MHz (25 °C). Whether this value is representative of the instantaneous relative permittivity of this glass remains to be seen. k_g is the geometric cell constant of the segment of glass in direct contact with the electrodes. By ignoring edge effects (i.e., the fringing fields) the cell constant may be estimated from $k_g = h \cdot w/d_g$, where d_g is the thickness of the glass ($d_g = 1.1$ mm for the Adelphi VC010-20C vial) and the area of the electrode is ($h \cdot w$) is 190 mm^2 (10 mm × 19 mm). However, given that the glass segment on which the electrode is attached comprises a curved surface rather than a planar one (Fig. 7), then the effective width of the glass segment that contributes to the cell constant is more likely to be closer to the average of the length of the external arc (19 mm) and the internal arc (17.28 mm) of the glass segment, i.e., $w = 18.14$ mm.

In a further refinement of the calculation of the theoretical capacitance of the glass-wall, one should also allow for the influence on the effective capacitance of the adhesive layer (C_a) in the composite assembly by applying the inverse sum rule of two capacitors in series [25].

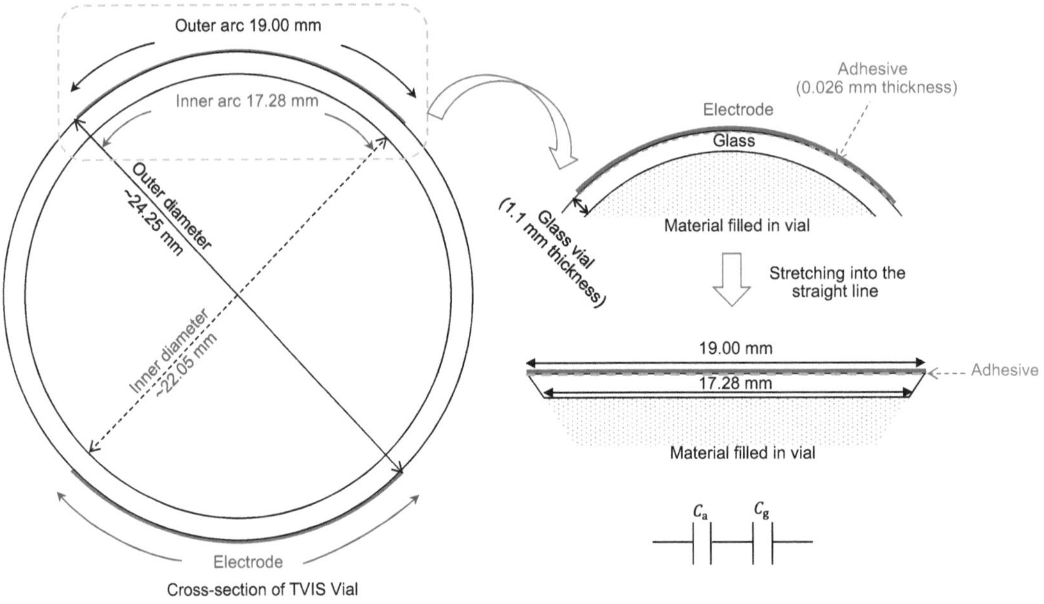

Fig. 7 Schematic showing the methodology for the estimation of the glass wall capacitance (C_g) from the geometric shape of the segment of the glass bounded by the external electrode and the literature value for the dielectric constant of the Fiolax® glass ($\varepsilon_g = 5.7$) and the adhesive ($\varepsilon_a = 3.2$). The curvature of glass vial and the dielectric constant of adhesive are taken into account for the calculation of the capacitance of the glass-composite segment (C_g = 8.32 pF, C_a = 197.7 pF, C_{a-g} = 7.98 pF) with an electrode of dimension 10 × 19 mm)

$$\frac{1}{C_{a-g}} = \frac{1}{C_a} + \frac{1}{C_g} \tag{6}$$

$$C_{a-g} = \frac{C_a \cdot C_g}{C_a + C_g} \tag{7}$$

In each case, the capacitance of the respective elements is given by an appropriate form of the parallel plate capacitor equation ($C = \varepsilon_0 \varepsilon_r k$) such that $C_a = 197.7$ pF and $C_g = 8.32$ pF. The estimated capacitance (C_{a-g}) of the composite of the glass wall and adhesive segment is therefore 7.98 pF. Therefore, a predicted value of C_{a-G} would be $C_{a-g}/2 = 3.99$ pF.

Figure 8 shows a typical capacitance spectrum for a TVIS-modified Adelphi VC010-20C glass tubing vial (nominal fill volume 10 mL) containing 7 g double distilled water and with a pair of external electrodes of height 10 mm and width 19 mm (separated from the base of the vial by 3 mm). The points on the graph are the data points (C' and C'') recorded by the TVIS instrument and the line is the result of fitting the equivalent circuit in Fig. 6 using proprietary software (e.g., RelaxIS or Zview®), to give C'_{fit} and C''_{fit}.

In a number of applications for TVIS, for example the determination of the product temperature, the extent of data analysis may be restricted to the scrutiny of the amplitude of the dielectric loss peak (C''_{PEAK}) and the frequency on which the loss peak is centered (F_{PEAK}). See Appendix 1 for a description of a simple peak finding

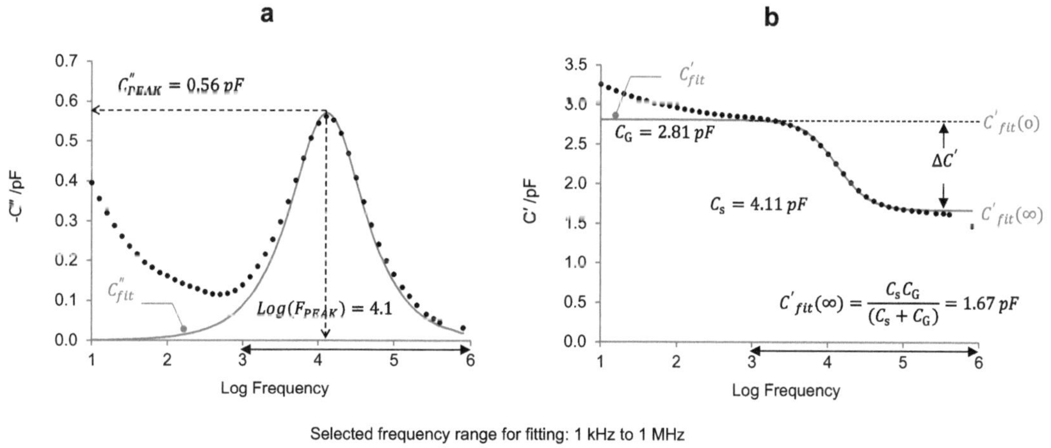

Fig. 8 A typical capacitance spectrum of 7 g double distilled water in a 10 mL Type I glass tubing vial (Adelphi VC010-20C) which has been modified with a pair of external copper electrodes of dimensions 10 × 19 mm and positioned 3 mm from the base of the vial. The temperature of the liquid is 22 °C. The *gray line* shows the fit to the equivalent circuit model shown in Fig. 6 and the symbols (*black dots*) show the data points. The horizontal line with double headed arrow marks the frequency range for fitting. The disagreement between the fit and the data at the lower frequencies is due to the presence of a separate dielectric process which is thought to arise from Maxwell-Wagner (space charge) polarization within the glass wall of the vial

approach used in our LyoView™ software. This provides a more pragmatic approach to the otherwise more complex procedures involved in fitting an equivalent circuit model to the data. However, in order to extract some physical meaning from these empirical parameters, it is necessary to consider the relationships between the empirical parameters (C''_{PEAK} and F_{PEAK}) and the underlying changes in the equivalent circuit elements (C_s, R_s, C_G) that define the characteristics of the impedance spectrum. These relationships will be explored here for the case of a simple solvent, i.e., water. Further basic explanations of impedance spectroscopy, as it applies to a liquid filled TVIS vial, are given in Appendix 2.

Figure 8a shows the imaginary-part capacitance (i.e., dielectric loss) spectrum of the TVIS vial containing liquid water. As the frequency tends toward zero ($\omega \rightarrow 0$) the value for C''_{fit} from the equivalent circuit model also tends to zero. As the frequency increases, C''_{fit} increases to a maximum (C''_{PEAK}) at a frequency F_{PEAK} then decreases to zero as the frequency increases above F_{PEAK} (i.e., $\omega \rightarrow \infty$).

$$C''_{\mathrm{PEAK}} = \frac{C_{\mathrm{G}}^2}{2(C_{\mathrm{s}} + C_{\mathrm{G}})} \tag{8}$$

$$F_{\mathrm{PEAK}} = \frac{1}{2\pi R_{\mathrm{s}}(C_{\mathrm{s}} + C_{\mathrm{G}})} \tag{9}$$

The corresponding real part is shown in Fig. 8b. In the limit of low frequency ($\omega \rightarrow 0$) the real part capacitance of the equivalent circuit, C'_{fit}, tends toward a value equal to the capacitance of the glass-sample interface, i.e., C_G. As the frequency increases ($\omega \rightarrow \infty$) then C'_{fit} decreases to a plateau of

$$C'_{\mathrm{fit}}(\infty) = \frac{C_{\mathrm{s}} C_{\mathrm{G}}}{(C_{\mathrm{s}} + C_{\mathrm{G}})} \tag{10}$$

Note that the increment in the real part capacitance, $\Delta C'$ (Eq. 11, is twice that of the amplitude of the dielectric loss peak (Eq. 8).

$$\Delta C' = \frac{C_{\mathrm{G}}^2}{C_{\mathrm{s}} + C_{\mathrm{G}}} \tag{11}$$

Using expressions Eqs. 8 and 9 it is possible to rationalize the changes in both F_{PEAK} and C''_{PEAK} as the liquid within the vial is cooled to lower temperatures:

The parameter F_{PEAK} depends on the inverse of both the solution resistance and the sum of the solution capacitance and the glass wall capacitance. However, given the much greater temperature coefficient of electrical resistance over electrical capacitance F_{PEAK} is particularly sensitive to the temperature of the product via changes in the solution resistance.

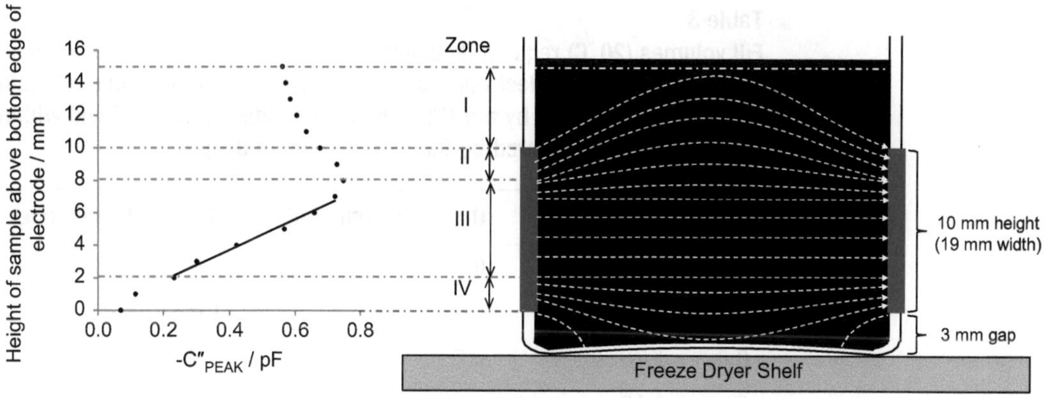

Fig. 9 The dependence of C''_{PEAK} on the height of liquid water from bottom edge of the electrode. *Zone I* is the fringing field region above the electrode which continues to contribute to the overall capacitance despite the fact that the liquid in this region is above the top edge of the electrode; *Zone II* is the nonlinear response region to the liquid at the top of the volume of liquid bounded by the electrodes; *Zone III* is the quasi-linear response region to the liquid in the region bounded by the electrodes; *Zone IV* is the nonlinear response region to the liquid at the top of the bottom of liquid bounded by the electrodes

The magnitude of the peak (C''_{PEAK}) is a function of the height of the liquid layer within the region bounded by the electrodes and in intimate contact with the inside of the vial. Figure 9 shows the relationship between C''_{PEAK} and the fill volume/height of the liquid in the TVIS vial. The dependence of C''_{PEAK} on the height of liquid in the region bounded by the electrodes is only quasi-linear in the mid band of this region. For this vial, of internal diameter 22.05 mm, the linear region starts at ~2 mm above the bottom edge of the electrode and finishes approximately 2 mm from the top edge of the electrode.

Another way of expressing the height of the sample within the volume bounded by the external electrodes (i.e., the electrode space) is to state this quantity in relative terms, in the format of a fill factor (Ø) which is ratio of the height of the liquid in the electrode space to the height of the electrode. Table 3 shows the volumes of liquid water at 20 °C which provide fill factors of 0–1.2.

2.3.4 Enhanced Model for the TVIS Spectrum of the Liquid State

The basic model, which assumes that the glass wall behaves like a simple capacitor, with a frequency independent response, does not adequately account for the dielectric response of the glass wall toward the lower frequencies of the TVIS spectrum which, rather than having a flat frequency response, is characterized by an increase in both the real and imaginary impedance (For example, see the real part capacitance spectra at frequencies below 1 kHz or Log Frequency = 3, Fig. 8b). This feature of the low-frequency response (which is observed for many micro-structured materials containing semi-mobile charge carriers) is often referred to as an anomalous low-frequency dispersion (abbreviated to LFD in the dielectric

Table 3
Fill volumes (20 °C) required to deliver fill factors from Ø = 0 (the liquid fill to the bottom of the electrode) to Ø = 1.2 (the maximum volume of liquid that can be measured by the TVIS system, i.e., the volume of liquid within the field lines propagated by the external electrodes)

Ø	Volume (mL)	Ø	Volume (mL)	Ø	Volume (mL)
0	0.5	0.5	2.60	0.9	4.28
0.2	1.34	0.6	3.02	1.0	4.70
0.3	1.76	0.7	3.44	1.1	5.12
0.4	2.18	0.8	3.86	1.2	5.54

Data is for the Adelphi VC010-20C vial
Note that on freezing the fill factor will increase given that the density of ice is lower than that of liquid water. The density of water is 0.99819 g cm^{-3} (20 °C) and the density of ice at a range of sub-zero temperature can be estimated from $\rho = 917 - 0.13 \times T$ (kg m^{-3}), where T is given in °C [26]. For example ρ(ice) = 0.9196 g cm^{-3} at −20 °C such that a liquid fill factor of 0.7 at 20 °C will increase to 0.76

literature) and in the case of glass results from proton percolation (space charge polarization) within the porous/hydrated silica. Because the extent of charge migration (i.e., the numbers of charges and the length of the percolation path) is dependent on time (and hence frequency of the applied field) the magnitude of the induced polarization also increases as the frequency of the applied field decreases, resulting in the ever-increasing contribution to the glass wall capacitance and dielectric loss.[3] This percolation of protonic charges, through the glass wall microstructure, provides an additional admittance to that associated with the atomic and electronic polarizations that define the instantaneous capacitance of the glass. In the impedance community this low-frequency dispersion is often modeled using another circuit element, known as a constant phase element (*CPE*) which, given the additionality of its admittance, is positioned in parallel with the instantaneous capacitance of the glass wall (C_G).

The admittance (Υ) and hence impedance (Z) of a constant phase element (*CPE*) is given by

$$\Upsilon_{\mathrm{CPE}} = \frac{1}{Z_{\mathrm{CPE}}} = Q_{\mathrm{o}}(i\omega)^{p} \tag{12}$$

where Q_o has the numerical value of the admittance at the angular frequency of $\omega = 1$ rad s^{-1}, and units of F·s$^{(p-1)}$ *or* S·s^{p}, and p defines the impedance phase angle (ϑ) according to the expression $\vartheta = -(90 \times p)$ degrees. If the object behaves more like a capacitor

[3] A more comprehensive treatment of the dielectric properties of glass (porous silica) can be found in the publication of Ryabov et al. [27].

then p tends to 1 (for a pure capacitor, $p = 1$ hence $1/Z_C = \Upsilon_C = Q_o(i\omega)^1 = i\omega C$ and $\vartheta = -90°$) whereas if the object behaves more like a resistor then p tends to 0 (for a pure resistor $p = 0$ hence $1/Z_R = \Upsilon_R = Q_o(i\omega)^0 = 1/R$ and $\vartheta = 0°$). The Nyquist plot of the impedance spectrum (where $-Z''$ is plotted against Z') and the Cole-Cole plot of the capacitance spectrum (where $-C''$ is plotted against C') provide useful ways to display the characteristics of this low-frequency dispersion (Fig. 10). For the CPE_G alone, i.e., without the instantaneous capacitance of the glass wall, one can see how the increase in the negative of the imaginary impedance, $-Z''$ toward low frequency is directly proportional to the increase in the real part impedance, Z' (Fig. 10a gray line). In other words, the ratio of the two parameters is invariant with frequency, hence the name constant phase element (CPE). The phase angle can be determined from the slope of the impedance phasor against the axis for the real part impedance of the Nyquist plot, according to Eq. 13:

$$\vartheta = a \tan\ (\text{slope}) \tag{13}$$

On the Cole-Cole plot (Fig. 10b) the angle (α) between the capacitance scalar and the axis for real part capacitance (C')

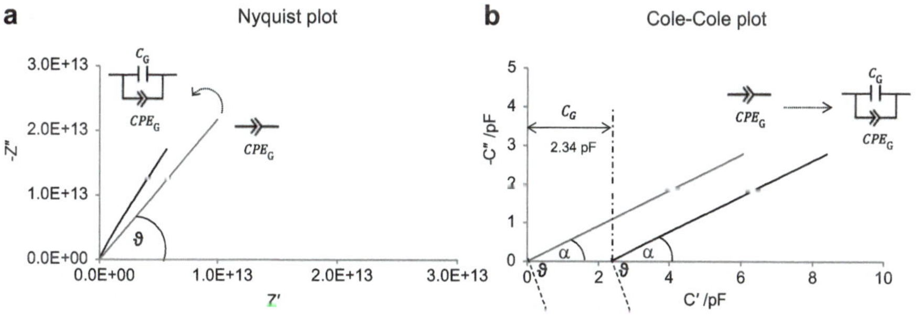

Fig. 10 (**a**) Nyquist plot of imaginary part impedance vs. real part impedance for a CPE_G alone (*gray line*) and a CPE_G in parallel with a capacitor (C_G) (*black line*); (**b**) Cole-Cole plot of imaginary part capacitance vs. real part capacitance for the same CPE_G (*gray line*) and the CPE_G in parallel with a capacitor (C_G) (*black line*); On the Nyquist plot, for the CPE_G alone (*gray line*) the phase angle, in radians, is given by a tan (slope). On the Cole-Cole plot the phase angle for the CPE_G (in radians) is given $\pi/2 - a$ tan (slope), irrespective of whether the model contains the additional capacitance element or not. Each data set for this figure has been created from values for a constant phase element (CPE_G) and capacitor (C_G) that are typical to those observed from experimental data for liquid water at 20.1 °C in an Adelphi VC010-20C glass tubing vial (of nominal volume 10 mL) and with 10 × 19 mm electrodes at a height of 3 mm from the base of the vial. Those value are $Q_o = 1.587 \times 10^{-12}\ S{\cdot}s^p$ and $p = 0.725$ for the magnitude and phase of the glass wall CPE_G and $C_G = 2.34$ pF for the glass wall capacitance. The frequency range over which the impedance has been simulated is 0.001 Hz to 1 MHz

provides an alternative assessment of the impedance phase angle (where $\alpha = 90 - \vartheta$).

In this example (Fig. 10a) the slope of the impedance vector with the axis for real part impedance is 2.173 (note that $-Z''$ is plotted against Z' so the slope is positive). It follows that $\vartheta = 1.1395$ rad or 65.29° and therefore $p = 0.725$ (from $p = \vartheta/90$).

When the capacitor is added in parallel (Fig. 10a *black line*) then the line for the impedance magnitude on the Nyquist curve appears to have a steeper gradient, and when examined more closely is in fact slightly curved. Therefore, it is not possible to estimate the phase angle of a constant phase element directly from the Nyquist plot when there is a capacitor in parallel. Fortunately, the impact of the additional capacitance (C_G) on the Cole-Cole plot (Fig. 10b) is more straightforward, given that C_G only has a real part and that capacitances in parallel can be added together to get the total capacitance. As a consequence, the net effect of the C_G on the Cole-Cole plot is to shift the complex capacitance along the real part axes by an amount which is equal to the value of C_G. The phase angle may still be determined from the slope of the capacitance vector with the axis for the real part capacitance.

The Bode plot of the imaginary vs. real parts of the impedance (Fig. 11) provides a convenient way to predict the magnitude of the constant phase element, Q_o, given that it has a numerical value of $1/|Z|$ at an angular frequency of $\omega = 1$ rad s^{-1} (or $f = \omega/2\pi = 0.16$ Hz). Figure 11a, b highlight the opportunity to "read" off the magnitude of the constant phase element at a frequency of $\omega = 1$ (or $\log \omega = 0$). In the example of the CPE_G without C_G (Fig. 11a) $\log |Z| = 11.8$, $Z = 630$ GΩ and therefore $Q_o = 1.587 \times 10^{-12}$ $S{\cdot}s^p$. When the capacitor is added in parallel (Fig. 11b, d) there is a moderate change in the value of $\log |Z|$ at $\log \omega = 0$, from $\log |Z| = 11.8$ to $\log |Z| = 11.4$, i.e., $|Z|$ changes from 630 to 251 GΩ. This intercept value is close enough (i.e., within one order of magnitude) of the intercept value for CPE_G without C_G such that it provides an acceptable starting parameter estimate when fitting data with a $CPE_G = C_G$ model.

The frequency range of the Bode plots in Fig. 11c, d has been extended way below that achievable by any available commercial impedance or broad band dielectric spectrometer, in order to demonstrate the complete frequency response of a parallel combination of a constant phase element and a capacitor. At low frequency ($<10^{-2}$ Hz) the impedance of the CPE_G is lower than that of the capacitor C_G and so the CPE_G begins to dominate the total impedance and hence the phase angle converges on that of CPE_G, i.e., =65.29°. At high frequency ($<10^2$ Hz) the impedance of the capacitor is lower than that of the CPE_G element and so the capacitance C_G begins to dominate the impedance spectrum and the phase angle therefore converges on a value of −90°.

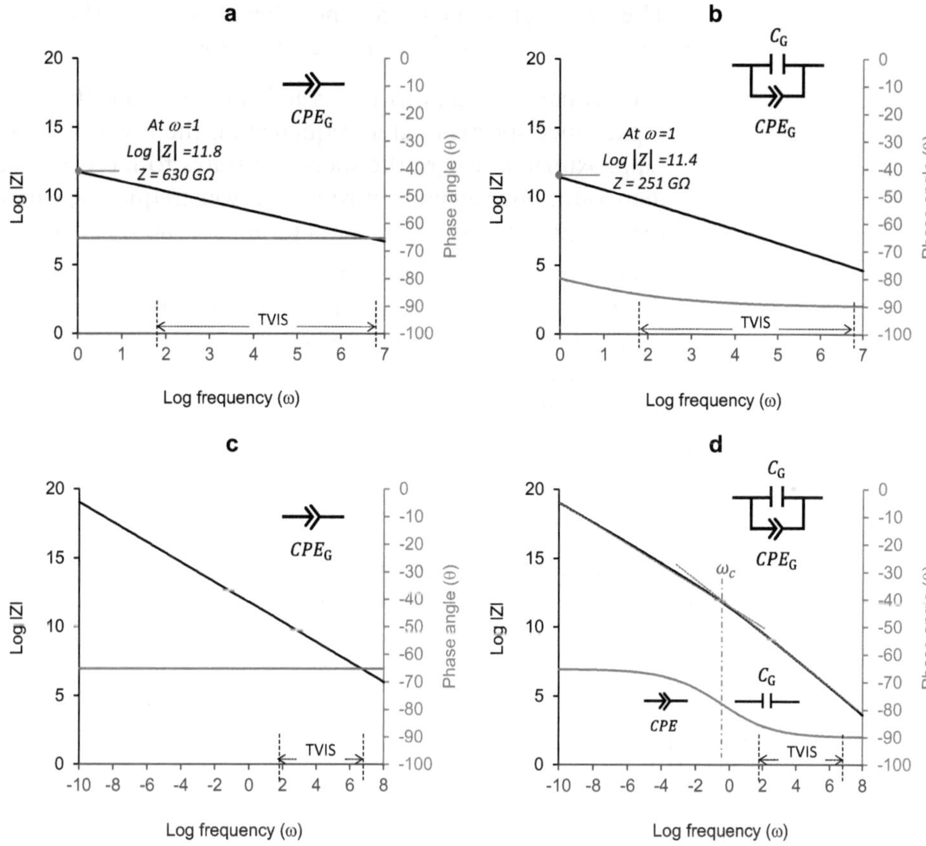

Fig. 11 Bode plot of impedance magnitude and phase angle for a CPE_G alone (**a** and **c**) and for a CPE_G in parallel with a capacitor C_G (**b** and **d**). The frequency scale on the top graphs has been set to show the range of frequencies which are accessible to the TVIS instrument (log $\omega = 1.8$–6.8) while extending the range to $\omega = 1$ in order to demonstrate how an estimate for Q_o might be derived from the intercept with the *y*-axis (at log $\omega = 0$, i.e., $\omega = 1$ rad s^{-1} or 0.16 Hz). The frequency range marked by the two dotted lines immediately above the frequency axis shows the experimental frequency range accessible to the TVIS instrument (10 Hz to 1 MHz). The frequency range for the bottom two graphs has been extended to ultra-low frequencies in order to "capture" the dominance of the *CPE* element (CPE_G) at those frequencies (well below the frequency range achievable by commercial instrumentation)

The transition frequency (ω_c) between the dominance of one element and the other is marked by the vertical dot-dashed line (Fig. 11d).

This understanding of how to "read" the Cole-Cole plot to determine the phase angle of a CPE_G element, and the Bode plot to determine the magnitude of the CPE_G element, is helpful when trying to find starting parameters (estimates) for fitting an equivalent circuit model using modeling software such as Zview® or RelaxIS.

The starting parameters for the other elements in the enhanced model (C_s, R_s, C_G) can be estimated as follows:

1. An estimate for C_G can be "read" directly from the real part capacitance spectrum at a frequency on the low side of F_{PEAK} (approximately where the spectrum states to level out, before increasing once again toward even lower frequency, where the low-frequency dispersion starts to impact the spectrum).
2. An estimate for C_s is determined by "reading" an estimate for $C'(\infty)$ from the real part capacitance spectrum at a frequency on the high side of F_{PEAK}, where the spectrum starts to level out, and then substituting the estimate for $C'(\infty)$ along with the estimate for C_G from (1) above into Eq. 10.
3. Once C_G and C_s are known an estimate for R_s can be determined from Eq. 9 where the value for F_{PEAK} is estimated from reading the peak frequency off the dielectric loss spectrum.

Figure 12 shows the result of fitting the *enhanced model* to the totality of the impedance response from the vial, including the

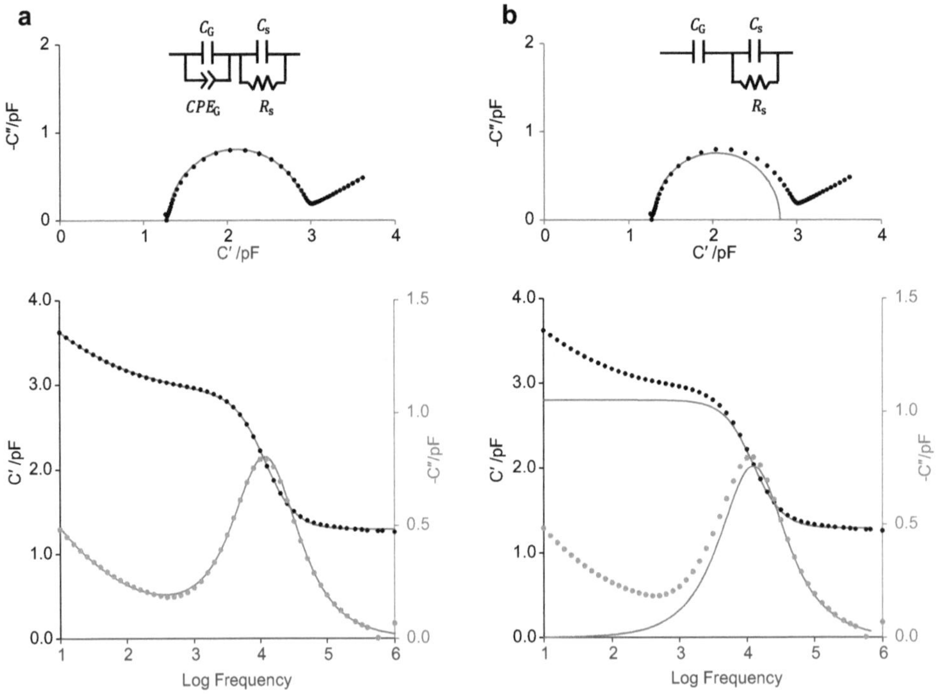

Fig. 12 Enhanced model for the MW process of a Adelphi VC010-20C glass tubing vial with 10 × 19 mm electrodes at a distance of 3 mm from the base of the vial, containing 3.4 g of ultrapure water (Ø = 0.7). The temperature of the water is ~22 °C. (**a**) Shows the enhanced model that includes a CPE_G for the low-frequency response associated with the glass wall impedance whereas (**b**) has the CPE_G removed and the impedance response from the other elements simulated. The fit parameters determined by the software are $Q_o = 3.94 \times 10^{-12}$ $S{\cdot}s^p$, $p = 0.658$, $C_G = 2.34$ pF, $R_s = 2.49$ MΩ, $C_s = 2.38$ pF

CPE_G element which models the dispersive nature of the glass wall. The graphs on the left show the results from fitting the enhanced model, where $CPE_G = C_G$ represents the glass wall impedance and $C_s = R_s$ represents the sample impedance (The symbol "=" means two elements in parallel). The graphs on the right show the contribution to the enhanced model from the elements included in the simplified model, i.e., $C_G - C_s = R_s$. These graphs have been created by a process involving the fit to the enhanced model, followed by the exclusion of the CPE element and running a simulation of the reduced model but keeping the same parameters that were determined when fitting the enhanced model.

It is clear from Fig. 12b that the simulated response, in the absence of the *CPE* element, does not perfectly match the data on the low-frequency side of the Maxwell-Wagner peak and that the influence of the low-frequency dispersive characteristics of the glass extend to frequencies as high as 10 kHz.

2.3.5 Cell Constant Determination

An alternative approach to determining the geometric cell constant of the sample space (Eq. 3), which is ideally suited to a parallel plate capacitor equation, is to express the cell constant in terms of the empty cell capacitance (C_o). A convenient experimental approach for determining this parameter is to plot values of the sample capacitance C_s, as a function of the dielectric constant of a range of polar liquids with sufficient conductivity to give relaxation to a MW process and then the empty cell capacitance (C_o) can be estimated straight from the slope of the graph, according to Eq. 14:

$$C_{\mathrm{s}} = k\varepsilon_{\mathrm{o}}\varepsilon_{\mathrm{s}} = C_{\mathrm{o}}\varepsilon_{\mathrm{s}} \tag{14}$$

Values for C_s are taken from fitting the enhanced model to the complex capacitance spectrum for each liquid at a fill height in excess of 15 mm from the internal base of vial (in the case of an Adelphi VC010-20C vial with a single electrode pair of dimensions 10×19 mm ($h \times w$) and positioned at 3 mm from the base of vial). At this fill height, the electric field lines between electrodes are fully contained within the liquid volume and therefore give the maximum value of capacitance (Fig. 9). Figure 13 shows the plot of C_s against dielectric constant of various samples (i.e., water, methanol and acetone) at room temperature. The slope from this plot is 0.0525 and the units are in pF, given that the dielectric constant is a dimensionless parameter.

Once the empty cell capacitance (C_o) is known, then it is straightforward to estimate the sample capacitance for any other liquid or indeed solid, provided one has an estimate for dielectric constant for that material. This is exploited later in the case of measurements on ice; for example if the permittivity of ice at −40 °C is 111.4, then one expects a sample capacitance, $C_{\mathrm{s}}(\mathrm{ice}_{-40^{\circ}\mathrm{C}})$, to be 5.81 pF.

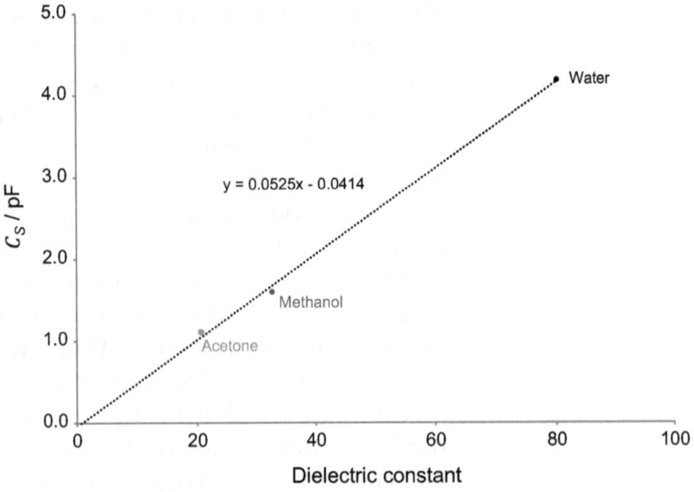

Fig. 13 The sample capacitance as the function of dielectric constant. The slope of the line of best fit is 0.0525 pF and represents the cell constant. Note that this capacitance is lower than the measured capacitance of the TVIS vial when empty (i.e., 0.07 pF, Fig. 5) suggesting that there is a small stray capacitance of the order of 0.02 pF. Theoretically, one would expect this stray capacitance to show as the value of the intercept on the *y*-axis. However, the uncertainty in the measured values for the three solvents has probably resulted in some uncertainty in the intercept value such that the stray capacitance is not quantifiable by that approach

Note that the corresponding values for C_G lie within the range 2.98–3.07 pF; (C_G (water) = 3.07 pF, C_G (methanol) = 2.98 pF and C_G (acetone) = 3.03 pF). The fact that these values are all lower than the theoretical value C_{a-G} of 3.99 pF which has taken into account the additional capacitance of the adhesive (Fig. 7 and Eq. 7) is most likely due to the presence the capacitance associated with the glass-sample interface. This capacitance in series with the glass and adhesive capacitance will inevitably reduce the effective capacitance of the glass wall by an amount which appears to depend on the specific nature of the liquid-glass interaction.

It is clear from what has been said here about the characteristics of the composite capacitance (Fig. 14) that its impedance response is somewhat complex and difficult to predict due to the limited understanding of the individual layers that make up this complex impedance, especially the uncertainty in our understanding of the glass-sample interface and the dependency on the nature of the contact with the fill material. This issue will be discussed later in the chapter when a method for determining the interfacial capacitance from measurements on ice, at different temperatures, is explored.

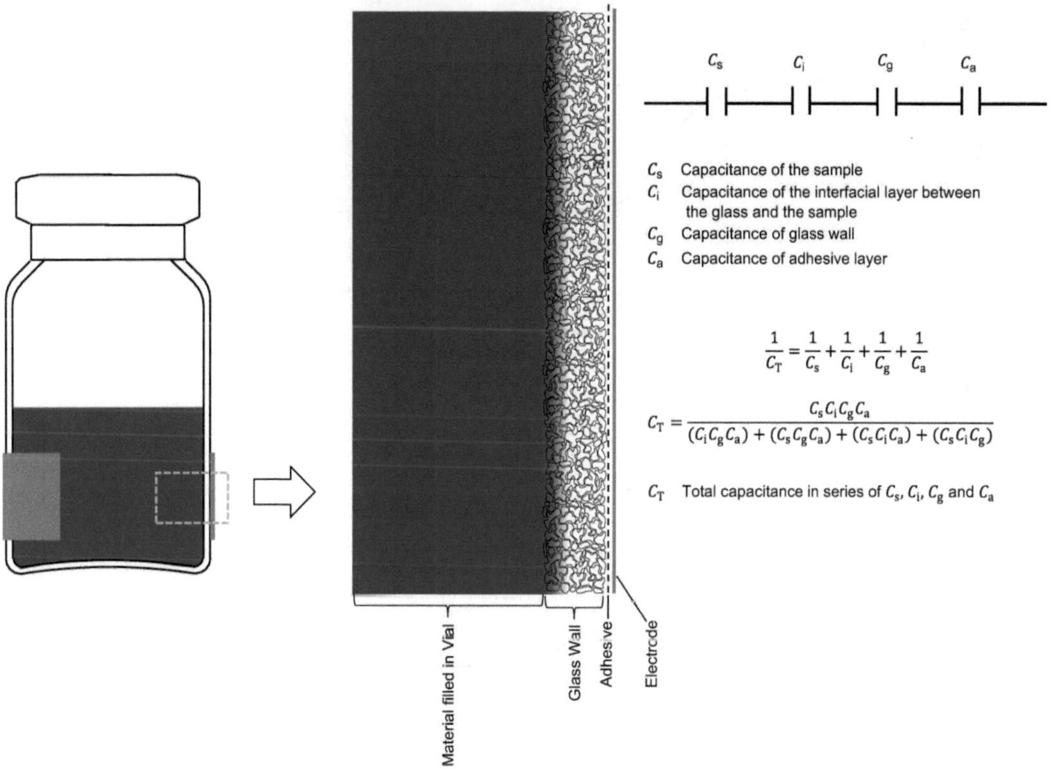

Fig. 14 Illustration showing a close-up schematic of the composite capacitance resulting from a layer of adhesive (C_a) in contact with the glass wall of the vial (C_g) which has a microstructure that supports a capacitance (C_i) of an interfacial layer of hydrated glass in contact with the bulk liquid (C_s)

2.3.6 Frozen Water and the Dielectric Relaxation of Ice

As soon as the water in the vial begins to freeze then the dielectric loss peak moves to lower frequencies. Figure 15 shows the capacitance spectrum of a TVIS-modified Adelphi VC010-20C glass tubing vial (with an electrode pair of dimensions 10 × 19 mm) containing double distilled water, at three temperatures of +20, −20, and −40 °C. The figure has been created partly from experimental data (solid line) and partly from the anticipated response in the microwave range, and beyond, in order to include the dielectric relaxation of water (dotted line). Note that the shape of the dielectric loss peak in the frozen state is rather like that one observes for the MW process in the liquid state and so one might think that it is simply the Maxwell-Wagner process but shifted to lower frequencies because of an increase in the resistance of the sample. However, this observation is not because the electrical resistance of ice is higher than that of water (although that in itself would be expected to shift the peak to lower frequencies) but rather because of the appearance of a new process which is fundamentally different to MW polarization, namely the dielectric relaxation of ice. The dielectric relaxation of ice means that the sample capacitance (C_s)

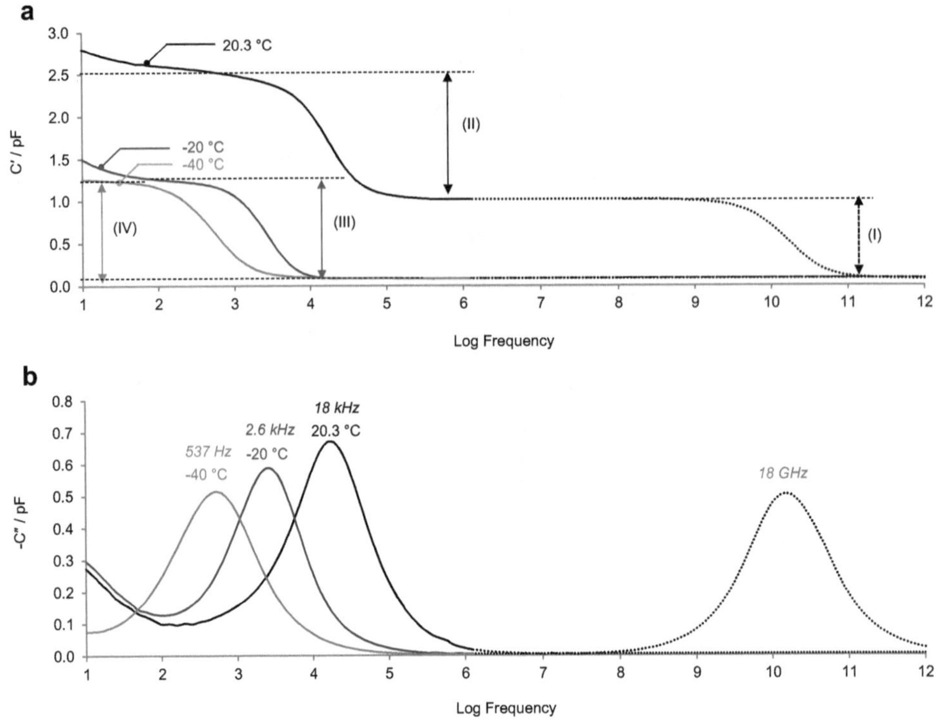

Fig. 15 Part simulation and part real data for double distilled water in a TVIS-modified Adelphi VC010-20C glass tubing vial (with electrodes of dimension 10 × 19 mm and positioned 3 mm from the base). The real (**a**) and imaginary (**b**) parts of capacitance at three temperatures of +20, −20, and −40 °C are shown. Approximate increments in the real part capacitance spectrum (**a**) for each temperature are marked with Roman numerals: (*I*) is the simulated contribution to the capacitance resulting from polarization of the water dipole in liquid water,+20 °C, with a loss peak frequency of ~18 GHz; (*II*) is the contribution to the measured capacitance resulting from the Maxwell-Wagner polarization of the glass wall of the TVIS vial, +20 °C, with a loss peak frequency of 17.8 kHz; (*III*) and (*IV*) are the contribution to the measured capacitance resulting from dielectric polarization of ice at −20 °C and −40 °C respectively, for which the dielectric loss peak frequencies are 2.57 kHz and 537 Hz

is no longer constant over the experimental frequency range of the TVIS instrument but has taken on a frequency dependence, whereby the permittivity of the frozen water changes from a value between 120 and 97 at low frequency (which is known as the static relative permittivity (ε_s of ice)[4] to a value between 3.03 and 3.09 at high frequency (which is known as the instantaneous relative permittivity ε_∞) [28]. The values given for ε_s and ε_∞ are for the limits of temperature ~−70 to 0 °C that are most relevant to freeze-drying applications. There are also changes in the width of the dielectric relaxation for ice, with the dielectric loss peak becoming

[4] "Static" refers to the low-frequency value of capacitance at which all polarization mechanisms have had sufficient time to respond fully to the applied field.

broader at the lower temperatures of −40 °C, whereas the width at −20 °C is similar to that for the Maxwell-Wagner process of the liquid state.

Dielectric relaxation is a phenomenon which is manifest in the frequency response of the dielectric permittivity, and the dielectric loss, or in the decay of the electric field inside a dielectric on removal of the external field. It results from the change in polarization state of a dielectric component in the system. For example, the water molecule has a permanent dipole which is highly mobile in the liquid state, with its polarization being characterized by a time constant of the order of 9 ps (at 20 °C). This translates to: (1) a contribution to the dielectric permittivity at low frequencies when the dipoles have sufficient time to follow the changing polarity of the external field, which stores energy from the external field, (2) a loss of that contribution and reduction in the dielectric permittivity as the dipoles relaxation to a randomized state as the frequency of the applied field exceeds the response time for the dipolar system, and (3) a peak in the dielectric loss during the transition between the ordered/polarized state and the relaxed state as the dipoles absorb energy from the field rather than store it.

The relaxation of liquid water at 20 °C is centered in the microwave range, close to 18 GHz and way above the experimental range of the TVIS instrument; hence the use of a dotted line on Fig. 15 to indicate that the liquid water relaxation is just a simulation of the theoretical response one might observe if it were possible to extend the frequency range of the TVIS instrument to these high frequencies. And so far as TVIS measurements are concerned, the dielectric permittivity of liquid water can be considered to be constant over the frequency range of the instrument, which then justifies the choice of a simple capacitor to model the liquid state of water. However, in the frozen state, water molecules form a regular architecture with oxygen atoms positioned in a repeating tetrahedral arrangement and with the hydrogen atoms randomly arranged within the crystal according to the Bernal–Fowler–Pauling rules [29–31] such that the rotational motion of a water molecule is significantly restricted, in ice, relative to the degrees of freedom that water molecules have in the liquid state. As a result the experimental relaxation time is reduced by six orders of magnitude. For example, the relaxation time of ice is 162 μs (at −20 °C) which translates to a relaxation peak centered on ~1 kHz (in contrast to ~18 GHz at 20 °C). At the limits of the temperatures encountered in a freeze-drying process (e.g., −70 °C) this relaxation frequency is expected to be low as 100 Hz. However, that frequency is well within the experimental frequency range of the TVIS instrument.

The dielectric properties of ice have been studied in some detail for well over 60 years. However, the most accurate investigation of ice Ih (for both D_2O and H_2O) was reported by Johari and Whalley [28] with ice Ih ice being revisited later by Shinyashiki et al. [32]. From these works, the main features of the dielectric relaxation of ice can be summarized as follows [33]: (1) the relaxation is characterized by a single relaxation time at temperatures above 250 K (which can be described by a Debye function, Eq. 15) but there is a symmetrical broadening of the peak as the temperature is lowered below 250 K (which can be described by a Cole–Cole function, Eq. 16); (2) the high-frequency limit of the dielectric permittivity (ε_∞) is almost independent of temperature, whereas the static permittivity (ε_s) obeys the Curie–Weiss law $\varepsilon_s - \varepsilon_\infty) = A/(T - T_{CW})$, where T_{CW} tends to zero [28]; (3) The temperature dependencies of the relaxation times (τ) above and below 250 K obey the Arrhenius law with activation energies of ~53 kJ mol^{-1} and ~19 kJ mol^{-1}, respectively.

$$\varepsilon^*(\omega) = \frac{(\varepsilon_s - \varepsilon_\infty)}{(1 + i\omega\tau)} + \varepsilon_\infty \tag{15}$$

$$\varepsilon^*(\omega) = \frac{(\varepsilon_s - \varepsilon_\infty)}{\left(1 + (i\omega\tau)^{1-\alpha}\right)} + \varepsilon_\infty \tag{16}$$

α is an exponent that models the width of the relaxation peak. When $\alpha < 1$ the relaxation is said to be stretched; In other words it extends over a wider range of frequencies than a Debye relaxation. When $\alpha = 0$ the Cole-Cole model (Eq. 16) reduces to the Debye model (Eq. 15). For example, at the temperatures of −20 and −40 °C the Cole-Cole parameter changes from 1.00 to 0.97.

Only recently has a definitive, mechanistic model emerged which begins to explain the features of dielectric broadening in terms of a transition from one charge propagation mechanism, to another [34], i.e., orientation charge propagation transferring L-D defects through the ice matrix to ionic charge propagation of H_3O^+ and OH^- ion pairs, whereby protons hop through the like matrix in a similar manner to the Grotthus mechanism. This is interesting from a freeze-drying point of view because it potentially provides a mechanism by which changes in ice crystal structure might be elucidated.

2.3.7 Model for the TVIS Spectrum of Frozen Water

In the literature, the majority of dielectric spectroscopy measurements of ice have been undertaken using parallel plate electrodes made of metal (invariably gold-coated) and appropriate models developed for the overall measured response which incorporate the impedance of the electrode-sample interface (namely electrode polarization). In the case of the TVIS vial, the interfacial properties of the system are defined by the glass wall-sample impedance which, in a basic equivalent circuit model, may be approximated by a simple capacitance (C_G). In reality, the glass will retain the constant phase element behavior that was described by the enhanced model for the TVIS vial containing liquid sample (where the CPE_G models the fractal polarization mechanism associated with the percolation of protonic charge) (Fig. 12a).

In the new model for frozen water (ice) the sample capacitance (C_s) is no longer constant across the frequency range of the instrument (10 Hz to 1 MHz) but undergoes a step-like change in the real part capacitance and a peak in the imaginary capacitance due to the dielectric relaxation of ice. The sample capacitance, C_s, (which in the liquid state is based on the assumption that the dielectric properties of the liquid are independent of frequency, i.e., C_s was the static capacitance of the sample) is now replaced by a distributed element (DE_s) in parallel with an instantaneous capacitance $C_s(\infty)$. The distributed element (DE_s) represents the dispersive part of the Cole-Cole function (which models the dielectric relaxation of ice) whereas the instantaneous capacitance $C_s(\infty)$ represents the very fast induced polarization processes associated with electronic and atomic charge distortions in ice. The sample resistance (R_s) is presumed to be so high that it can be ignored, i.e., removed from the model (Fig. 16). The frequency dependence of the sample

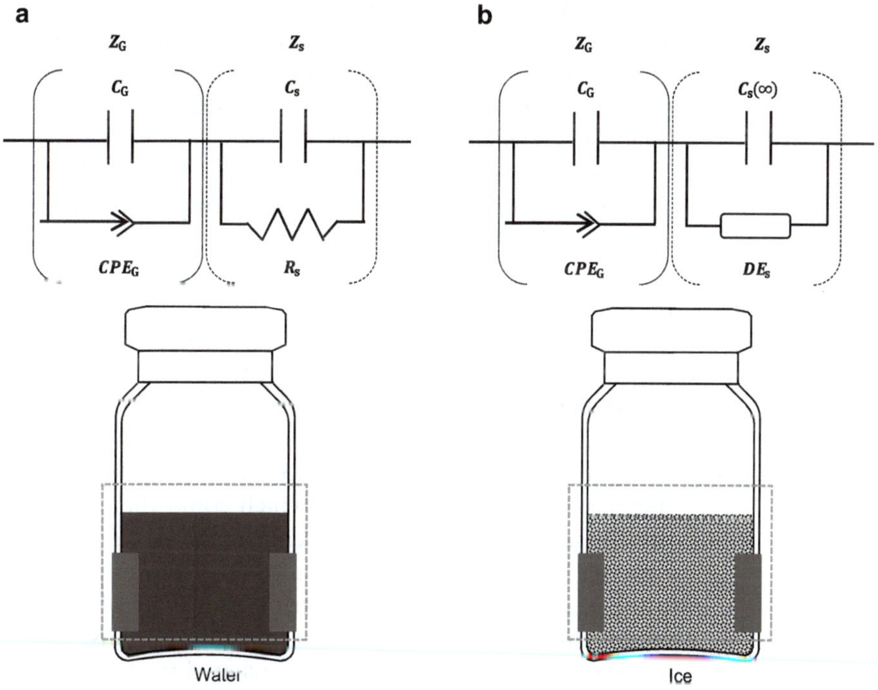

Fig. 16 Model for the TVIS vial containing (**a**) liquid water where the polarization mechanism association with percolation of protonic charge through the glass wall is modeled by the CPE_G element and the impedance of the water is represented by a resistor (R_S) and capacitor (C_S); and (**b**) frozen water where the impedance of the sample includes the dielectric relaxation of ice (as modeled by the distributed element DE_S of the Cole-Cole type) and an instantaneous capacitance $C_S(\infty)$. The glass wall impedance is assumed to behave like a capacitor (C_G) with a low-frequency dispersive attribute, modeled by the constant phase element, CPE_G

capacitance, $C_s(f)$, which is due to the dielectric relaxation of ice, results in the sample capacitance changing from a value of $C_s(0)$ at low frequency (the static capacitance) to a value of $C_s(\infty)$ at high frequency (the instantaneous capacitance). As a consequence, the capacitance of the model, $C'_{\mathrm{fit}}(f)$, is also frequency dependent changing from a value of $C'_{\mathrm{fit}}(0)$ at low frequency to a value of $C'_{\mathrm{fit}}(\infty)$ at high frequency.

In the example fit to the TVIS spectrum of frozen water at −20 and −40 °C (Fig. 17) the low-frequency data, from where the CPE_G element starts to manifest in the spectrum, has been excluded from the fitting process and so the CPE_G element has also been removed from the model (The horizontal line with the double arrow heads marks out the frequency range used for the fitting process). This simplified model then provides a good fit to the dielectric relaxation spectrum of ice at frequencies close to, and on the high frequency side of, the dielectric loss peak. Therefore, using this approach, i.e., by excluding *CPE* from the fitting, it might be possible to extract reasonable estimates for the relaxation time (τ) and distribution parameter (α) from fitting the Cole-Cole function over the middle to high-frequency range of the TVIS spectrum.

Having modeled the impedance spectrum of the ice filled vial, it is interesting to see what the spectrum would look like if the fit parameters for the ice relaxation and instantaneous capacitance were simulated in the absence of the glass wall capacitance (Fig. 18). It is clear from the differences between the simulated spectrum (gray line) and the experimental data (black dots) that the glass wall capacitance shifts the relaxation peak to higher frequencies and reduces it in size.

2.3.8 Determination of the Glass Wall Capacitance (C_G)

In the section on liquids, it was demonstrated how one could determine the cell constant ($C_o = 0.0525$ pF) from the measurement of a range of liquids and how the interfacial capacitance (C_G) varied slightly between the liquids (in the range 2.98–3.07 pF). These calculations were based on the fact that the low-frequency end of the real part capacitance spectrum provided an estimate for the glass wall capacitance (C_G) which could then be inserted into the equation for the high-frequency response (Eq. 10) to find an estimate for the sample capacitance (C_s). Plotting sample capacitance as a function of the dielectric permittivity of a range of polar liquids then provided the estimate for the cell constant.

For ice, the response is somewhat different, given that the dispersion is due to a dielectric relaxation rather than the Maxwell-Wagner polarization of the glass wall capacitance. Here, in the limit of low frequency ($f \rightarrow 0$) the capacitance of the model for ice (Fig. 17) can be written as:

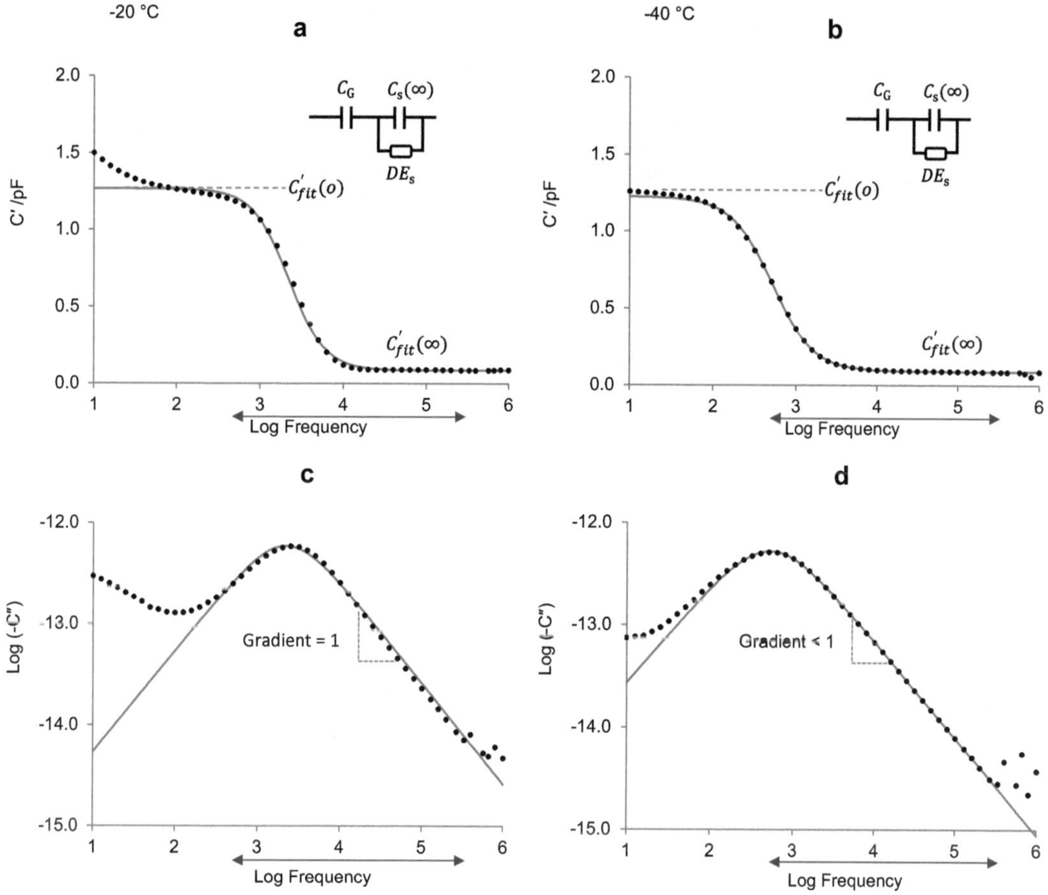

Fig. 17 Measured sample capacitance $C_s(f)$ as a function of frequency (*black dots*) and fitting results (*gray line*) to the simplified model for the dielectric relaxation of ice and the glass wall capacitance (which ignores the CPE_G response of the glass) (**a–d**) for the TVIS vial containing 3.5 g of double distilled water (fill factor 0.7) with electrodes of dimensions 19 × 10 mm and a 3 mm gap between the bottom of the electrode and base of the vial. The frequency range used for the fitting process is marked by the *double-headed arrow.* The real part capacitance of ice at (**a**) −20 °C and (**b**) −40 °C, and the imaginary part capacitance of ice at (**c**) −20 °C and (**d**) −40 °C are shown. Both temperatures were arrived at on reheating of frozen water from −45 °C. Note that the imaginary permittivity is plotted on a log scale in order to demonstrate more clearly the broadening of the relaxation peak as the temperature is reduced from −20 to −40 °C. This broadening is manifest in the Cole-Cole distribution parameter α which has a value of $\alpha = 1$ at −20 °C (which means that the relaxation has a Debye-like characteristics) and a value of $\alpha = 0.945$ at −40 °C, which is consistent with the change in polarization mechanism from orientation charge propagation transferring L-D defects through the ice matrix to ionic charge propagation of H_3O^+ and OH^- ion pairs

$$C'_{\text{fit}}(0) = \frac{C_s(0) \cdot C_G}{C_s(0) + C_G} \tag{17}$$

where $C_s(0)$ has a value equal to the sum of the magnitude of DE_s and $C_s(\infty)$. Incidentally, in the limit of high frequency ($f \to \infty$) the capacitance of the model in Fig. 17 can be written as:

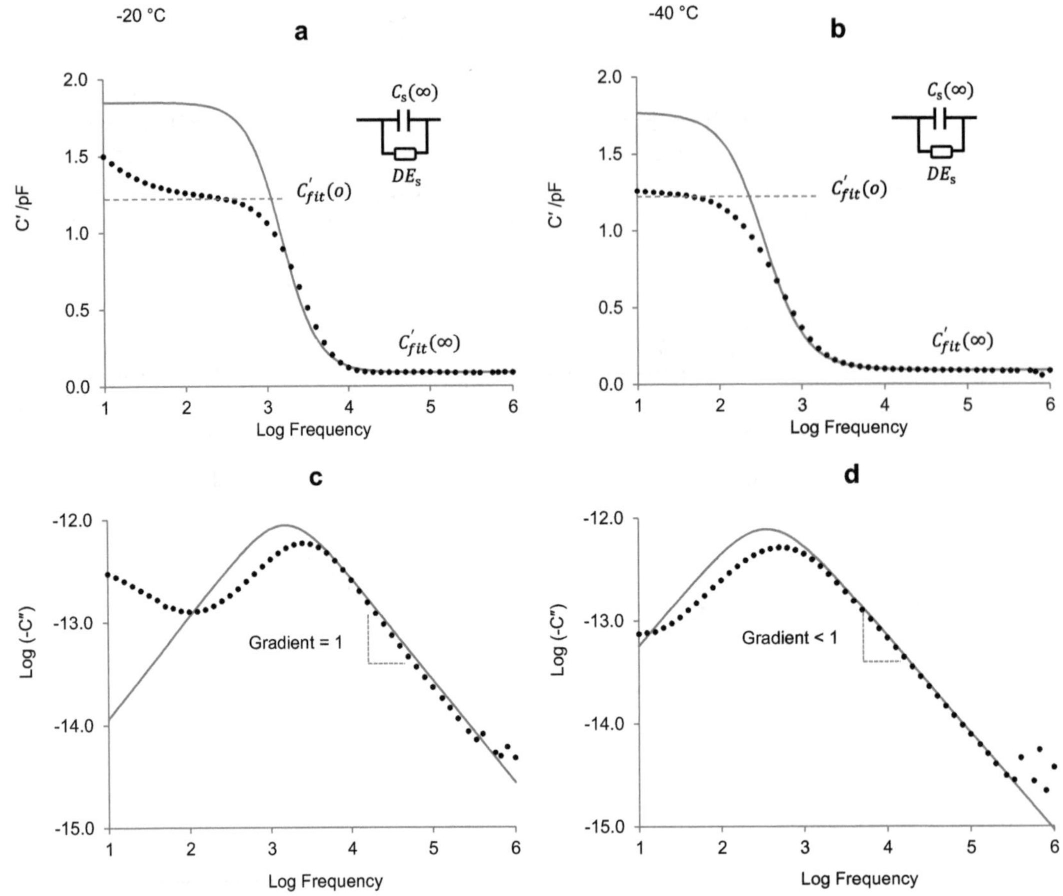

Fig. 18 The capacitance spectrum of 3.5 g frozen water at −20 °C (**a** and **c**) and −40 °C (**b** and **d**) in a TVIS vial with electrode dimensions of 10 × 19 mm and positioned at 3 mm from the base of vial are shown. The *black dots* represent the measured data points whereas the *gray line* shows the simulation results when the C_G element is removed from the simplified model ($C_G - C_s(\infty) = DE_s$) to illustrate the impact of glass capacitance (C_G) on the peak frequency and peak amplitude of ice at (**c**) −20 °C and (**d**) −40 °C

$$C'_{\text{fit}}(\infty) = \frac{C_s(\infty) \cdot C_G}{C_s(\infty) + C_G} \tag{18}$$

An expression for the glass wall capacitance C_G (Eq. 22) can be found by re-arranging Eq. 17 as follows:

$$C'_{\text{fit}}(0) = \frac{C_s(0) \cdot C_G}{C_s(0) + C_G} \cdot \frac{C_s(0) - C_G}{C_s(0) - C_G} \tag{19}$$

$$C'_{\text{fit}}(0) = \frac{C_s^2(0) C_G - C_s(0) C_G^2}{C_s^2(0) - C_G^2} \tag{20}$$

$$\left(C_s(0) - C'_{\text{fit}}(0)\right) C_G^2 - C_s^2(0) C_G + C'_{\text{fit}}(0) C_s^2(0) = 0 \tag{21}$$

Table 4
Estimate for the instantaneous capacitance of the glass wall (C_G) during the re-heating of ice (for ultrapure water 6.5 g is filled in an Adelphi VC010-20C Type I glass tubing vial attached with a pair of electrodes of dimensions 19 × 10 mm and 3 mm gap between the bottom of the electrode and base of the vial) [34]

Temperature (°C)	$C'(0)$ (pF)	$\varepsilon_s(0)$	$C_s(0)$ (pF)	C_G1 (pF)	C_G2 (pF)
−51.8	1.65	117.6	6.17	2.25	6.17
−50.1	1.65	116.7	6.12	2.26	6.12
−45.1	1.65	114.0	5.99	2.28	5.99
−39.9	1.65	111.4	5.85	2.31	5.85
−35.1	1.66	109.1	5.73	2.33	5.73
−29.9	1.66	106.7	5.60	2.37	5.60
−24.9	1.67	104.5	5.49	2.40	5.49
−20.1	1.67	102.5	5.38	2.42	5.38

The value of C_G taken from Eq. 22 has two values (C_G1 and C_G2). However, C_G1 is selected as a parameter for $C_G - C_s = \mathrm{DE}_s$ model because it has the correct temperature dependency (i.e., C_G increases with temperature) as shown in Fig. 19 and its values are also lower than both the theoretical (C_G = 3.99 pF) and experimental values (C_G = 2.98–3.07 pF). Moreover, a linear extrapolation of these low-temperature values to +20 °C (i.e., the temperature at which the liquid water measurements were made) predicts a value for C_G of ~2.65 pF which is close to that obtained experimentally for liquid water (C_G = 3.07 pF). A second order polynomial fit to the low-temperature values of C_G provides an estimate (C_G = 2.75 pF) which is even closer to that obtained for liquid water

$$C_G = \frac{-\left(C_s^2(0)\right) \pm \sqrt{\left(C_s^2(0)\right)^2 - 4\left(C'_{\mathrm{fit}}(0) - C_s(0)\right)\left(C'_{\mathrm{fit}}(0) C_s^2(0)\right)}}{2\left(C'_{\mathrm{fit}}(0) - C_s(0)\right)} \tag{22}$$

One can then estimate the dielectric properties of the ice-glass wall interface (C_G) by first fitting the complex capacitance spectrum to find estimates for the low-frequency capacitance ($C'_{\mathrm{fit}}(0)$) at various temperatures and then inserting those estimates into Eq. 22 along with estimates for the low-frequency capacitance of the ice, which have been calculated from literature values of the dielectric properties of ice ($\varepsilon_s(0)$) [34] as shown in Table 4 and the cell constant that has been determined in the section on liquids.

Estimate for the glass capacitance C_G at different temperatures during the re-heating of ice is shown in Table 4 and Fig. 19.

2.3.9 Freezing of Solutions

As ice forms during the freezing stage, the remaining water becomes concentrated into an unfrozen fraction which contains the solutes from the original solution. The solutes are either in an

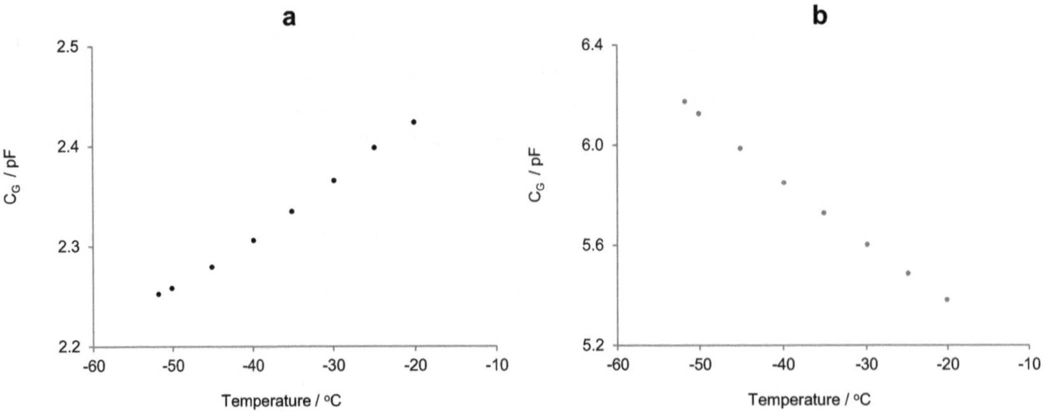

Fig. 19 Estimates for the instantaneous capacitance of the glass wall over the temperature range −20 to −50 °C; (**a**) is C_G1 and (**b**) is C_G2

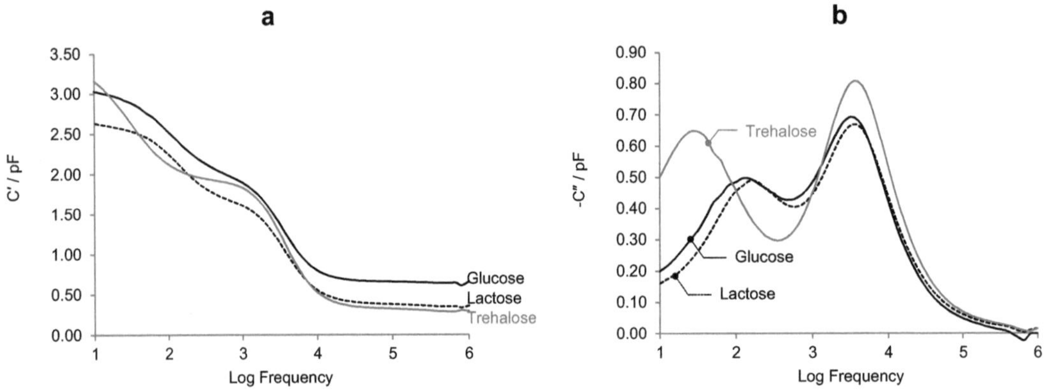

Fig. 20 The capacitance spectra of 3% solutions of glucose (*black solid line*), lactose (*black dash line*), and trehalose (*gray solid line*) contained in the TVIS vial with electrode dimension of 10 × 19 mm and at a height of 3 mm from vial base during re-heating process. The temperature of the samples is −18 °C. The real part and imaginary part capacitance are shown in (**a**) and (**b**), respectively

amorphous super-cooled liquid/glass (depending on whether the temperature of this fraction is below its glass transition temperature) or will have precipitated from solution (crystallized) as they exceed their solubility limit. Given the high viscosity of this phase and the tortuosity of the path length for the conduction of ionic charges its conductivity is expected to be dramatically lower than that of the original liquid phase (even allowing for the fact that the concentration of ionic conductors in this phase is higher that of the original solution). However, the conductivity of the unfrozen fraction is likely to be higher than ice and so there is potential for the re-introduction of a Maxwell-Wagner process to the complex capacitance spectrum of a frozen solution. Figure 20 shows an example of such a response.

Two possible mechanisms provide feasible explanations of the origin of this second process. The first is that the juxtaposition of ice crystals with the thin interstitial spaces of the unfrozen results in Maxwell-Wagner polarization at the mesoscale. The second is that the conductivity pathways for charges migrating through the unfrozen fraction to the extremities of the sample result in a Maxwell-Wagner process that is manifest at the macroscopic scale of the glass-sample interface. The reason why it is manifest in the lower frequency part of the spectrum is a consequence of the much higher resistance of the unfrozen fraction compared with that of the original solution.

The equivalent circuit must then be modified to account for this second process by re-introducing a resistance, R, in parallel with the Cole-Cole element for the relaxation of ice (Fig. 21).

Complete solidification of all components (not just that of the ice) is achieved by cooling the contents of the vial to temperatures lower than the eutectic temperature of the crystalline solutes and/or the glass transition temperatures of the non-crystallizing solutes. Combinations of non-crystallizing excipients and crystallizing excipients have been used to suppress the crystallization of the latter and it has been demonstrated that TVIS may be used to witness the crystallization of an eutectic material while being able to monitor the suppression of the eutectic by the addition of another agent such as sucrose [6].

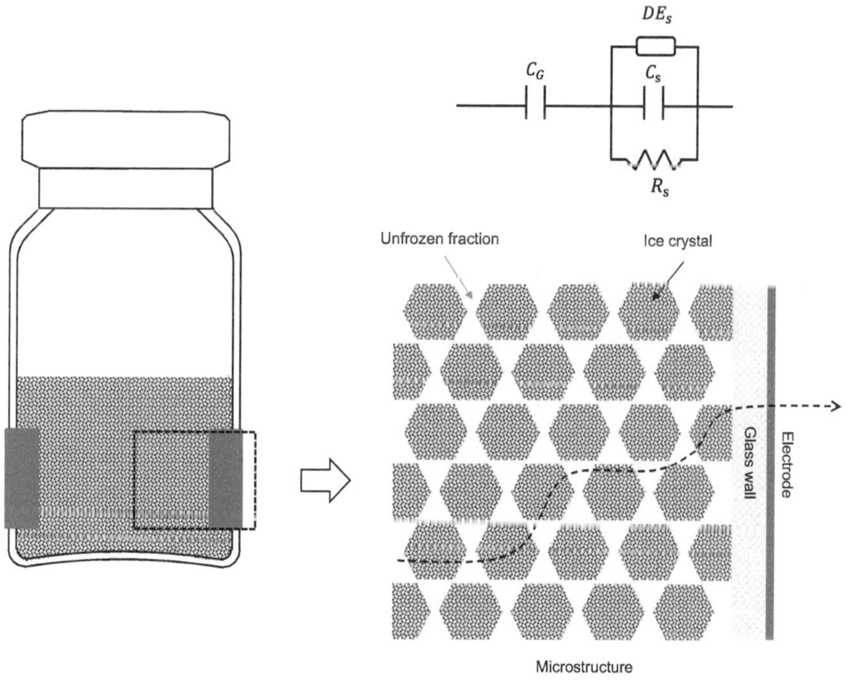

Fig. 21 A more complex equivalent circuit model is required for the two phase system comprising ice fraction and unfrozen fraction

Previous publications on various applications of TVIS technology for frozen solutions, describe the uses of TVIS for determining (1) the glass transition temperature of maltodextrin solutions [19]; (2) the potential application of TVIS in mini pilot studies [18]; (3) the impact of annealing on primary drying rate [11].

3 Future Prospects

The TVIS technology described in this chapter is currently being developed further for the purpose of establishing new approaches for determining a number of critical process parameters:

1. The distribution of temperature, in the vertical direction within the vial, such that the sublimation interface temperature and the base temperature inside the vial might be predicted.
2. The sublimation rate in primary drying.
3. The heat transfer coefficient (K_v) and the dry layer resistance (R_p).
4. The impact of microcollapse.

A commercial system has now been developed by Sciospec GmbH which replicates the capability of De Montfort University's laboratory demonstrator that has been used to create the data throughout this book chapter, but with the additional benefit of an extended frequency range to 10 MHz and a temperature stabilized operational amplifier to reduce instrumentation drift.

Further developments in the instrumentation, with ever-increasing sensitivity to small capacitances, will enable the electrode system to be removed from the vial and a new single electrode to be placed over a small cluster of vials in a non-contact or stand-off mode. A "non-contact" through vial impedance spectrometer of this type (NC-TVIS) would be compatible with the automatic vial loading system. Its limitation is that it may not be compatible with the vial stoppering system unless the electrode system is integrated within the dryer, e.g., built into the underside of the shelf above the vials. In order to provide compatibility with both automatic vial loading and vial stoppering a further development of the TVIS system is envisaged that can be pushed into the dryer along with the other vials, in a similar way to the operation of the Lyo Shuttle that was developed by Ellab for thermocouple measurements. The operation principles of a "TVIS Shuttle" would be similar to the TVIS system described in this book chapter and would rely on modified vials with electrodes attached to the outside surface. The instrument (which is now located inside the dryer) would need to be stable within the environment of low temperature and pressure, while generating minimal heat so as to have an insignificant impact on the heat transfer to the nearest neighbor vials, including the

TVIS measurement vial. Data from the device could be downloaded after the completion of the process, and the instrument removed from the dryer, or transmitted by RF or some other protocol during the freeze-drying process.

4 Further Reading

While applications for impedance spectroscopy in the pharmaceutical sciences are quite limited in scope and application, there are more generalized applications for impedance spectroscopy and its sister technique of broadband dielectric spectroscopy, in a wide range of applications, including electrochemistry, materials science, and biology.

1. Raicu V, Feldman Y (eds) (2015) Dielectric relaxation in biological systems: physical principles, methods, and applications. Oxford University Press, Oxford
2. Orazem ME, Tribollet B (2008) Electrochemical impedance spectroscopy. Wiley, Hoboken, NJ
3. Barsoukov E, Macdonald JR (eds) (2005) Impedance spectroscopy: theory, experiment, and applications, 2nd edn. Wiley-Interscience, a John Wiley & Sons, Inc., Hoboken, NJ
4. Kremer F, Schönhals A (eds) (2003) Broadband dielectric spectroscopy. Springer, Berlin

Acknowledgments

The original TVIS system used to generate the spectra within this book chapter was developed by Evgeny Polygalov and Geoff Smith (from De Montfort University) in a collaboration with GEA Pharma Systems (Eastleigh, UK) and was part-funded by a UK government, Innovate UK Collaborative R&D project called Lyo-DEA (Project Reference: 100527).
Special thanks go to Yowwares Jeeraruangrattana (from the Government Pharmaceutical Organization, in Thailand and one of De Montfort University's PhD students from 2015 to 2018) for creating the majority of the images, drawings and figures, and assisting in formatting of the text and bibliography.

Appendix 1: Analysis of Peak Frequency and Peak Magnitude

The relative simplicity of the imaginary capacitance spectrum means that it is possible to follow two features of the peak using proprietary LyoView™ data viewing software, namely the peak frequency (F_{PEAK}) and the peak amplitude (C''_{PEAK}).

LyoView™*PeakFindingProcedure* :
This procedure is intended for the determination of the Maxwell-Wagner peak parameters such as peak amplitude and frequency position for individual dielectric spectra obtained during the freeze-drying cycle.

There are four stages in peak search procedure:

1. Preparation of the spectrum: (a) Smoothing of the dielectric loss spectrum to eliminate sharp spikes originating from scattering due to finite sensitivity or from electromagnetic interference. For this purpose the RMS deviation throughout the curve is calculated. For each point deviation from average of previous and next point is calculated and if the deviation is larger than half of RMS the value point is replaced by the average of previous and next point. After that moving average filter with aperture 3 is applied twice and using free cubic spline the number of points N is increased to $10 \times N$); followed by (b) interpolation by free cubic spline in order to increase the number of points and accuracy of peak parameters determination.
2. Differentiation of the spectrum obtained in step 1 and finding all negative peaks (zero first derivative and positive second derivative) and all positive peaks (second derivative negative) peaks which are present in the smoothed spectrum.
3. Rejection of any narrow peaks that originate from residual spikes which are not completely suppressed by curve smoothing.
4. Selection of the principle peak, if there is more than one peak that meets all previous criteria. Several criteria are applied depending on the stage of the freeze-drying: (a) at freezing and early stages of primary drying the peak with the largest amplitude is selected, (b) at the middle and late stage of primary drying, the peak with frequency position closest to frequency position of principal peak in previous spectrum is selected.

The F_{PEAK} parameter can be used to predict the product temperature whereas the C''_{PEAK} parameter can be used to determine the amount of ice remaining during the primary drying phase from which one can then predict both drying rate and end point. Both parameters lend themselves to the determination of phase behavior (ice formation, eutectic formation, and glass transition events).

Appendix 2: Basic Principles of Impedance Spectroscopy as It Applies to a Liquid Filled in TVIS Vial

The impedance of most real objects (i.e., those which have a combination of characteristics, for example, some resistance and some electrical capacitance) takes on a frequency-dependence largely because the impedance of a capacitance (Fig. 22a) is dependent on the frequency of the applied field, whereas an ideal resistor has zero frequency dependence (Fig. 22b). The impedance spectrum of a capacitor (in terms of the impedance magnitude and phase angle) displays a characteristic negative slow of −1 in the plot of log impedance magnitude vs. log frequency. This is because the impedance is an inverse function of the capacitance and the applied frequency.

$$Z = \frac{1}{i\omega C} \tag{23}$$

In the case of a composite object which has capacitance and resistance then the impedance spectrum that results will be dominated by one or the other element, depending on whether the elements are in series or in parallel and how the frequency of the applied field defines the relative magnitude of the impedance of the capacitance and the resistance.

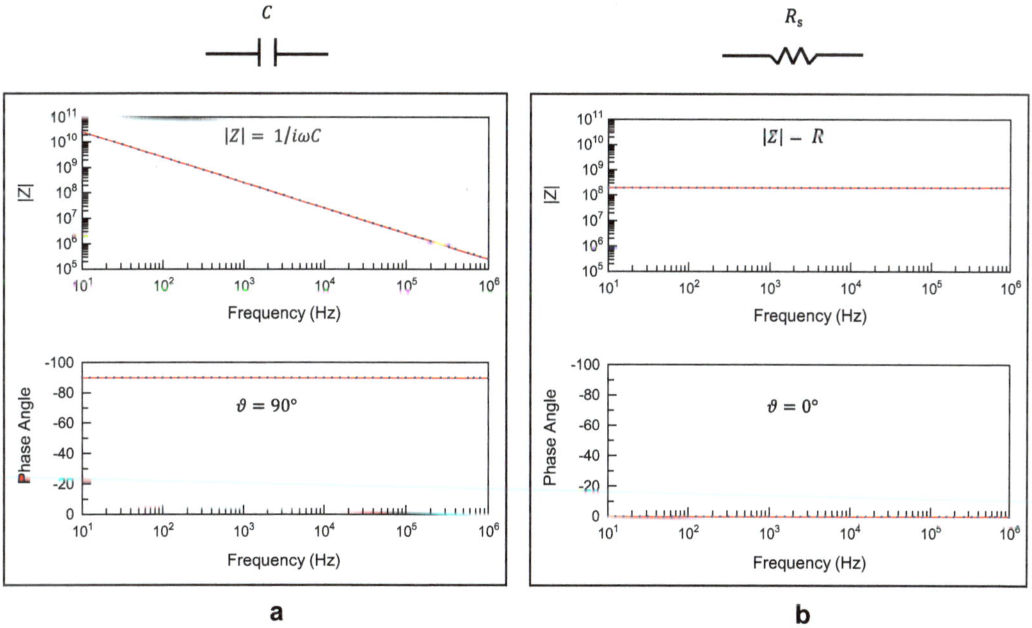

Fig. 22 Bode plots (impedance magnitude (|Z|) and phase angle (ϑ)) for the impedances of a capacitor (**a**) and a resistor (**b**)

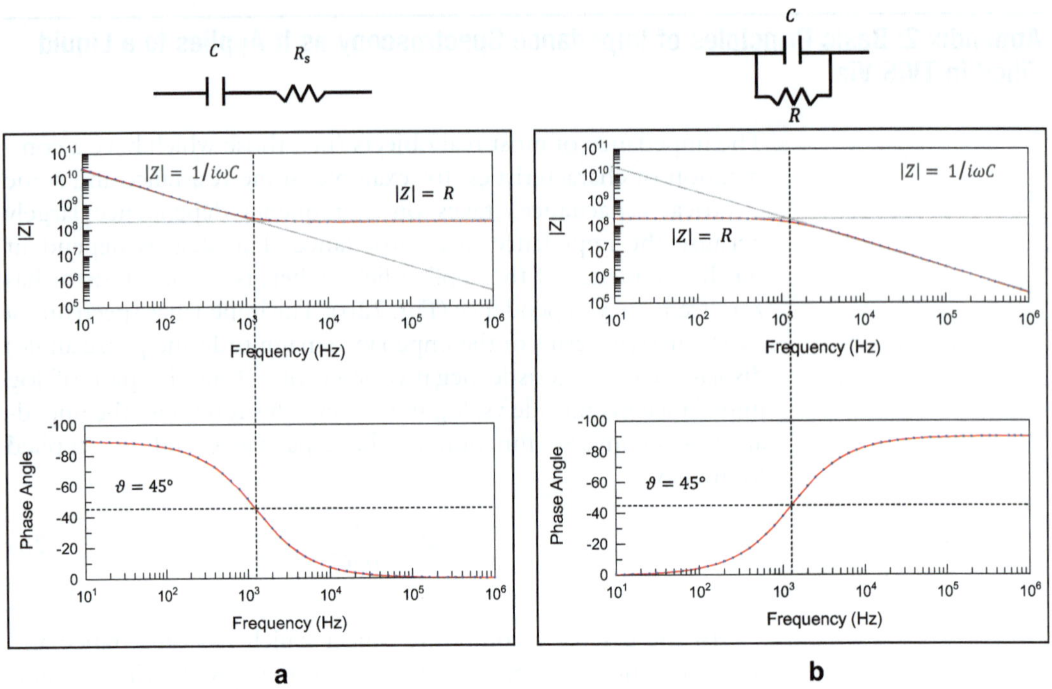

Fig. 23 Bode plots (impedance magnitude (|Z|) and phase angle (ϑ)) for the impedances of a series circuit (**a**) and a parallel circuit (**b**)

In a Series Circuit

At low frequency the capacitor dominates the spectrum (Fig. 23a) because the impedance of the capacitance is so high that the capacitor effectively controls the current that flows through the circuit.

At high frequency the resistor dominates the spectrum (Fig. 23a) because the impedance of the capacitor has fallen below that of the resistor such that the resistor effectively controls the current that flows through the circuit.

In a Parallel Circuit

At low frequency the resistor dominates the spectrum (Fig. 23b) because the impedance of the capacitance is so high that all the current flows through the resistor.

At high frequency the capacitor dominates the spectrum (Fig. 23b) because the impedance of the capacitance is now lower than the resistor such that all the current now flows through the capacitor.

More complex composite objects can be considered combinations of impedances. Again, the impedance spectrum that results will be dominated by one or the other impedance.

In a Complex Circuit

At low frequency (<1 kHz) the resistor R (Fig. 24) dominates the impedance of the RC_1 circuit, because this circuit is in series with a capacitor, C_2 (which has a high impedance at low frequency) then C_2 effectively controls the current that flows through the entire circuit.

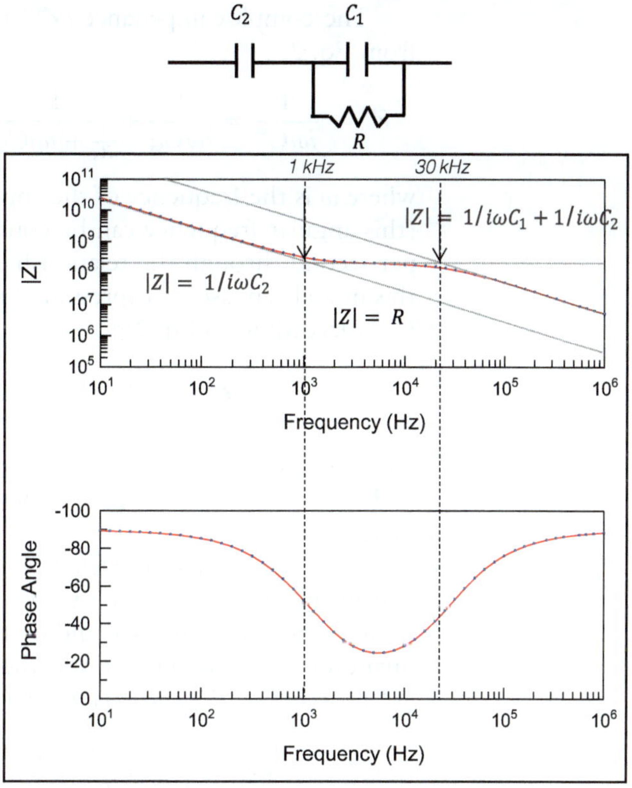

Fig. 24 Bode plots (impedance magnitude (|Z|) and phase angle (ϑ)) for the impedances of a complex circuit

At intermediate frequency (1–30 kHz) the impedance of C_2 drops below that of the resistor (Fig. 24), such that the resistor begins to dominate the impedance and therefore the phase angle tends to increase from −90 to 0 (Fig. 24).

At high frequency (>30 kHz) the impedance of the capacitor (C_1) in parallel with the resistor, decreases below that of the resistor (Fig. 24) such that the resistor no longer dominates the impedance of the parallel RC_1 circuit and as a result the circuit behaves like two capacitors in series. The high-frequency impedance is therefore dominated by the inverse of the sum of the capacitances

$$Z = \frac{1}{i\omega(C_1 + C_2)} \tag{24}$$

The above model can be mapped onto the physical characteristic of the liquid filled vial, where C_2 is the glass wall capacitance (C_G), C_1 is the sample capacitance (C_s), and R is the sample resistance (R_s).

The complex impedance (Z^*) of the model can be calculated from Eq. 25:

$$Z^* = \frac{1}{i\omega C^*} = \frac{1}{i\omega C_G} + \frac{1}{\frac{1}{R_S} + i\omega C_S} = \frac{1 + i\omega R_S(C_G + C_S)}{i\omega C_G - \omega^2 R_S C_G C_S} \quad (25)$$

where ω is the frequency of the applied field in radians per second (this angular frequency can be converted into frequency in cycles per second through the relationship $\omega = 2\pi f$). The impedance of this model can also be expressed in terms of a complex capacitance (C^*) according to Eq. 26:

$$C^* = C' + iC'' = \frac{1}{i\omega Z^*} = \frac{C_G + i\omega R_S C_G C_S}{1 + i\omega R_S(C_G + C_S)} \quad (26)$$

where C' is the real part capacitance (or simply, the capacitance) and C'' is the imaginary part capacitance (otherwise known as the dielectric loss).

From the complex capacitance formula, the expressions for real and imaginary capacitance can be calculated. This is achieved by multiplying the nominator and denominator by the complex conjugate of the denominator and then grouping to obtain the real (C') parts (Eq. 29) and imaginary (C'') parts (Eq. 30).

$$C^* = \frac{1}{i\omega Z^*} = \frac{(C_G + i\omega R_S C_2 C_G)(1 - i\omega R_S(C_S + C_G))}{(1 + i\omega R_S(C_S + C_G))(1 - i\omega R_S(C_S + C_G))} \quad (27)$$

$$= \frac{C_G + \omega^2 R_S^2 C_G C_S(C_S + C_G) - i\omega R_S C_G^2}{1 + (\omega R_S((C_S + C_G))^2} \quad (28)$$

$$C' = \frac{C_G + \omega^2 R_S^2 C_G C_S(C_S + C_G)}{1 + (\omega R_S((C_S + C_G))^2} \quad (29)$$

$$C'' = -\frac{\omega R_S C_G^2}{1 + (\omega R_S((C_S + C_G))^2} \quad (30)$$

References

1. Greaves RIN (1954) Theoretical aspects of drying by vacuum sublimation. In: Harris RJC (ed) Biological applications of freezing and drying. Academic, New York, pp 87–127
2. DeLuca PP (1977) Freeze drying of pharmaceuticals. J Vac Sci Technol 14(1):620–629
3. Deluca P, Lachman L (1965) Lyophilization of pharmaceuticals I. Effect of certain physical-chemical properties. J Pharm Sci 54 (4):617–624
4. Rey LR (1960a) Study of the freezing and drying of tissues at very low temperatures. In: Parkes AS, Audrey US (eds) Recent research in freezing and drying. Blackwell, Oxford, pp 40–62
5. Ward KR, Matejtschuk P (2010) The use of microscopy, thermal analysis, and impedance measurements to establish critical formulation parameters for freeze-drying cycle development. In: Rey L, May JC (eds) Freeze

drying/lyophilization of pharmaceutical and biological products, 3rd edn. Informa Healthcare, London, pp 111–135

6. Arshad MS, Smith G, Polygalov E et al (2014) Through-vial impedance spectroscopy of critical events during the freezing stage of the lyophilization cycle: the example of the impact of sucrose on the crystallization of mannitol. Eur J Pharm Biopharm 87(3):598–605. https://doi.org/10.1016/j.ejpb.2014.05.005
7. Evans SA, Morris KR, Mackenzie AP et al (1995) Dielectric characterization of thermodynamic first order events in model frozen systems intended for lyophilization. PDA J Pharm Sci Technol 49(1):2–8
8. Rey LR (1960b) Thermal analysis of eutectics in freezing solutions. Ann N Y Acad Sci 85 (1):510–534
9. Morris KR, Evans SA, Mackenzie AP et al (1994) Prediction of lyophile collapse temperature by dielectric analysis. PDA J Pharm Sci Technol 48(6):318–329
10. Her LM, Jefferis RP, Gatlin LA et al (1994) Measurement of glass transition temperatures in freeze concentrated solutions of non-electrolytes by electrical thermal analysis. Pharm Res 11(7):1023–1029
11. Smith G, Arshad MS, Polygalov E et al (2014b) Through-vial impedance spectroscopy of the mechanisms of annealing in the freeze-drying of maltodextrin: the impact of annealing hold time and temperature on the primary drying rate. J Pharm Sci 103(6):1799–1810
12. Mackenzie AP (1985) Changes in electrical resistance during freezing and their application to the control of the freeze-drying process. In: Anonymous (ed) Fundamentals and applications of freeze-drying to biological materials, drugs and foodstuffs. International Institute of Refrigeration, Paris, pp 155–163
13. Smith G, Polygalov E, Arshad M et al (2013a) An impedance-based process analytical technology for monitoring the lyophilisation process. Int J Pharm 449(1):72–83
14. Bandari S, Sesha Sai M, Reddy YR (2013) Optimization of lyophilization cycles for gemcitabine. Int J Pharm Pharm Sci 5(2):216–221
15. Alkeev N, Averin S, von Gratowski S (2015) New method for monitoring the process of freeze drying of biological materials. AAPS PharmSciTech 16(6):1474–1479
16. Smith G, Arshad MS, Nazari K et al (2014) Through-vial impedance spectroscopy: a new in-line process analytical technology for freeze drying. Pharm Technol 38(4):30–37
17. Smith G, Arshad MS, Polygalov E et al (2014a) Factors affecting the use of impedance spectroscopy in the characterisation of the freezing stage of the lyophilisation process: the impact of liquid fill height in relation to electrode geometry. AAPS PharmSciTech 15 (2):261–269
18. Smith G, Arshad MS, Polygalov E et al (2017) Process understanding in freeze-drying cycle development: applications for through-vial impedance spectroscopy (TVIS) in mini-pilot studies. J Pharm Innov 12(1):26–40
19. Smith G, Arshad MS, Polygalov E et al (2013b) An application for impedance spectroscopy in the characterisation of the glass transition during the lyophilization cycle: the example of a 10% w/v maltodextrin solution. Eur J Pharm Biopharm 85(3, Part B):1130–1140. https://doi.org/10.1016/j.ejpb.2013.08.004
20. Shen M, Ge S, Cao W (2001) Dielectric enhancement and Maxwell-Wagner effects in polycrystalline ferroelectric multilayered thin films. J Phys D Appl Phys 34(19): 2935–2938
21. Liu J, Duan CG, Mei WN et al (2005) Dielectric properties and Maxwell-Wagner relaxation of compounds $A\ Cu_3Ti_4O_{12}$(A = Ca, $Bi_{2/3}$, $Y_{2/3}$, $La_{2/3}$). J Appl Phys 98(9):093703
22. Foster KR, Schwan HP (1989) Dielectric properties of tissues and biological materials: a critical review. Crit Rev Biomed Eng 17:25–104
23. Stubbe M, Gimsa J (2015) Maxwell's mixing equation revisited: characteristic impedance equations for ellipsoidal cells. Biophys J 109 (2):194–208. https://doi.org/10.1016/j.bpj.2015.06.021
24. Jacob JM (2004) Sinusoidal waveforms. In: Anonymous (ed) Advanced AC circuits and electronics: principles & applications. Delmar Learning, New York, pp 3–28
25. Carlson G, Illman B (2002) Series capacitors and the inverse sum rule. Am J Phys 70 (11):1122–1128
26. Melinder Å (2010) Properties and other aspects of aqueous solutions used for single phase and ice slurry applications. Int J Refrig 33(8):1506–1512
27. Ryabov Y, Gutina A, Arkhipov V et al (2001) Dielectric relaxation of water absorbed in porous glass. J Phys Chem B 105 (9):1845–1850
28. Johari GP, Whalley E (1981) The dielectric properties of ice Ih in the range 272–133 K. J Chem Phys 75(3):1333–1340
29. Bernal J, Fowler R (1933) A theory of water and ionic solution, with particular reference to hydrogen and hydroxyl ions. J Chem Phys 1 (8):515–548
30. Hobbs PV (1974) Ice physics. Claredon press, Oxford

31. Pauling L, Brockway LO, Beach JY (1935) The dependence of interatomic distance on single bond-double bond resonance. J Am Chem Soc 57(12):2705–2709
32. Shinyashiki N, Yamamoto W, Yokoyama A et al (2009) Glass transitions in aqueous solutions of protein (bovine serum albumin). J Phys Chem B 113(43):14448–14456
33. Popov I, Puzenko A, Khamzin A et al (2015) The dynamic crossover in dielectric relaxation behavior of ice I h. Phys Chem Chem Phys 17 (2):1489–1497
34. Popov I, Lunev I, Khamzin A et al (2017) The low-temperature dynamic crossover in the dielectric relaxation of ice I h. Phys Chem Chem Phys 19(42):28610–28620

Chapter 12

Lyophilization of High-Concentration Protein Formulations

Patrick Garidel and Ingo Presser

Abstract

High-concentration protein formulations are in the focus of current pharmaceutical development because the required therapeutic doses of biologics, especially monoclonal antibodies, are extremely high, ranging between 5 and 750 mg per patient. Considering applications via the sub-cutaneous route, protein concentrations much above 300 mg/mL are often requested. At present, commercialized high-concentration biologics, with protein concentrations between 150 and 200 mg/mL, are launched as lyophilized (freeze-dried) products, while liquid protein formulations are available with concentrations around 100 mg/mL.

The current chapter will address specific topics linked to high-concentration lyophilized protein formulations. The term "high-concentration protein formulation" (HCPF) is often used, but hardly ever defined. We have therefore asked, how highly concentrated can a protein formulation become? We consider this question, particularly for monoclonal antibody drugs, along with the rationale for developing HCPF and the issues encountered during formulation.

Lyophilization is the technique of choice for stabilizing labile molecules. However, for the development of high-concentration, freeze-dried protein formulations (HC-FDPFs), new challenges appear, such as extremely prolonged reconstitution times or even stability issues. Therefore, new technologies such as controlled nucleation are introduced and presented as one option for reducing these unfavorable reconstitution times.

Key words High-concentration, Protein, Lyophilization, Freeze-drying, Controlled nucleation, Pharmaceutical development, Monoclonal antibody, Formulation, Packaging characteristics, Solubility, Colloidal properties

1 Introduction

Lyophilization, also known as freeze-drying, is the most valuable and accepted technology in the pharmaceutical industry for drug-product development, especially in cases where the active pharmaceutical ingredient lacks a reasonable stability under liquid conditions. A number of excellent monographs, books, and review papers are available, which cover the essentials of lyophilization such as formulation development, the process of freeze-drying, specific analytics for solid dosage forms, and instrumentation

Kevin R. Ward and Paul Matejtschuk (eds.), *Lyophilization of Pharmaceuticals and Biologicals: New Technologies and Approaches*, Methods in Pharmacology and Toxicology, https://doi.org/10.1007/978-1-4939-8928-7_12,

from lab-scale to the fully validated and qualified process freeze-dryer [1–13].

The terms lyophilization and freeze-drying are used in this chapter synonymously. The origins of these terminologies, as well as the history of the drying process, have been presented in depth by Louis Rey and Joan May [11] or Felix Franks and Tony Auffret [10], and will not be considered here.

Despite lyophilization's high costs and the complexity of adding another process step, freeze-drying offers a major advantage: improved stability allows lyophilized drug products to be stored even at room temperature. This advantage comes with challenges, however, such as the need for reconstitution prior to application, the development of specific reconstitution media, the general high costs of goods, the addition of another batch process, etc.

"High-concentration protein formulations" (HCPF) — whether the term is applied to a lyophilized or liquid formulation — is generally, but imprecisely, applied to preparations ranging between 50 and 150 mg/mL protein. The pharmaceutical community uses the term to highlight characteristic sets of solution properties that are more common among HCPFs than in formulations of, for example, 10 mg/mL protein. Characteristics of HCPFs include, for example, increased viscosities, high opalescence, liquid-liquid phase separation, gel formation, or the increased propensity for protein particle formation. Solutions of low-concentration protein formulations, on the other hand, usually behave more or less like solutions of the corresponding placebo formulations.

Some of the properties observed at high protein concentration impose particular challenges for developing a lyophilized drug product.

These aspects will be covered, the underlying challenges discussed, and potential solutions described in this contribution.

In summary, this chapter will consider:

1. The lack of definition of the term "high-concentration protein formulation," with potential methods for measuring protein solubility, and calculations for estimating the maximum achievable protein concentration, based on structural and molecular packing considerations.
2. Why process developers and clinicians consider high concentration protein formulations necessary or desirable.
3. The issues related to the development of high concentrated protein formulations, including molecular properties, formulation, primary packing/device, and process development as well as manufacturing constraints.
4. The specific demands for lyophilizing drug products with high protein concentration are more deeply discussed and various case studies presented. Detailed attention is given to the

prolonged reconstitution times of high-concentration protein freeze-dried proteins and specific stability issues.

5. Technologies that have been shown to provide some advantages for the lyophilization of high-concentration protein formulations.
6. Current trends and open topics in the field.

2 Why Do We Need High-Concentration Protein Formulations?

Most biologics are developed as parenteral drugs, and the most conventional delivery route is an intravenous administration via infusion. Subcutaneous injection is, however, a viable alternative for frequent and chronic administration of drug products, particularly when coupled with delivery to pre-filled syringes (PFS), pens, or auto-injector devices which allow self- and home-administration. Subcutaneous self-administration both increases patient compliance and avoids hospitalization, thus reducing treatment costs.

To avoid pain at the site of the injection, subcutaneous delivery volumes are usually restricted to just 1–1.5 mL [14, 15]. The challenge, then, is "dissolving" the whole therapeutic dose in that small volume.

Co-formulations with the enzyme hyaluronidase (which breaks down the subcutaneous matrix and lets the tissue accommodate larger volumes of fluid) have been developed that allow subcutaneous injections up to 10 mL (for more details, see for example: Frost [16], Tang et al. [17], Narasimhan et al. [18], Shpilberg and Jackisch [19], Leveque [20], Jackisch et al. [21], Mathaes et al. [22]. Such co-formulations may trigger additional stability issues, so this approach must be evaluated carefully and case-by-case.

Biologics like monoclonal antibodies are often administered at frequent dosing regimens and at very high doses of several mg of drug per kg of patient body weight. Delivering monoclonal antibodies in subcutaneous doses of 100–700 mg protein in a 1 mL PFS requires protein concentrations sometimes well above 100 mg/mL.

Kling [23] has summarized the discussions about clinicians' dosage requests, noting that "clinicians [are] asking for formulations containing 500 mg/mL of protein" and sometimes much more. Demands for such high protein concentrations ignore the basic physical properties of proteins, such as solubility and packing properties, which often make developing high-concentration protein formulations unfeasible.

Hyaluronidase co-formulation offers one approach to overcome the 1 mL volume limit. Ongoing work to develop a 2 mL auto-injector is another approach. The issues here are how much tissue back-pressure and injection pain the patient will tolerate.

Injection-site irritation and pain depend on composition of the injected formulation, needle size and geometry, injection performance, and, especially, the patient [24, 25].

Dias et al. [25] have recently tested the effect of dose volume and injection rate of a 5 mPa · s viscous placebo formulation on the tolerability of higher-volume subcutaneous injection. In a randomized, crossover, single-center study, they injected up to 3.5 mL. The results suggested "a single large-volume subcutaneous injection of a biotherapeutic agent could be used instead of multiple injections" [25]. Thus, an increase of the injected volume would somehow reduce the pressure on the development of high-concentration protein formulations.

3 High-Concentration Protein Formulations: What Is High?

The term high-concentration protein formulation (HCPF) is mostly used in the context of monoclonal antibody formulations and describes formulations at high protein concentrations. Such high protein concentrations are usually needed for subcutaneous delivery, to ensure the applied therapeutic dose.

Subcutaneously delivering antibodies in high concentrations — 50–150 mg/mL for monoclonal antibodies (Table 1), and 150–200 mg/mL for polyclonal antibodies [26] — can be particularly challenging because of the molecules' very large size, with hydrodynamic diameters around 10 nm [27].

Table 1
Lyophilized polyclonal and monoclonal antibody commercial products with protein concentration ≥30 mg/mL

Product name	Immuno-globulin	Protein concentration ($mg \cdot mL^{-1}$)	Delivery route	Company
Gammagard SD®	Polyclonal	50[a]	IV	Baxter
Synagis® (Palivizumab)	Monoclonal	100[a]	IM	Abbott, MedImmune
Raptiva® (Efalizumab)	Monoclonal	100[a]	SC	Serono, Genentech
Xolair® (Omalizumab)	Monoclonal	125[a]	SC	Genentech, Novartis
Cosentyx® (Secukinumab)	Monoclonal	150[a]	SC	Novartis
Ilaris® (Canakinumab)	Monoclonal	150[a]	SC	Novartis
Cimzia® (Certolizumab pegol)[b]	Monoclonal	200[a]	SC	UCB

IV intravenous, *SC* subcutaneous, *IM* intramuscular
[a]After reconstitution
[b]Recombinant humanised antibody-Fab′-fragment

Maximum achievable protein concentrations in a specific formulation under specific environmental conditions (e.g., pressure, temperature) are derived from solubility tests [28, 29]. However, determining protein solubility is not as straightforward as expected. Proteins are quite labile molecules that undergo unfolding. As a consequence, the solute (protein) can change its conformation and so its hydrophobicity. Thus, the solubility of native proteins differs from that of partially or fully unfolded proteins. Strictly speaking, a solution of proteins in different stages of unfolding now consists of a population of distinctly different solutes. Furthermore, proteins do not necessarily undergo a clear phase separation with the formation of a solid (protein precipitate) at the solubility limit. A number of highly concentrated protein solutions form an intermediate gel-like phase, making it difficult to determine a solubility limit. The researcher must also discriminate between kinetic solubility (forming an amorphous or crystalline phase) and thermodynamic solubility [30, 31].

Kinetic solubility is observed for a solute precipitation when the compound is added to a new solvent (solution) and thus determines the concentration of the remaining solute in solution (that does not precipitate). Such a solubility experiment is performed by dissolving the compound in a specific solvent and adding it to a new buffer system. After a certain equilibration time, and after phase separation is observed, the concentration of the compound in the tested buffer is determined [32]. Thermodynamic solubility, however, refers to a state of maximal dissolution of a solid compound in a solvent, meaning the transfer from a solid to a liquid phase. Solubility is therefore defined as the solute concentration that is reached in a specific solvent under specific environmental conditions. Often kinetic solubility is higher than thermodynamic solubility, because precipitates typically form an amorphous solid phase and not a crystalline solid phase [32].

Different solubility tests, based on the use of a precipitant such as PEG (polyethylene glycol), have been used to determine solubility or apparent solubility data. However, most of the proposed tests are not robust enough and do not provide reliable and comparable results (for more details see for example Middaugh et al. [33]; Trevino et al. [28]; Garidel [31]; Kalonia et al. [34]).

We have therefore estimated maximum achievable protein concentrations by considering the physical properties of proteins (especially the geometrical size) and using different packing models [26].

There are two principal steps in this analysis.

First, one must "model" the protein molecule itself. Assuming the molecule to be a sphere is the simplest first approximation. The antibody molecule can also be considered a Y-shaped structure, reflecting the most popular representation of an IgG1 monoclonal antibody structure. Cones and rectangular prisms may also be used to model the protein shape.

Current available structure data derived from solution SAXS (small-angle X-ray scattering) and SANS (small-angle neutron scattering) measurements reveal, however, quite compact solution structures with gyration radii around 4–4.5 nm [26, 35–41]. For example, Clark et al. [39] performed molecular simulations of a model antibody and suggested that a wide range of structural configurations are possible, adopting different molecule shapes, with radii of gyration values spanning from 3.9 to 5.5 nm.

The Y-shaped structure is an idealized form [42]. In the end, it makes sense in a first approximation to model the monoclonal antibody as a sphere (for more details about the impact of the different molecule models upon the estimation of the upper limit of protein concentration, see Garidel et al. [26]).

Second, one must choose a suitable packing model. The face centered cubic (fcc) model provides for the tightest packing of the spheres (Fig. 1). For such a model, each unit cell contains four protein molecules and the packing density (the fraction of volume that is occupied by the spheres) is close to 0.74. Free space around

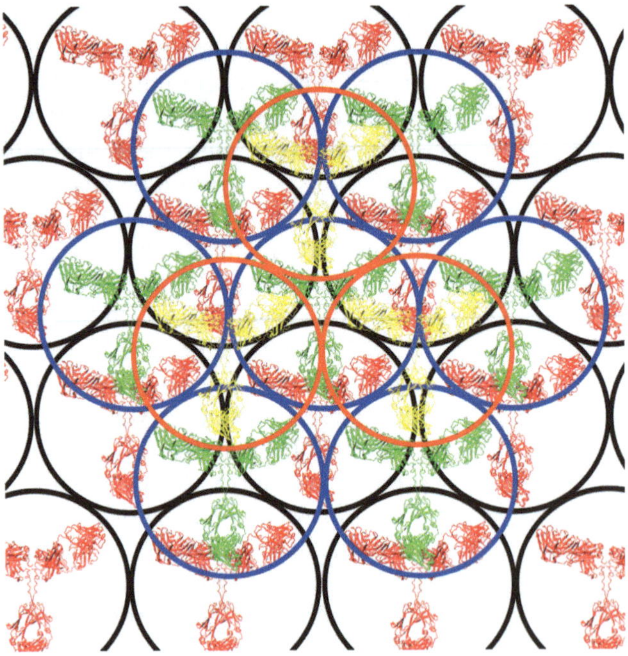

Fig. 1 Two-dimensional representation of monoclonal antibodies as spheres with radius of gyration. Face centred cubic (fcc) lattice was used for packing, which reaches the highest average density (0.74) for spherical packing. The size of the spheres is shown by the circles with the Padlan antibody model inside [42]. Circles in black, blue and orange represent the different layers of the fcc stack

the spheres accounts, therefore, for just 26% of total volume. In a maximally concentrated protein, this is the space that can be "filled" with water or other solvent molecules. Clearly, reduced "free space" might impose limits on hydration and colloidal stability, among other properties.

The literature includes discussions of other packing models, including the packing of rectangular antibody molecules [26]. Here, one can consider examples with one ($N = 1$) or two ($N = 2$) molecule per unit cell, for which the geometries of the molecules and unit cells were derived from data available from crystallographic studies [26].

These studies notwithstanding, we have recently shown that it is reasonable to assume protein molecules, even monoclonal antibodies, as spherical, and to assume the tightest fcc packing model. The resulting relationship between the monoclonal antibody concentration (molecular weight MW = 147,940 g/mol [42]) and the molecule (sphere) size is shown in Fig. 2. The calculated monoclonal antibody concentrations shown in Fig. 2 represent upper limits, because such a model assumes an idealized close packing and neglects all entropic, colloidal, hydration effects, and other constraints on idealized packing.

Even assuming a molecular radius of 4.5 nm, about the same as the gyration radius, the maximal protein concentration is still below 500 mg/mL (Fig. 2) and, in fact, solubility experiments have rarely produced monoclonal antibody concentrations much above 300 mg/mL (25 °C).

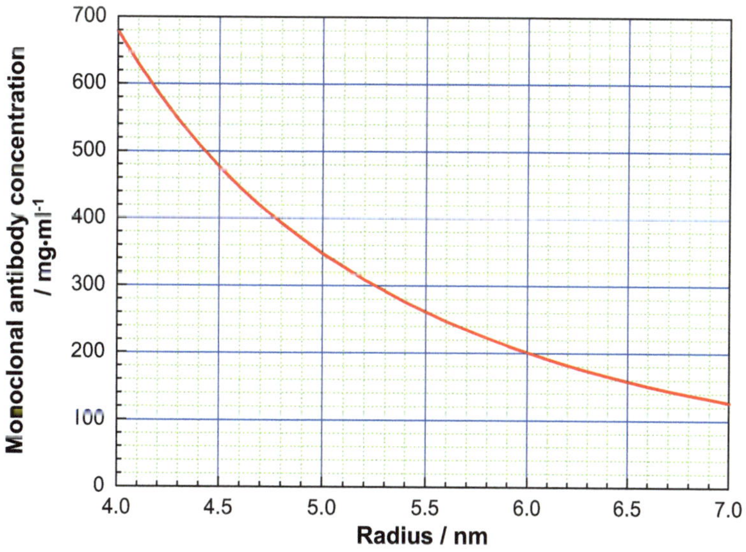

Fig. 2 Calculation of the protein concentration for spheres with radius *r* using a face centred cubic (fcc) packing model

This simplified approach, which is solely based on estimating the maximum antibody concentration by assuming idealized antibody geometries, packed in an idealized crystal lattice, shows that the maximum antibody concentration limit is below 500 mg/mL.

4 Challenges with High-Concentration Protein Formulations

Developing a lyophilized protein formulation requires reasonable product stability, preferably at room temperature, in the liquid formulation prior to the lyophilization step.

4.1 Manufacturing

The drug substance manufacturing of biologics ends with the last downstream process step, which delivers the protein in its final concentration and buffer. In the pharmaceutical industry, this step is most commonly ultra-filtration/dia-filtration (UF/DF) [43–47].

UF/DF has two main objectives, namely, (1) a buffer exchange to achieve the final formulation buffer, and (2) concentrating the protein solution to a concentration higher (generally about 25% higher) than that at which it will be administered to the patient. Though UF/DF strategies may differ, the dia-filtration buffer usually corresponds to the final product buffer, and formulators reach the final composition by such operations as spiking excipients into the protein solution so as to deliver the requested formulation composition.

Whatever the UF/DF strategy, dia-filtration and formulation buffers may show an unequal distribution of excipients. This phenomenon was described nearly a century ago by Frederick Donnan [48, 49] and Jacques Loeb [50]. In the Donnan effect, a membrane potential forms at the dia-membrane interface, which influences the removal and exchange of charged excipients during dia-filtration of high-concentration protein solutions [48–50]. In consequence, the composition of the formulation buffer differs from the composition of the dia-filtration buffer. The effect is more pronounced for high-concentration proteins than for lower protein concentrations (for more details see Steele and Arias [51], Bolton et al. [52], Neergaard et al. [46], Garidel et al. [46]).

As protein concentration increases, so usually does solution viscosity. In many cases, the viscosity increases exponentially (Fig. 3). The viscosity increase depends on the formulation composition and molecule properties [53]. Weak protein-protein interactions can cause large viscosity increases [54, 55]. Until now, formulators have had no generalized approach for reducing viscosity. The large, nonlinear increase of viscosity with rising concentration has imposed operating limits on UF/DF systems. High viscosity induces strong backpressures in the UF/DF systems, reducing filtration and making process development challenging, or even, impossible.

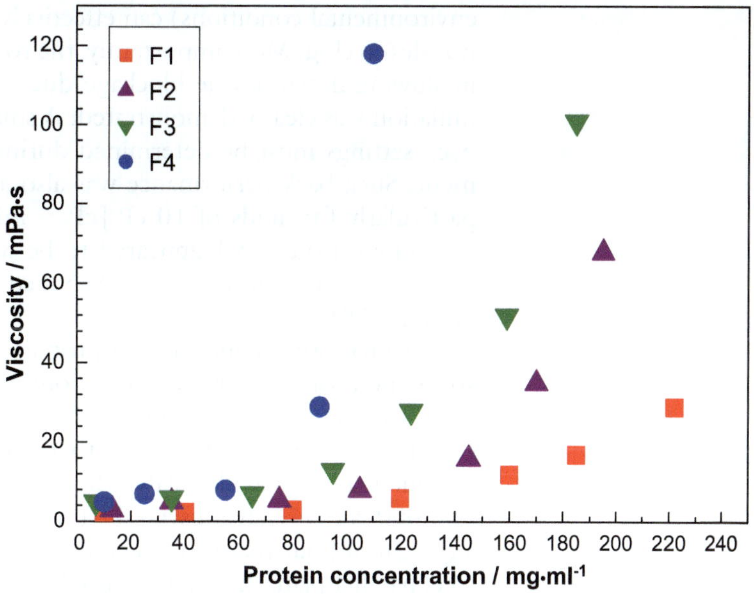

Fig. 3 Relationship between protein concentration and dynamic viscosity at 20 °C of various protein formulations (F1 to F4)

Recently, Luo et al. [56] have presented a case study of the formation of a liquid-liquid phase separation during downstream processing. During low pH elution in Protein A affinity chromatography, they observed high turbidity and increasing back pressure related to protein phase separation.

High viscosity might also impair such process steps as sterile filtration and the pumping of the liquid during fill-and-finish. Recent research has shown that the sterile filtration of highly concentrated protein formulations depends on (1) protein concentration, (2) formulation composition, and (3) filter material (e.g., polyvinylidene difluoride, PVDF, or polyethersulfone, PES) [57]. Allmendinger et al. [57] also observed formulation-dependent differences in the filtration behavior of concentrated protein formulations during aseptic biologic drug product manufacturing. The variations were particularly on the presence or absence of surfactants, but were also influenced by specific excipients and their interactions with the filter membrane. The same study showed a relationship between filtration properties and rheological non-Newtonian flow behavior.

A study by Shieu et al. [58] aimed to optimize filling of high-concentration monoclonal antibody formulations (bovine serum albumin: 370 mg/mL and mAB: 180 mg/mL) using a peristaltic pump. The researchers used glass nozzles in a bench-top syringe filling unit, as a down-scale model for understanding the effects of different fill parameters. They observed that increasing fill-nozzle size and decreasing water-evaporation rates (under appropriate environmental conditions) can effectively alleviate the tendency of nozzles to clog. More importantly, the role of the suck-back setting in slowing down nozzle blockage due to high-concentration formulation was clearly demonstrated. A small range of optimal suck-back settings must be determined during filling process development. Suck-back performance was also affected by fluid viscosity, particularly for fluids of 10 cP [cP = mPa · s]. The effect of the substrate on suck-back appeared to be weak, and so observations made with glass nozzles could be applied to standard stainless-steel nozzles [58].

In processing concentrated protein solutions, potential shear stress and protein interface interactions must be under control. Bee et al. [59] studied the response of a high-concentration antibody (ca. 100 mg/mL) formulation to high shear stress (shear rates obtained in a parallel-plate rheometer between 20,000 and 250,000 s^{-1}). They observed "that shear alone did not cause aggregation, but that prolonged exposure to shear in the stainless steel parallel-plate rheometer caused a very minor reversible aggregation (<0.3%)". The same study suggested that in many cases air-bubble entrainment, adsorption to solid surfaces (with possible shear synergy), contamination by particulates, or pump cavitation stresses could be much more important causes of aggregation than shear exposure during production.

4.2 Pharmaceutical Drug Product Development

Increasing protein concentration increases opalescence and the appearance of colored protein solutions, which usually are yellow and/or brown [53, 60]. Figure 4 illustrates the opalescence trend as a function of protein concentration for saccharose-succinate-based monoclonal antibody formulations. At 40 mg/mL protein the opalescence is ca. 8 FNU (formazin nephelometric units) and increases to 19 FNU at 210 mg/mL. The opalescence increase is not related to the formation of protein aggregates and particles, because the measured HPSEC (high performance size-exclusion chromatography) data show more or less constant monomer content; at 210 mg/mL, a slight monomer decrease of just 0.5% is observed (Fig. 4), which is in line with a small increase of high molecular species. Furthermore, subvisible particles, measured by means of light obscuration, showed no changes in the particle load (data not shown).

It must be remembered that the protein itself may act as a buffer component, and, in fact, the protein's self-buffering capacity dominates the buffer capacity of highly concentrated protein formulations [61, 62].

HCPF's rheological and syringeability (injectability) properties may limit the suitability of delivery via syringe or injection device [14, 63]. In most cases, the key parameter is solution viscosity (η), which must be considered along with injection volume, injection flow rate, and needle geometry in relation to subcutaneous

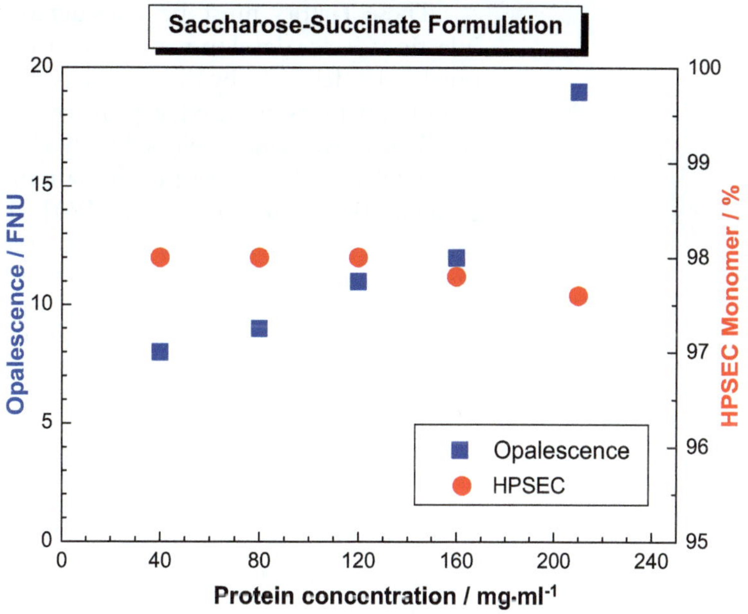

Fig. 4 Opalescence of a saccharose-succinate protein formulation with increasing protein concentration and the corresponding monomer content (*HPSEC* high performance size exclusion chromatography) after UF/DF manufacturing. *FNU* formazine nephelometry unit

injection tolerance [25, 64–66]. Doughty et al. [66], for example, studied subcutaneous tissue pressure in injection devices for large-volume protein delivery. They observed that the subcutaneous tissue can accommodate large-volume (up to 10 mL) injections with little back pressure, as long as low flow rates are used. Injecting 1 mL over 10 s (360 mL/h flow rate) generated ~24 kPa back pressure, while injecting 10 mL over 10 min (60 mL/h flow rate) generated lower back pressures of ~7 kPa. After the subcutaneous injection, the pressure decays to zero within several seconds. The researchers concluded that "the subcutaneous pressures and mechanical strain increased with increasing flow rate but not increasing dose volume" [66]. High-pressure and needle-free devices have also been evaluated in this context [67, 68]. However, developers must evaluate, whether a 10 min subcutaneous application is really practicable in a self-administered dosage; patients do not usually hold an auto-injector or pen device in place for more than 15–20 s for a full injection [69].

For subcutaneous administration one usually employs extremely thin needles, of 27–30 gauge. This increases patient convenience and reduces injection pain. Injecting high-concentration protein solutions with a viscosity around 20 mPa · s (20 °C) through a 30-gauge needle requires an injection force above 80 N, because the pressure decrease, ΔP, is correlated with $\Delta P \propto \eta \cdot r^{-4}$ (where r is needle radius).

These factors must be considered at the beginning of the injection-device development. Moreover, HCPFs are usually developed to be delivered by the subcutaneous route, so pre-filled syringes or cartridges are used as primary packaging. Double-chamber cartridges have been developed for lyophilized products: one chamber is filled with reconstitution medium, and the other chamber contains the freeze-dried drug [70]. The glass barrel must be lubricated (most commonly with 0.2–0.6 mg silicone oil per barrel, depending on manufacturer and type of syringe) to guarantee that these primary packaging-formulation combination devices function properly. Because silicone oil forms a hydrophobic surface at the glass barrel-to-liquid interface, protein degradation and aggregation might occur. Examples in the literature include Jones et al. [71], Liu et al. [72], Li et al. [73], Krayukhina et al. [74], Saggu et al. [75]. Li et al. [73] have shown that an interfacial syringe adsorption of abatacept (a 92 kDa fusion protein composed of the Fc region of the immunoglobulin IgG1 fused to the extracellular domain of CTLA-4) may be the key process responsible for soluble-protein loss when contacting silicone oil. Additionally, irreversible adsorption of protein may be associated with protein denaturation/aggregation [73]. It is expected that protein-silicone oil-induced aggregates should increase with increasing protein concentration.

Tungsten-induced protein degradation has also been observed in syringes used as primary packaging [76, 77]. This effect is also observed at low protein concentration [78, 79]. Liu et al. [77] have, however, presented a root-cause analysis of tungsten-induced protein aggregation in pre-filled syringes, tracing the problem to residue from the tungsten pin used to pierce the glass syringe barrel during the forming process. To keep the syringe clear of tungsten, the tungsten pin must be changed regularly during manufacturing. An improved washing process at the pre-filled syringe supplier has also considerably lowered the residual tungsten content and significantly reduced risks for protein aggregate formation due to the presence of tungsten [77].

Colloidal instability also increases at higher protein concentrations [44, 55, 80, 81]. Liquid-liquid phase separation of HCPF has been observed for such products as dual variable domain immunoglobulin or intrinsically disordered proteins (IDPs) [82–85]. Such a phase transition can be enhanced during the freezing step of lyophilization.

Phase separation of excipients during lyophilization can also impair protein stability [86–88]. Excipient phase-separation may be one of the reasons that the "glassy immobilization" concept, often used to explain protein stabilization in lyophilized solids, does not always hold. That is, the protein simply does not "see" the glass [86]. As a consequence, Pikal has proposed a modified version of the glassy immobilization hypothesis [89]. He suggests that an excipient acting as an effective protein stabilizer not only forms a chemically inert glass, but also "forms a single phase with the protein, which requires a 'moderate' interaction with the protein surface to resist separation but yet not denature the protein" [89]. According to Randolph, "in this version of the hypothesis, hydrogen bond replacement is a sufficient but unnecessary condition for stability; that is, an excipient that remains hydrogen bonded to the protein during drying cannot be phase-separated from the protein, but the reverse is not necessarily true. Thus, it can be seen that the 'water replacement' hypothesis for protein stabilization by excipients during lyophilization is just a special case of a broader hypothesis that we might call the 'single-phase glass' hypothesis" [86].

The protein's behavior during freezing is another important aspect of lyophilization. Figure 5 shows the effect of a freeze/thaw cycle of a protein formulation (in trehalose-histidine at pH 6) from room temperature to −50 °C at various protein concentrations. Between protein concentrations of 15 and 40 mg/mL, the freeze/thaw cycle has no impact on protein integrity. Increasing the protein concentration increased opalescence above 20 FNU, accompanied by the formation of visible particles and a decrease in monomer content from 99% to less than 96% (Fig. 5). Whether the damage to the protein is due to freezing or thawing is not yet clear.

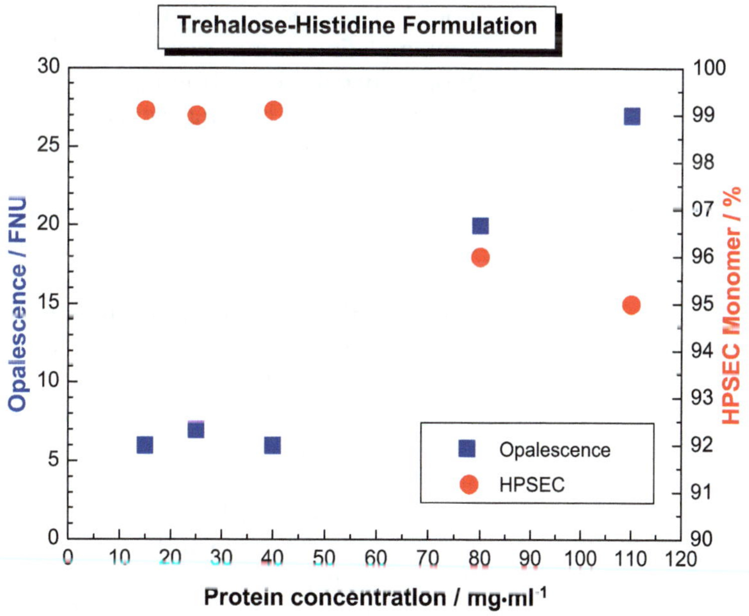

Fig. 5 Opalescence and the corresponding monomer content (*HPSEC* high performance size exclusion chromatography) of a trehalose-histidine monoclonal antibody formulation (pH 6) with increasing protein concentration after 1× freeze/thaw cycle from room temperature to −50 °C. Thawing was performed at ambient temperature. *FNU* formazine nephelometry unit

Recently, Awotwe-Otoo and collaborators [90] investigated how freezing methods affect glycation and protein aggregation of a lyophilized monoclonal antibody formulation. Using controlled nucleation as a specific method to induce sample freezing, they observed a higher residual moisture content and significantly lower specific surface areas for the two monoclonal antibody concentrations (1 and 20 mg/mL), compared with uncontrolled nucleation. They also observed chemical degradation, namely glycation, by excipient sucrose. The uncontrolled nucleation process resulted in significantly higher levels of glycation (from 4 to 7%) after reconstitution compared with controlled nucleation samples. They also found that incubation at higher storage temperatures (25 °C/60% RH) resulted in higher rates of glycation than did storage at 5 °C. Spectroscopic protein characterization using circular dichroism revealed no differences in secondary antibody structure for either of the two concentrations after lyophilization. Awotwe-Otoo et al. [90] concluded: “The freezing step method impacted the extent of glycation in lyophilized samples and the hydrolyzed component of sucrose was critical for increasing glycation. Even though some level of glycation was observed in lyophilized samples, the native structure of the protein was not affected. Further, it was demonstrated that storage of both lyophilized cakes and reconstituted formulations at higher temperatures could increase the extent of glycation in monoclonal antibody formulations.” Thus, potential glycation must be investigated by those contemplating using sucrose (saccharose) as a bulking agent. More generally, formulation developers should carefully investigate the impacts of all bulking agents and excipients on the stability of a lyophilized monoclonal antibody [91–96].

4.3 Analytic

Most analytical assays used to characterize protein formulations rely on a dilution step prior to the analytical investigation. Only a limited number of methods, such as Fourier-transform spectroscopy, specific calorimetric and fluorescence spectroscopic applications, allow the characterization of high-concentration formulations without a prerequisite of a dilution step [97–100]. For specific investigations, such as the quantification of polysorbate, the presence of large amounts of proteins can cause some challenges for the recovery of polysorbate [101, 102]. Consequently, specific tests have to be developed for the characterization of HCPF. Wuchner et al. [103], for example, presented a microflow digital imaging assay for monoclonal antibody formulation that can characterize protein particulates at 90 mg/mL. They also discussed the issues related to current methods [103].

4.4 Protein Physico Chemical Properties

Protein solubility, protein hydration, colloidal and structural stability, as well as solution properties are key factors that drive HCPF development strategies [26, 34, 55, 104, 105]. At high protein concentration >100 mg/mL, the solution becomes crowded, and protein-protein self-interactions dominate. Our current understanding relies on protein-protein self-interaction and the formation of a protein network at high protein concentration that translates into increased opalescence and/or increased viscosity [60, 83, 104, 106].

The propensity of a high-concentration protein formulation to form gels or undergo liquid-liquid phase separation is well observed, and depends on the antibody's amino acid sequence and chemical structure (Reiche et al. [84] and references cited therein, Kalonia et al. [34], Trainor et al. [105], van der Kant et al. [107]). Various studies have investigated monoclonal antibodies that differ just slightly in the amino acid sequence, yet demonstrate pronounced differences in solution properties at high concentrations [35, 44, 108].

Most solubility assays are not very robust, generating solubility data that often show large variabilities. Surrogate parameters, such as opalescence or protein-protein interaction measurements, can aid in deriving apparent solubility data. At best, these data might allow a ranking of different solution conditions with regards to protein solubility [28, 29, 31, 109, 110].

5 Lyophilization of High-Concentration Protein Formulations

Table 1 summarizes some commercially available high-concentration freeze-dried protein formulations (HCFDPF) with protein concentrations ranging between 50 and 200 mg/mL. The corresponding chemical compositions of these formulations are listed in Table 2. As can be seen, the formulations contain various excipients with specific functionalities — such as a buffer, cryo/lyoprotectant, and in most cases a detergent — to stabilize the protein in the dried state as well as to prevent protein aggregation on reconstitution [6].

Spitznagel and colleagues have investigated the lyophilization of a high-concentration monoclonal antibody formulation from 25 to 100 mg/mL [111]. The focus of the study was the development of a lyophilization cycle for a formulation lacking a crystalline agent. The study investigated a monoclonal antibody formulation composed of 10 mM citrate at pH 6.5, 8% sucrose and 0.04 w% polysorbate 80. Colandene et al. [111] observed that — at low protein concentrations, below 50 mg/mL — the glass transition temperature T'_g (measured by differential scanning calorimetry) of the maximally freeze-concentrated solution was similar to the collapse temperature T_C. The collapse temperature is determined by

Table 2
Lyophilized polyclonal and monoclonal antibody commercial products with protein concentration ≥30 mg/mL

Product name	Buffer	Excipients	pH	Container
Gamma-gardSD®	22.5 mg/mL glycine	20 mg/mL glucose 8.5 mg/mL sodium chloride 3 mg/mL albumin (human) 2 mg/mL polyethylene glycol (PEG) 1 μg/mL tri-n-butyl phosphate 1 μg/mL octoxynol 9 0.1 mg/mL Polysorbate 80	6.8 ± 0.4	Vial for a 5 g bottle: reconstituted with 100 mL SWFI
Synagis®	8.7 mg histidine	67.5 mg mannitol 0.3 mg glycine	6.0	Single-use vial Reconstituted with 1.0 mL SWFI
Raptiva®	4.3 mg L-histidine 6.8 mg L-histidine hydrochloride monohydrate	123.2 mg Sucrose 3 mg Polysorbate 20	6.2	Single-use vial Reconstituted with 1.3 mL SWFI
Xolair®	1.8 mg L-histidine 2.8 mg L-histidine hydrochloride monohydrate	145.5 mg Sucrose 0.5 mg Polysorbate 20	6.0 ± 0.5	Single-use vial Reconstituted with 1.4 mL SWFI
Cosentyx®	4.656 mg L-histidine/L-histidine hydrochloride monohydrate	92.43 mg Sucrose 0.6 mg Polysorbate 80	5.8	Single-use vial Reconstituted with 1 mL sterile water
Laris®	L-Histidine L-Histidine HCl monohydrate	Sucrose Polysorbate 80	6.5 ± 0.3	Single-use vial Reconstituted with 1 mL preservative-free SWFI
Cimzia®[a]	0.9 mg lactic acid	100 mg Sucrose 0.1 mg Polysorbate 20	5.2	Single-dose vial Reconstituted with 1 mL SWFI

SWFI sterile water for injection
[a]Recombinant humanised antibody-Fab′-fragment

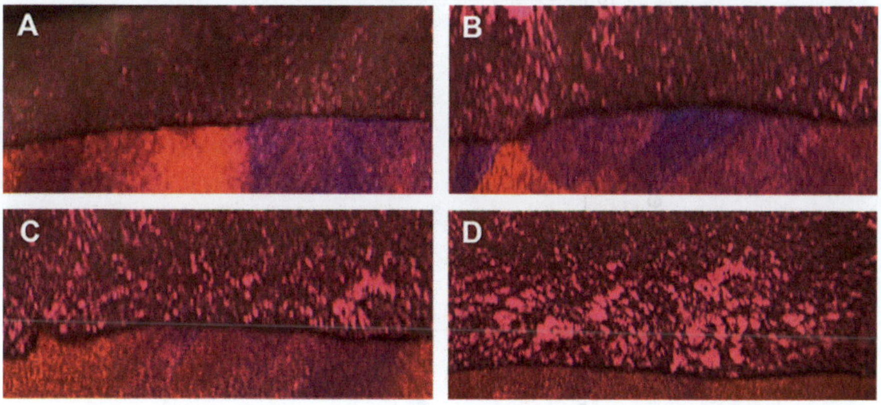

Fig. 6 Freeze-dry-microscopic pictures of the freeze-drying process of a 10 μL aliquot of a 1:4 (m:m) mannitol-saccharose solution at −40.0 °C (**A**), −38.0 °C (**B**), −37.0 °C (**C**) and −36.0 °C (**D**). At −40 °C (**A**) first signs of loss of structure can be seen. At −36 °C (**D**), the product forms no coherent product layer adjacent to the sublimation front, indicating full collapse. Thus the collapse temperature $T_C = -36$ °C

freeze-dry microscopy; Fig. 6 shows an example of the freeze-drying and the collapse of a cake. With increasing protein concentration, the difference between the glass transition and collapse temperature becomes progressively larger [111].

This statement corresponds to our observations of 0–210 mg/mL monoclonal antibody formulated in 10 mM succinate at pH 5.5, with 220 mM saccharose (sucrose) and 0.04 w% polysorbate 80. As can be seen from Fig. 7, T'_g and T_C of the formulation in the absence of protein is between −34 and −35 °C. With increasing protein concentration, T'_g increases to about −30 °C. For the formulation with 210 mg/mL, T'_g could not be accurately detected (marked as * in Fig. 7). However, increasing protein concentration from 40 to 210 mg/mL has a strong impact on the collapse temperature, with a nonlinear increase from −34 to −15 °C. Thus, at high protein concentration, the difference between T'_g and T_C is about 15 K. This difference corresponds to the observations of Colandene et al. [111].

Based on this finding, Spitznagel and his coworkers [111] have developed a lyophilization cycle with shortened primary drying; this is an advantage, due to the increase of T_C with increasing protein concentration. They used the observed difference between T'_g and T_C and adjusted the conditions so that product temperature during primary drying greatly exceeded the glass transition temperature without impairing product quality.

In certain cases, to improve protein stability, high concentration freeze-dried formulations were used as alternatives to liquid [112]. It was observed, however, that reconstitution times of freeze-dried HCPF are extremely prolonged, up to 30 min and longer [113]. Figure 8 illustrates the reconstitution times of a saccharose-based monoclonal antibody HCPF from 40 to

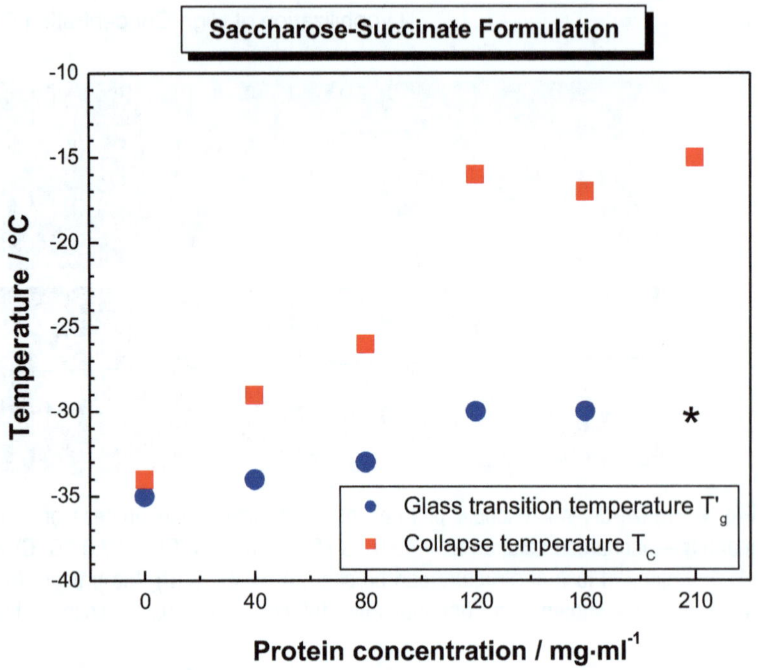

Fig. 7 Comparison of determined glass transition temperatures T_g' (differential scanning calorimetry) with collapse temperatures T_C (freeze-dry microscope) at different protein concentrations in 220 mM Saccharose, 10 mM Succinate, 0.04 w% polysorbate 80, pH 5.5. *: T_g' could not be detected at 210 mg/mL

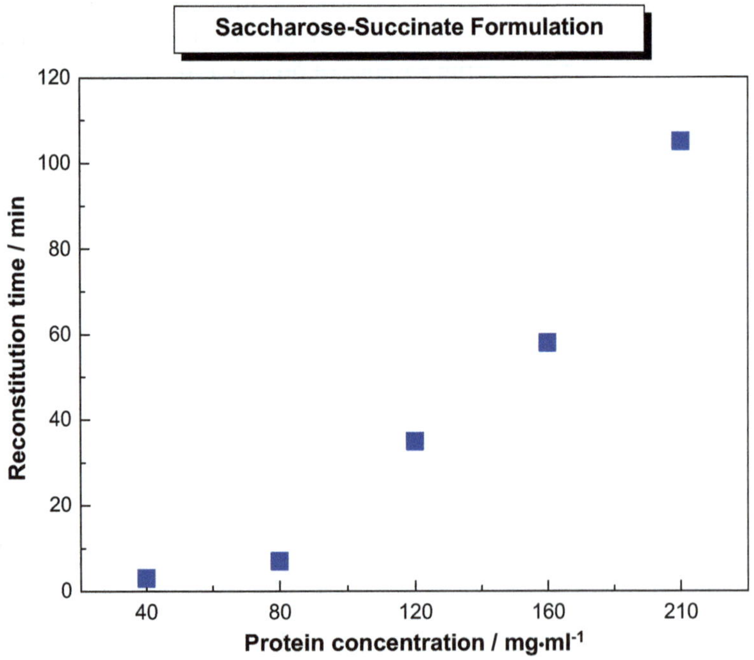

Fig. 8 Reconstitution time of lyophilized monoclonal antibody formulations for protein concentrations ranging from 40 to 210 mg/mL. All lyophilisates are reconstituted with 5 mL of water for injection and gently shaken (200–250 rpm) at 25 °C until the cake solid is completely dissolved

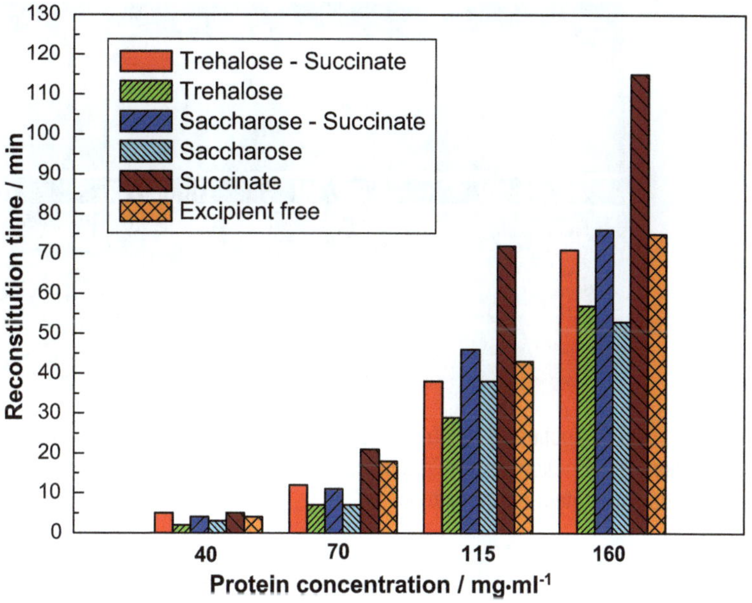

Fig. 9 Reconstitution time of lyophilized monoclonal antibody formulations for protein concentrations ranging from 40 to 160 mg/mL. All lyophilisates are reconstituted with 5 mL of water for injection and shaken (200–250 rpm) at 25 °C until the cake solid is completely dissolved. Reconstitution time is measured using a stopwatch. Excipient concentrations used: Trehalose: 220 mM, succinate: 20 mM, saccharose: 220 mM

210 mg/mL. At high protein concentration, reconstitution at 20 °C is close to 2 h.

The general trend seems to be obvious: as protein concentration increases, so does reconstitution time (Fig. 9). However, optimizing the formulation can reduce reconstitution time. For example, while a protein at 160 mg/mL in succinate shows reconstitution close to 2 h, reconstitution time for the same protein concentration can be cut in half if it is formulated in trehalose or saccharose in the absence of salt (Fig. 9).

Visual inspection of the lyo cake shows increasing protein concentration is associated with larger cracks and cake fragments (Fig. 10). One would expect that such cracks would allow a faster wetting of the cake and thus reduce reconstitution time. This does not appear to happen in practice. Therefore, further investigations are necessary (of specific surfactants, for example) to understand this phenomenon.

As mentioned before, for specific proteins and formulations, viscosity increases with protein concentration. Usually, the pre-lyophilization solution viscosity corresponds more or less to the viscosity of the reconstituted solution (post-lyophilization) (Fig. 11). In one case, however, we observed pre-lyo dynamic viscosity around 4–5 mPa s (20 °C) for a 60 mg/mL monoclonal

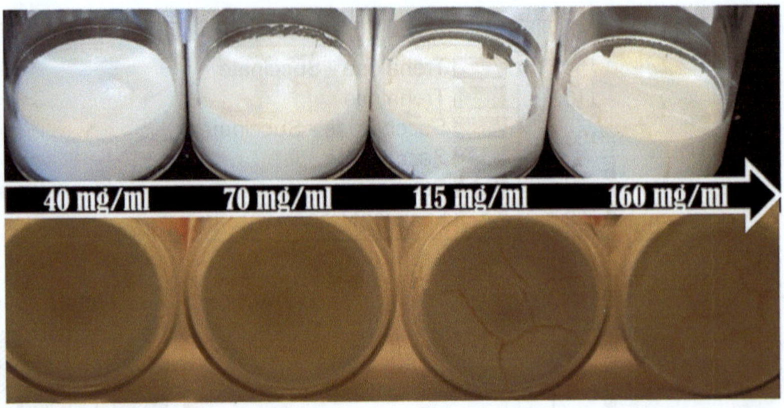

Fig. 10 Visual inspection of lyophilized 20 R vials containing a saccharose-succinate monoclonal antibody formulation as a function of protein concentration. The formation of larger cracks and cake fragments occurs with increasing protein concentration

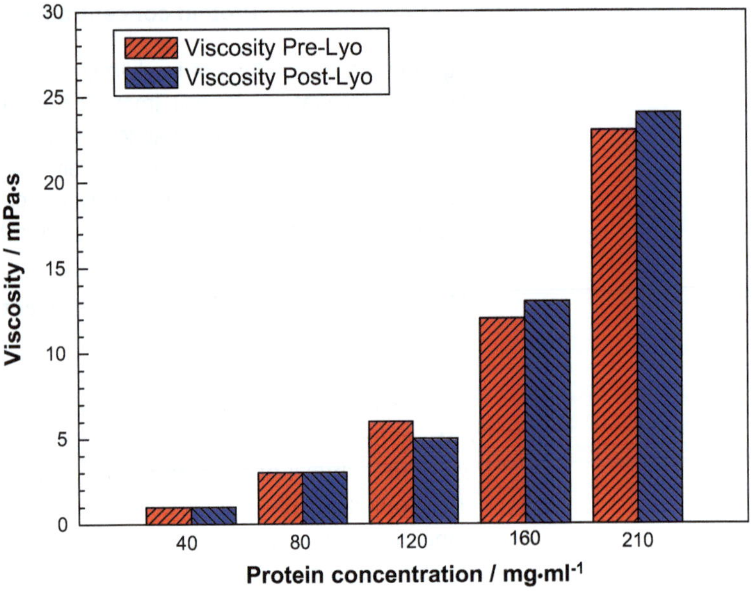

Fig. 11 Dynamic viscosity at 20 °C of a saccharose-succinate-based monoclonal antibody protein formulation as a function of protein concentration prior to lyophilization (pre-lyo) and after reconstitution (post-lyo). The viscosity was measured 3 h after reconstitution at 20 °C

trehalose-based formulation, and, after freeze-drying and reconstitution with the same water volume, a dynamic viscosity close to 10 mPa s (20 °C) (data not shown).

For another unusual case, changes in dynamic viscosity pre- and post-lyophilization were observed for a single chain variable region domain fragment. After reconstituting the lyophilisate cake with water (same volume as the initial volume prior to lyophilization),

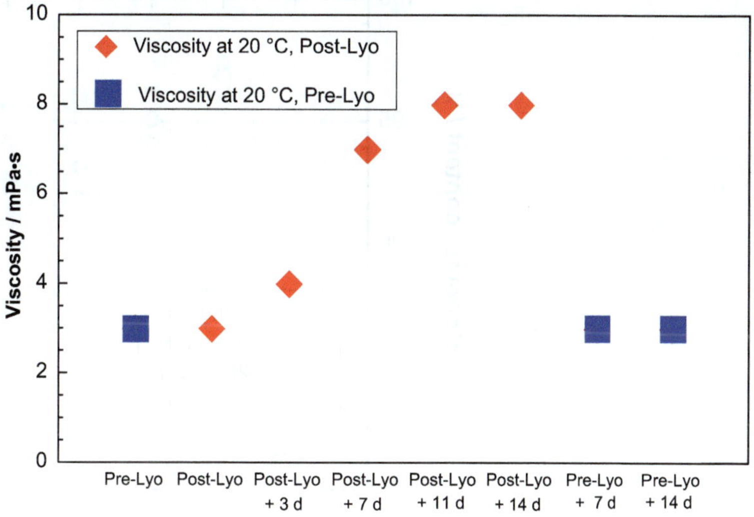

Fig. 12 Dynamic viscosity at 20 °C of a single chain variable fragment (scFv) pre- and post-lyophilization. After reconstitution, the protein formulations were stored up to 14 days at 20 °C. Protein concentration was 35 mg/mL and did not change during the experiment

the dynamic viscosity was similar to the viscosity before lyophilization. After a certain hold time at 20 °C, the reconstituted solution's viscosity, increased from 3 to about 8 mPa s (20 °C) (Fig. 12). In contrast, samples that were not lyophilized showed no change in viscosity after a hold time of up to 14 days at 20 °C (Fig. 12). Investigating protein integrity and protein concentration showed no significant changes compared to the initial sample. This example shows that the freeze-drying process can have an impact on the reconstituted solution properties.

Freeze-drying is often used to stabilize protein formulations, to reduce formation of high-molecular-weight species (aggregates), for example. Figure 13 summarizes an accelerated stability study of liquid formulations at 40 °C. The formulation composition was 220 mM saccharose, 10 mM succinate, 0.04 w% polysorbate 80 at pH 5.5 for all tested formulations; protein concentration varied from 40 to 210 mg/mL. Figure 13 shows a decrease of the monomer content as a function of time and protein concentration. The higher the protein concentration, the faster aggregates form and the greater the drop in monomer content—a common observation.

Freeze-drying these formulations and performing the same accelerated stability study (6 months at 40 °C) shows the following monomer trends (Fig. 14): For protein concentrations up to 80–120 mg/mL, monomer content decreases more slowly over time that it did in the corresponding liquid formulations (compare Figs. 13 and 14). For protein concentrations above 160 mg/mL, however, monomer fraction in the lyophilized samples decreases

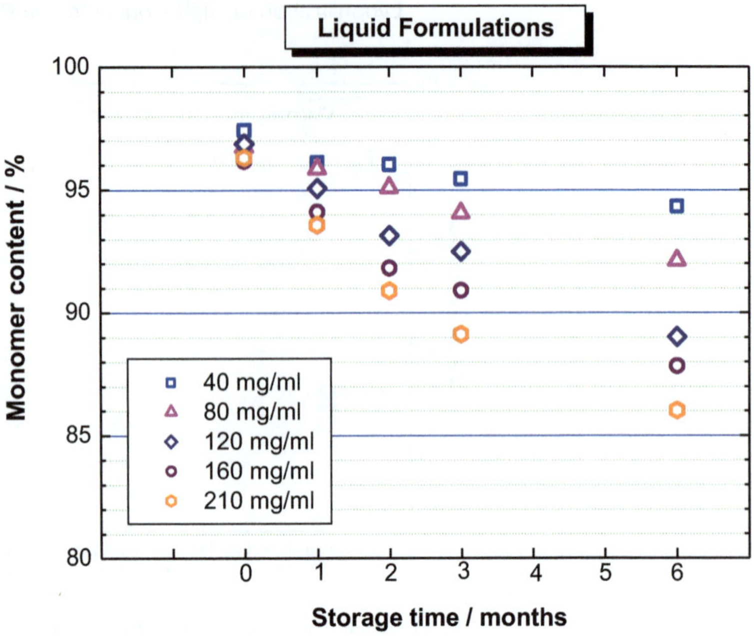

Fig. 13 Stability studies of a liquid formulated monoclonal antibody formulation (220 mM saccharose, 10 mM succinate, 0.04 w% polysorbate 80, pH 5.5, in vials, type 1 glass) at 40 °C at various protein concentrations. Monomer decrease is assessed by HPSEC (high performance size exclusion chromatography)

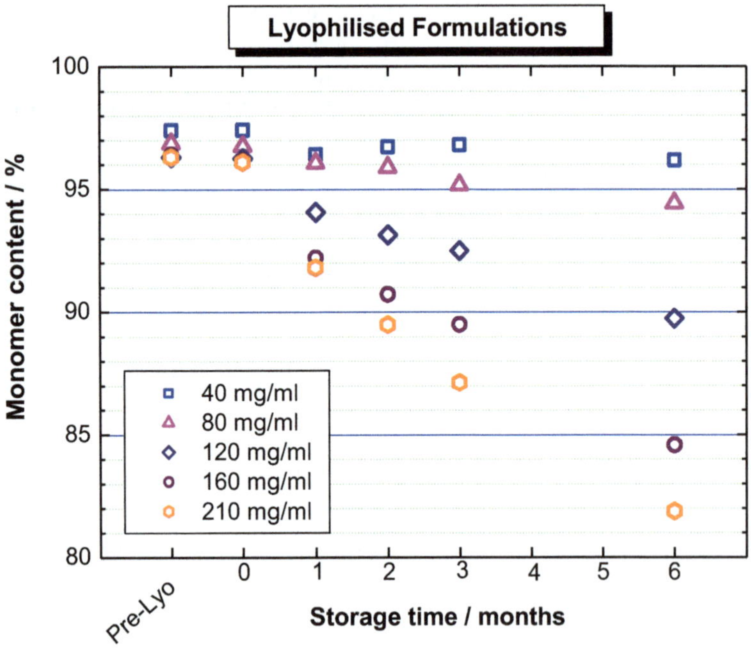

Fig. 14 Stability studies of a lyophilized monoclonal antibody formulation (220 mM saccharose, 10 mM succinate, 0.04 w% polysorbate 80, pH 5.5, in vials, type 1 glass) at 40 °C at various protein concentrations. Monomer decrease is assessed by HPSEC (high performance size exclusion chromatography)

faster over time than in the corresponding liquid formulations (compare Figs. 13 and 14).

This result was surprising. Since residual moisture has a strong impact on aggregate formation in freeze-dried formulations, we measured residual moisture using Karl-Fischer and near-infrared spectroscopy [114–116]. For all formulations, the residual moisture was below 1%. For the lyophilized formulations with 40–120 mg/mL, residual moisture was 0.5–0.6%; for the two lyophilized formulations at 160 and 210 mg/mL, the residual moisture was 0.6–0.8%. Whether this small difference in residual moisture is the reason for the reported trend in the stability of the lyophilized formulations, is unclear. In general, freeze-drying of protein formulations improves drug-product stability; there are, however, clear exceptions (Figs. 13 and 14).

The impact of residual moisture and excipient sorbitol on the stability of lyophilized antibodies was studied by Chang et al. [117], who elaborated their observations into a proposed mechanism of protein stabilization in the solid state. To generate different residual moistures from less than 1 w% to 5 w% for different plasticizer systems (composed of various mixtures of sorbitol and/or sucrose or trehalose), lyophilized samples were equilibrated at different relative humidities. Their structural relaxation time (alpha-relaxation) was measured by means of thermal activity monitor (TAM), showing a strong decrease with increasing the residual moisture. The stability data presented by Chang et al. [117] suggested a minimum in degradation rate at 2 w% to 3 w% water content. Addition of a small amount of sorbitol to a sucrose-based formulation resulted in greater retention of native structure, lower relaxation time, and improved stability. In trehalose-based formulations, however, adding sorbitol had no effect on protein structure, but the decrease in relaxation time and the improvement in stability were qualitatively similar to the corresponding data obtained with the sucrose-based formulation [117]. The results showed that glass dynamics could not explain the stability results. "Stability correlated best with the preservation of native structure for sucrose-based formulations, but with the trehalose-based formulation, neither structural relaxation time nor extent of native structure was predictive of stability." As a potential working hypothesis, they proposed that it is possible that the β-relaxations rather than the α-relaxation are critical to the stability [6, 117].

6 Controlled Nucleation and Impact on Properties of High-Concentration Protein Formulations

The development and introduction of controlled nucleation has received a lot of attention in the biologics freeze-drying community. This technology enables much better control of the ice nucleation temperature, which depended previously on stochastic events. The technique also let process developers change physical properties and quality aspects of the product, and to optimize the freeze-drying process times.

In the field of pharmaceutical freeze-drying, heterogeneous nucleation of ice is a reality [118]. One reason is the presence of impurities, which affect the average formation of the ice nucleation temperature in a batch. Still, super-cooling pharmaceutical formulations up to −20 or −30 °C could be observed. The inevitable environmental differences between lab-scale development and aseptic production also affect the nucleation temperature, due to the amount of submicron particles in the up-scaling process. It may be concluded that, at production scale, ice nucleation temperatures are on average lower than in early development, and that modifications of the freeze-drying process are therefore necessary [119].

All freeze-drying processes start with the freezing step, either within the freeze dryer or externally, and the literature clearly demonstrates an understanding of how important the freezing process is [6]. It defines the structure and texture of the product, and significantly affects later drying behavior. Besides the process influences and the optical appearance of the cake, structure also affects biological stability and can therefore be described as the foundation for the whole freeze-drying cycle.

To understand the advantage of controlled nucleation, it is worth taking a closer look at the nucleation process. Searles et al. [120] summarized the effects on protein aggregation, primary and secondary drying rate, crystallinity, and surface areas. He described different nucleation phases moving through the liquid phase, referred to the crystallization until the freezing is completed by the solidification phase. For process control, this means that in addition to the nucleation temperature, the time and temperature slopes following primary nucleation are also essential for structure formation.

The nucleation temperature and the degree of supercooling are the most important parameters. The lower the solution temperature, the more crystallization heat can be absorbed: more ice can form instantly, and faster freezing produces smaller ice crystals. At higher temperatures (with lesser degrees of supercooling), ice forms more slowly, with the formation of larger crystals. Thus, by controlling the degree of supercooling, the process developer can choose the desired ice crystal morphology.

Some freeze-drying processes include an annealing step. This step comes directly after the ramp freezing, at temperatures above T'_g. Annealing improves sample homogeneity and primary drying speed. The ice/water interface around many small crystals is initially large; it reduces as smaller ice crystals melt in favor of larger ice crystals (Ostwald ripening process) [120]. This can be considered an advantage for interfacial-sensitive drugs. The downside for active ingredients that are sensitive to freeze-concentration is a long isothermal hold time, which may be detrimental; for these, a faster ramp cooling may result in better protein stability. Unwanted crystallization—of buffer components, for example—may also occur and result in pH shifts [121].

Homogeneity over the whole freeze-drying batch is always relevant to clinical or commercial production. Good knowledge of the lyophilization equipment, and thoughtful freeze-drying cycle development (possibly including an annealing step) are necessary.

Now the ability to control the ice nucleation temperature (and thereby eliminate the variations caused by random ice nucleation) brings within range a more elegant way to achieve a homogeneous frozen structure.

Note, though, that one recently published comparison of controlled-nucleated samples and uncontrolled, randomly nucleated samples does not fully show the expected difference [122]; the reported results may not result solely from initial ice crystal distribution. Different post-nucleation freezing rates due to spatial variations in intra shelf temperature distribution, variations of vial heat transfer coefficients, various heat inputs during primary and secondary drying, pressure inhomogeneities during primary drying, the edge-vial effect, and product temperature variations may have big impacts on the process and therefore on the product characteristics. Since commercial controlled nucleation is relatively new, there are as yet no lyophilized products produced via controlled ice nucleation on the market.

As may be anticipated, the idea of controlling ice nucleation is not new. What is new is the technology for controlling ice nucleation at the different scales, as well as under aseptic conditions in a GMP environment. These ease the way for applying controlled nucleation in commercial process development. Nevertheless, the maturity and comparability of the different technologies is still under investigation. Geidobler et al. [123] reviewed all then available methods (Table 3 and Fig. 15) and defined the requirements:

- Success of nucleation: ideal independent of the freeze-drying equipment.
- Robustness and controllability: free selection of nucleation temperature.
- Product quality: aseptic conditions must be maintained.

In this context, the two most interesting methods are (briefly):

Ice fog generation and depressurization technique. The ice fog methods are based on the most straightforward way to induce ice nucleation of super-cooled solutions, by using ice crystal as seeds. There are several ways to generate the ice-crystal seeds, either internally or externally, and then introduce and distribute them

Table 3
Selected overview of methods that allow to control and determine the ice nucleation temperature [122, 123]

Method	Scalability	Retrofit needed
Ice fog (original)	Difficult	Yes
Ice fog (commercial scale)	Yes	Yes
Ice fog (ice seed generator)	Yes	Yes
Ice fog (ventilation through cold condenser)	Not yet proven	No
Depressurization technique	Yes	Yes
Vaccum induced surface freezing	Difficult	No
Pre-cooled shelf method	Difficult	No

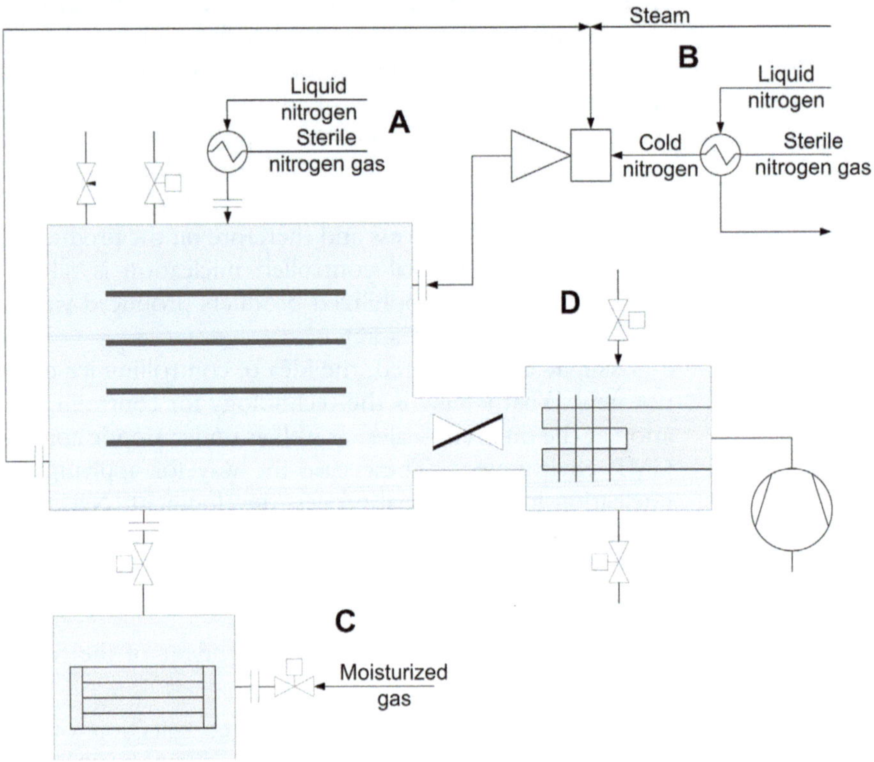

Fig. 15 Schematic representation of the technical set ups for the generation of ice fog (kindly provided with permission by Dr. R. Geidobler)

within in the freeze-drying chamber. A fast and complete distribution is supported by a depressurization step, which must be precisely controlled to keep the solutions from boiling. Depending on the method, the freeze-dryer may require minor adaptions, a retrofit, and/or additional equipment [123].

High-pressure/depressurization technique. The high-pressure/depressurization technique was adopted by Gasteyer et al. [124] and transferred to the field of freeze-drying. The product chamber, which contains the product vials, is pressurized. The shelf temperature is then lowered to the desired product nucleation temperature, and ice nucleation is induced by de-pressurizing the product chamber down to 1 bar. The mode of action is not completely understood, and the authors speculated that cooling of the liquid product surface by expansion of the gas induces ice nucleation [122]. One advantage is that commercial freeze-dryers are typically steam sterilized and can withstand high overpressure. The downside is that lab freeze-dryers are not built to withstand the same high pressures.

How could controlled nucleation be advantageous for high-concentration protein formulations?

As already mentioned, high concentration is often a consequence of clinicians' demands for high protein doses within a limited injection volume. This is not an ideal starting point for developing an efficient freeze-drying cycle. High concentration and high density of solids hinder water-vapor transport and result in longer drying times. There is also the correlation between protein concentration in the lyophilizate and increasing reconstitution time.

Awotwe-Otoo et al. [125] showed the general advantage of controlled nucleation for monoclonal antibodies at lower concentration. In a direct comparison of both freezing processes, controlled nucleation reduced primary drying time by 19%, due to the formation of larger ice crystals. The cake produced with controlled nucleation appeared more acceptable, showing less shrinkage and no visible collapse. The reconstitution time was also decreased, again due to the pores caused by the large ice crystals.

On the other hand, this structural difference resulted in higher residual moisture of the final product. This can be explained with a significant lower specific surface area (0.46 m^2/g controlled nucleation vs. 0.90 m^2/g without controlled nucleation). Thus, besides the freezing an identical freeze-drying cycle was used, the secondary drying conditions are not suitable to cope with the denser structure. There were no observed differences in aggregates or subvisible particle size distribution.

Geidobler et al. [123] focused on high-concentration protein formulations from 100 mg/mL up to nearly 200 mg/mL. The work confirmed the observations of Awotwe-Otoo et al. [125], but at higher protein concentrations. Figure 16 shows a reduction of the specific surface and the increased residual moisture for cakes produced with controlled nucleation. Especially for the monoclonal antibody, Geidobler et al. [126] showed much lower specific surface and reduced reconstitution time. Thus, controlled nucleation may reduce reconstitution time by improving cake-wetting and gas displacement (thanks to larger pores).

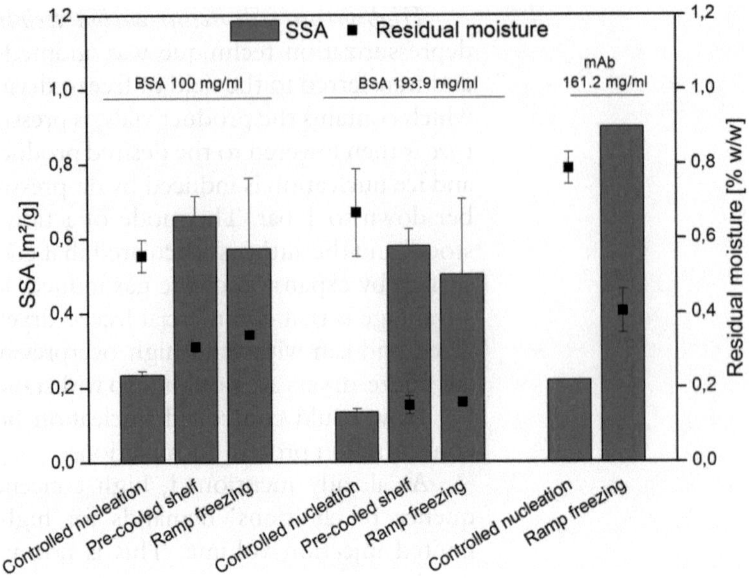

Fig. 16 Specific surface area and residual moisture for BSA at 100 mg/mL and at 193.9 mg/mL and a mAb formulation at 161.2 mg/mL (kindly provided with permission by Dr. R. Geidobler)

Current scientific work focuses on comparing different freeze-drying methods; these studies therefore use identical freeze-drying cycles. To take full advantage of controlled nucleation for high-concentration protein formulations, an optimized process needs to be developed. Developers should focus on the residual moisture level with the secondary drying, and on rapid freezing after nucleation to avoid having the process spend any time above T'_g.

To summarize, various and well-engineered techniques that allow further control of the freeze-drying process are now available to control ice nucleation temperature in pharmaceutical formulations. It is still unknown if different methods will result in a similar product with comparable ice crystal size and distribution, even if they induce ice nucleation at the same product temperature. Apart from these open technical questions, controlled nucleation can be clearly recommended as part of freeze-drying cycle development. No negative impact on product quality has so far been reported, and the noted issues of higher residual moisture can be addressed with a freeze-drying cycle optimized to control nucleation. Unacceptably long reconstitution times can be reduced for high concentration protein formulations and it is essential to do so, even while improving cake appearance and, on the process side, reducing primary drying times.

7 Conclusions

The descriptor "high-concentration protein formulation" should not be defined in terms of specific protein concentrations, but instead should refer to specific solution properties that become more relevant with increasing protein concentration: viscosity, opalescence, colloidal instabilities, liquid-liquid phase separation, gel formation, etc.

In developing lyophilized high-concentration protein formulations, one must first address all issues related to high-concentration *liquid* protein formulations. The main challenge is to reduce reconstitution times for high-concentration freeze-dried protein formulations. This appears to be possible, and one option is controlled nucleation.

Acknowledgments

The authors thank the following people for supporting the current study: Alexander Kuhn, Torsten Schultz-Fademrecht, Andreas Langer, Ortrud Betz, Regina Ziegler, Heidrun Schott, Sven Bahrenburg, Robert Mader, Douglas McCormick and Raimund Geidobler.

References

1. Rey L (1962) Progrés récents en lyophilisation. Band 1299, Actualités scientifiques et industrielles, pp 1–196
2. Essig D (1993) Lyophilisation. Wiss Verlag-Ges Stuttgart, Stuttgart, pp 1–158
3. Jennings TA (1999) Lyophilization. Taylor & Francis, Boca Raton, FL, pp 1–664
4. Wang W (2000) Lyophilization and development of solid protein pharmaceuticals. Int J Pharm 203(1–2):1–60
5. Nail SL, Chongprasert S (2002) Fundamentals of freeze-drying. In: Nail SL, Akers MJ (eds) Development and manufacture of protein pharmaceuticals, vol 6. Kluwer Academic, New York, pp 281–360
6. Constantino HR, Pikal MJ (2004) Lyophilization of biopharmaceuticals. AAPS Press, Arlington, pp 1–686
7. Oetjen H-W, Haseley P (2004) Freeze-drying, 2nd edn. Wiley-VCH, Weinheim, pp 1–394
8. Roy I, Gupta MN (2004) Freeze-drying of proteins: some emerging concerns. Biotechnol Appl Biochem 39:165–177
9. Matejtschuk P (2007) Lyophilisation of proteins. In: Day JG, Stacey GN (eds) Cryopreservation and freeze-drying protocols, Chapter 4, Methods in molecular biology, vol 368, 2nd edn. Humana Press Inc, Totowa, NJ, pp 59–72
10. Franks F, Auffret T (2009) Freeze-drying of pharmaceuticals and biopharmaceuticals. Principles and practice. RSC Publishing, Cambridge, UK, pp 1–206
11. Rey L, May JC (2010) Freeze drying/lyophilization of pharmaceutical and biological products, vol 206, 3rd edn. Informa Heathcare, London, pp 1–564
12. Varshney D, Singh M (eds) (2015) Lyophilised biologics and vaccines modality-based approaches. Springer, New York, pp 1–401
13. Wolkers WF, Oldenhof H (eds) (2015) Cryopreservation and freeze-drying protocols, methods in molecular biology, vol 1257, 3rd edn. Humana Press, New York, pp 1–509
14. Cilurzo F, Selmin F, Minghetti P, Adami M, Bertoni E, Lauria S, Montanari L (2011) Injectability evaluation: an open issue. AAPS PharmSciTech 12(2):604–609

15. Hallouët P, Eggers J, Malaquin-Pavan E (2007) L'injection sous-cutanée. Soins Gérontologie 12(65):45–46
16. Frost GL (2007) Recombinant human hyaluronidase (rHuPH20): an enabling platform for subcutaneous drug and fluid administration. Expert Opin Drug Deliv 4(4):427–440
17. Tang L, Persky AM, Hochhaus G, Meibohm B (2004) Pharmacokinetic aspects of biotechnology products. J Pharm Sci 93:2184–2204
18. Narasimhan C, Mach H, Shameen M (2012) High-dose monoclonal antibodies via the subcutaneouy route: challenges and technical solutions, an industry perspective. Ther Deliv 3(7):889–900
19. Shpilberg O, Jackisch C (2013) Subcutaneous administration of rituximab (MabThera) and trastuzumab (Herceptin) using hyaluronidase. Br J Cancer 109:1556–1561
20. Leveque D (2014) Subcutaneous administration of anticancer agents. Anticancer Res 34:1579–1586
21. Jackisch C, Müller V, Maintz C, Hell S, Ataseven B (2014) Subcutaneous administration of monoclonal antibodies in oncology. Geburtshilfe Frauenheilkd 74(4):343–349
22. Mathaes R, Koulov A, Joerg S, Mahler HC (2016) Subcutaneous injection volume of biopharmaceuticals—pushing the boundaries (short Survey). J Pharm Sci 105:2255–2259
23. Kling J (2014) Highly concentrated protein formulations. BioProcess Int 12(5):2–11
24. Gatlin LA, Gatlin CAB (1999) Formulation and administration techniques to minimize injection pain and tissue damage associated with parenteral products. In: Gapta PK, Brazeau GA (eds) Injectable drug development: techniques to reduce pain and irritation. Interpharm Press, Denver, pp 401–425
25. Dias C, Abosaleem B, Crispino C, Cao B, Shaywitz A (2015) Tolerability of high-volume subcutaneous injections of a viscous placebo buffer: a randomized, crossover study in health subjects. AAPS PharmSciTech 16 (5):1101–1107
26. Garidel P, Kuhn AB, Schäfer LV, Karow-Zwick AR, Blech M (2017) High-concentration protein formulations: how high is high? Eur J Pharm Biopharm 119:353–360
27. Garidel P, Kebbel F (2010) Protein therapeutics and aggregates characterised by photon correlation spectroscopy: an application for high-concentration liquid formulations. BioProcess Int 8(3):38–46
28. Trevino SR, Scholtz JM, Pace CN (2008) Measuring and increasing protein solubility. J Pharm Sci 97:4155–4166
29. Bye JW, Platts L, Falconer RJ (2014) Biopharmaceutical liquid formulation: a review of the science of protein stability and solubility in aqueous environments. Biotechnol Lett 36:869–875
30. Arakawa T, Timasheff SN (1985) Theory of protein solubility. Methods Enzymol 114:49–77
31. Garidel P (2013) Protein solubility from a biochemical, physicochemical and colloidal perspective. Am Pharm Rev. http://wwwamericanpharmaceuticalreviewcom/Featured-Articles/152568-Protein-Solubility-from-a-Biochemical-Physicochemical-and-Colloidal-Perspective/
32. Saal C (2010) Optimising the solubility of research compounds. Am Pharm Rev:12–15
33. Middaugh CR, Tisel WA, Haire RN, Rosenberg A (1979) Determination of the apparent thermodynamic activities of saturated protein solutions. J Biol Chem 254:367–370
34. Kalonia C, Toprani V, Toth R, Wahome N, Gabel I, Middaugh CR, Volkin DV (2016) Effects of protein conformation, apparent solubility, and protein–protein interactions on the rates and mechanisms of aggregation for an IgG1 monoclonal antibody. J Phys Chem B 120(29):7062–7075
35. Yearley EJ, Zarraga IE, Shire SJ, Scherer TM, Gokarn Y, Wagner NJ, Liu Y (2013) Small-angle neutron scattering characterization of monoclonal antibody conformations and interactions at high concentrations. Biophys J 105:720–731
36. Shatz W, Hass PE, Mathieu M, Kim HS, Leach K, Zhou M, Crawford Y, Shen A, Wang K, Chang DP, Maia M, Crowell SR, Dickmann L, Scheer JM, Kelley RF (2016) Contribution of antibody hydrodynamic size to vitreal clearance revealed through rabbit studies using a species-matched Fab. Mol Pharm 13:2996–3003
37. Weeks ER, Weitz DA (2002) Properties of cage rearrangements observed near the colloidal glass transition. Phys Rev Lett 89(9):4 pages. https://doi.org/10.1103/PhysRevLett89095704
38. Pathak JA, Sologuren RR, Narwal R (2013) Do clustering monoclonal antibody solutions really have a concentration dependence of viscosity? Biophys J 104:913–923
39. Clark NJ, Zhang H, Krueger S, Lee HJ, Ketchem RR, Kerwin B, Kanapuram SR, Treuheit MJ, McAuley A, Curtis JE (2013) Small-angle neutron scattering study of a monoclonal antibody using free-energy constraints. J Phys Chem B 117:14029–14038

40. Rayner LE, Hui GK, Gor J, Heenan RK, Dalby PA, Perkins SJ (2014) The Fab conformations in the solution structure of human immunoglobulin G4 (IgG4) restrict access to its Fc region. Implications for functional activity. J Biol Chem 289(30):20740–20756
41. Hui GK, Wright DW, Vennard OL, Rayner LE, Pang M, Yeo SC, Gor J, Molyneux K, Barratt J, Perkins SJ (2015) The solution structures of native and patient monomeric human IgA1 reveal asymmetric extended structures: implications for function and IgAN disease. Biochem J 471:167–185
42. Padlan EA (1994) Anatomy of the antibody molecule. Mol Immunol 31(3):169–217
43. Jacobi A, Enenkel B, Garidel P, Eckermann C, Knappenberger M, Presser I, Kaufmann H (2014) Process development and manufacturing of therapeutic antibodies, Chapter 22. In: Dübel S, Reichert JM (eds) Handbook of therapeutic antibodies, Technologies, vol 1. Wiley VCH, Weinheim, pp 603–663
44. Shire SJ, Shahrokh Z, Liu J (2004) Challenges in the development of high protein concentration formulations. J Pharm Sci 93 (6):1390–1402
45. Shire SJ (2009) Formulation and manufacturability of biologics. Curr Opin Biotechnol 20 (6):708–714
46. Neergaard MS, Kalonia D, Parshad H, Nielsen AD, Møller EH, van de Weert M (2013) Viscosity of high concentration protein formulations of monoclonal antibodies of the IgG1 and IgG4 subclass – prediction of viscosity through protein-protein-interaction measurements. Eur J Pharm Sci 49:400–410
47. Flickinger MC (2013) Downstream Industrial Biotechnology. Wiley, Hoboken, NJ, pp 1–858
48. Donnan FG (1927) Concerning the applicability of thermodynamics to the phenomena of life. J Gen Physiol 8:685–688
49. Donnan FG (1932) Die Membrangleichgewichte. Kolloid-Zeitschrift 61:160–167
50. Loeb J (1921) La cause de l'influence des électrolytes sur certaines propriétés physiques des protéines. Arch Int de Physiol 18 (1):521–534
51. Steele A, Arias J (2014) Accounting for the Donnan effect in diafiltration optimisation for high-concentration UFDF applications. BioProcess Int 12(1):50–54
52. Bolton GR, Boesch AW, Basha J, Lacasse DP, Kelley BD, Acharya H (2011) Effect of protein and solution properties on the Donnan effect during the ultrafiltration of proteins. Biotechnol Prog 27:140–152
53. Salinas BA, Satish HA, Bishop SM, Harn N, Carpenter JF, Randolph TW (2014) Understanding and modulating opalescence and viscosity in a monoclonal antibody formulation. J Pharm Sci 99(1):82–93
54. Connolly BD, Petry C, Yadav S, Demeule B, Ciaccio N, Moore JMR, Shire SJ, Gokarn YR (2012) Weak interactions govern the viscosity of concentrated antibody solutions: high throughput analysis using the diffusion interaction parameter. Biophys J 103(1):69–78
55. Garidel P, Blume A, Wagner M (2015) Prediction of colloidal stability of high concentration protein formulations. Pharm Dev Technol 20(3):367–374
56. Luo H, Lee N, Wang X, Li Y, Schmelzer A, Hunter AK, Pabst T, Wang WK (2017) Liquid-liquid phase separation causes high turbidity and pressure during low pH elution process in Protein A chromatography. J Chromatogr A 1488:57–67
57. Almendinger A, Müller R, Huwyler J, Mahler HC, Fischer S (2015) Sterile filtration of highly concentrated protein formulations: impact of protein concentration, formulation composition, and filter material. Pharm Biotechnol 104:3319–3329
58. Shieu W, Torhan SA, Chan E, Hubbard A, Gikanga B, Stauch OB, Maa YF (2014) Filling of high concentration monoclonal antibody formulations into pre-filled syringes: filling-paramter investigation and optimization. PDA J Pharm Sci Technol 68(2):153–163
59. Bee JS, Stevenson JL, Mehta B, Svitel J, Pollastrini J, Platz R, Freund E, Carpenter JF, Randolph TW (2009) Response of a concentrated monoclonal antibody formulation to high shear. Biotechnol Bioeng 103 (6):936–943
60. Salinas BA, Sathish HA, Bishop SM, Harn N, Carpenter JF, Randolph TW (2010) Understanding and modulating opalescence and viscosity in a monoclonal antibody formulation. J Pharm Sci 99(1):82–93
61. Karow AR, Bahrenburg S, Garidel P (2013) Buffer capacity of biologics--from buffer salts to buffering by antibodies. Biotechnol Prog 29:480–492
62. Bahrenburg S, Karow AR, Garidel P (2015) Buffer-free therapeutic antibody preparations provide a viable alternative to conventionally buffered solutions: from protein buffer capacity prediction to bioprocess applications. Biotechnol J 10:610–622

63. Burckbuchler V, Mekhloufi G, Paillard Giteau A, Grossiord JL, Huille S, Agnely F (2010) Rheological and syringeability properties of highly concentrated human polyclonal immunoglobulin solutions. Eur J Pharm Biopharm 76:351–356
64. Berteau C, Filipe-Santos O, Wang T, Rojas HE, Granger C, Schwarzenbach F (2015) Evaluation of the impact of viscosity, injection volume, and injection flow rate on subcutaneous injection tolerance. Med Devices 8:473–484
65. Thomsen M, Hernandez-Garcia A, Mathiesen J, Poulsen M, Sørensen DN, Tarnow L, Feidenhans R (2014) Model study of the pressure build-up during subcutaneous injection. PLoS One 9(8):e104054
66. Doughty DV, Clawson CZ, Lambert W, Subramony JA (2016) Understanding subcutaneous tissue pressure for engineering injection devices for large-volume protein delivery. J Pharm Sci 105:2105–2133
67. Ravi AD, Sadhna D, Nagpaal D, Chawla L (2015) Needle free injection technology: a complete insight. Int J Pharm Investig 5 (4):192–199
68. Gupta J, Park S, Bondy B, Felner EI, Prausnitz MR (2011) Infusion pressure and pain during microneedle injection into skin of human subjects. Biomaterials 32 (28):6823–6831
69. Fry A (2014) Injecting highly viscous drugs. PharmTech 38(11). http://www.pharmtech.com/injecting-highly-viscous-drugs
70. Werk T, Ludwig IS, Lümkemann J, Mahler HC, Huwyler J, Hafner M (2016) Technology, applications and process challenges of dual chamber systems. J Pharm Sci 105 (1):4–9
71. Jones LS, Kaufmann A, Middaugh CR (2005) Silicone oil induced aggregation of proteins. J Pharm Sci 94(4):918–927
72. Liu L, Ammar DA, Ross LA, Mandava N, Kahook MY, Carpenter JF (2011) Silicone oil microdroplets and protein aggregates in repackaged bevacizumab and ranibizumab: effects of long-term storage and product mishandling. Invest Ophathalmol Vis Sci 52:1023–1034
73. Li J, Pinnamaneni S, Quan Y, Jaiswal A, Andersson FI, Zhang X (2012) Mechanistic understanding of protein-silicone oil interactions. Pharm Res 29:1689–1697
74. Krayukhina E, Tsumoto K, Uchiyama S, Fukui K (2015) Effects of syringe material and silicone oil lubrication on the stability of pharmaceutical proteins. J Pharm Sci 104:527–535
75. Saggu M, Patel AR, Koulis T (2017) A random forest approach for counting silicone oil droplets and protein particles in antibody formulations using flow microscopy. Pharm Res 34:479–491
76. Jiang Y, Nashed-Samuel Y, Li C, Liu W, Pollastrini J, Mallard D, Wen Z-Q, Fujimori K, Pallitto M, Donahue L, Chu G, Torraca G, Vance A, Mire-Sluis T, Freund E, Davis J, Narhi L (2009) Tungsten-induced protein aggregation: solution behaviour. J Pharm Sci 98:4695–4710
77. Liu W, Swift R, Torraca G, Nashed-Samuel Y, Wen Z-Q, Jiang Y, Vance A, Mire-Sluis A, Freund E, Davis J, Narhi L (2010) Root cause analysis of tungsten-induced protein aggregation in pre-filled syringes. PDA J Pharm Sci Technol 64(1):11–19
78. Bee JS, Nelson SA, Freund E, Carpenter JF, Randolph TW (2009) Precipitation of a monoclonal antibody by soluble tungsten. J Pharm Sci 98(9):3290–3301
79. Seidl A, Hainzl O, Richter M, Fischer R, Böhm S, Deitel B, Hartinger M, Windisch J, Casadevall N, London GM, Macdougall I (2012) Tungsten-induced denaturation and aggregation of Epoetin Alfa during primary packaging as a cause of immunogenicity. Pharm Res 29:1451–1467
80. Warne NW (2011) Development of high concentration protein biopharmaceuticals: the use of platform approaches in formulation development. Eur J Pharm Biopharm 78:208–212
81. Wagner M, Reiche K, Blume A, Garidel P (2012) The electrokinetic potential of therapeutic proteins and its modulation: impact on protein stability. Colloids Surf A Physicochem Eng Aspects 415:421–430
82. Raut AS, Kalonia DS (2015) Liquid-liquid phase separation in a dual variable domain immunoglobulin protein solution: effect of formulation factors and protein-protein interactions. Mol Pharm 12(9):3261–3271
83. Raut AS, Kalonia DS (2015) Opalescence in monoclonal antibody solutions and its correlation with intermolecular interactions in dilute and concentrated solutions. J Pharm Sci 104:1263–1274
84. Reiche K, Hart J, Blume A, Garidel P (2017) Liquid-liquid phase separation of a monoclonal antibody at low ionic strength: influence of anion charge and concentration. Biophys Chem 220:7–19

85. Lin Y-H, Chan HS (2017) Phase Separation and Single-Chain Compactness of Charged Disordered Proteins Are Strongly Correlated. Biophysical J 112(10):2043–2046
86. Randolph TW (1997) Phase separation of excipients during lyophilisation: effects on protein stability. J Pharm Sci 86 (11):1198–1203
87. Heller MC, Carpenter JF, Randolph TW (1997) Manipulation of lyophilisation-induced phase separation: implications for pharmaceutical proteins. Biotechnol Prog 13:590–596
88. Padilla AM, Pikal MJ (2011) The study of phase preparation in amorphous freeze-dried systems, Part 2: Investigation of Raman mapping as a tool for studying amorphous phase separation in freeze-dried protein formulations. J Pharm Sci 100(4):1497–1474
89. Pikal MJ (1994) Freeze-drying of proteins. In: Cleland JL, Langer R (eds) Stability, formulation and delivery of peptides and proteins, ACS Symposium series. American Chemical Society, Washington, DC, pp 120–133
90. Awotwe-Otoo D, Agarabi C, Read EK, Lute S, Brorson KA, Khan MA (2015) Product and process understanding to relate the effect of freezing method on glycation and aggregation of lyophilized monoclonal antibody formulations. Int J Pharm 490 (1–2):341–350
91. Ressing ME, Jiskoot W, Talsma H, van Ingen CW, Beuvery EC, Crommelin DJA (1992) The influence of sucrose, dextran, and hydroxypropyl-β-cyclodextrin as lyoprotectants for a freeze-dried mouse IgG_{2a} monoclonal antibody (MN12). Pharm Res 9(2):266–270
92. Meyer JD, Nayar R, Manning MC (2009) Impact of bulking agents on the stability of a lyophilized monoclonal antibody. Eur J Pharm Biopharm 38(1):29–38
93. Park J, Nagapudi K, Vergara C, Ramachander R, Laurence JS, Krishnan S (2013) Effect of pH and excipients on structure, dynamics, and long-term stability of a model IgG1 monoclonal antibody upon freeze-drying. Pharm Res 30(4):968–984
94. Stärtzel P, Gieseler H, Gieseler M, Abdul-Fattah AM, Adler M, Mahler HC, Goldbach P (2015) Freeze-drying of L-arginine/sucrose-based protein formulations, Part I: Influence of formulation and arginine counter ion on the critical formulation temperature, product performance and protein stability. J Pharm Sci 104(7):2345–2358
95. Stärtzel P, Gieseler H, Gieseler M, Abdul-Fattah AM, Adler M, Mahler HC, Goldbach P (2015) Freeze-drying of L-arginine/sucrose-based protein formulations, Part 2: Optimization of formulation design and freeze-drying process conditions for an L-arginine chloride-based protein formulation system. J Pharm Sci 104(12):4241–4256
96. Stärtzel P, Gieseler H, Gieseler M, Abdul-Fattah AM, Adler M, Mahler HC, Goldbach P (2016) Mannitol/L-arginine-based formulation systems for freeze drying of protein pharmaceuticals: effect of the L-arginine counter ion and formulation composition on the formulation properties and the physical state of mannitol. J Pharm Sci 105 (10):3123–3135
97. Matheus S, Friess W, Mahler HC (2006) FTIR and nDSC as analytical tools for high-concentration protein formulations. Pharm Res 23(6):1350–1363
98. Garidel P, Bassarab S (2008) Impact of formulation design on stability and quality. In: Lyscon N (ed) Quality for biologics: critical quality attributes, process and change control, production variation, characterisation, impurities and regulatory concerns. Biopharm Knowledge Publishing, London, UK, pp 94–113
99. Garidel P, Schott H (2006) Fourier-transform midinfrared spectroscopy for the analysis and screening of liquid protein formulations. Part 1: Understanding infrared spectroscopy of proteins. BioProcess Int 4(5):40–46
100. Garidel P, Schott H (2006) Fourier-transform midinfrared spectroscopy for the analysis and screening of liquid protein formulations. Part 2: Detailed analysis and applications. BioProcess Int 4(6):48–55
101. Kim J, Qiu J (2014) Quantitation of low concentrations of polysorbates in high protein concentration formulations by solid phase extraction and cobalt-thocyanate derivatisation. Anal Chem 806:144–151
102. Savjani N, Babcock E, Khor HK, Raghani A (2014) Use of ferric thiocyanate derivatization for quantification of polysorbate 80 in high concentration protein formulations. Talanta 130:542–546
103. Wuchner K, Büchler J, Spycher R, Dalmonte P, Volkin DB (2010) Development of a microflow digital imaging assay to characterize protein particulates during storage of a high concentration IgG1 monoclonal antibody formulation. J Pharm Sci 99 (8):3343–3361

104. Saluja A, Badkar AV, Zeng DL, Kalonia DS (2007) Ultrasonic rheology of a monoclonal antibody (IgG2) solution: implications for physical stability of proteins in high concentration formulations. J Pharm Sci 96 (12):3181–3195
105. Trainor K, Broom A, Meiering EM (2017) Exploring the relationship between protein sequence, structure and solubility. Curr Opin Struct Biol 42:136–146
106. Woods JM, Nesta D (2010) Formulation effects on opalescence of a high-concentration mAb. BioProcess Int 10:48–59
107. van der Kant R, Karow-Zwick AR, Van Durme J, Blech M, Gallardo R, Seeliger D, Aßfalg K, Baatsen P, Compernolle G, Gils A, Studts JM, Schulz P, Garidel P, Schymkowitz J, Rousseau F (2017) Prediction and reduction of the aggregation of monoclonal antibodies. J Mol Biol 429 (8):1244–1261
108. Yearley EJ, Godfrin PD, Perevozchikova T, Zhang H, Falus P, Porcar L, Nagao M, Curtis JE, Gawande P, Taing R, Zarraga IE, Wagner NJ, Liu Y (2014) Observation of small cluster formation in concentrated monoclonal antibody solutions and its implications to solution viscosity. Biophys J 106:1763–1770
109. LeBrun V, Friess W, Bassarab S, Mühlau S, Garidel P (2010) A critical evaluation of self-interaction chromatography as a predictive tool for the assessment of protein-protein interactions in protein formulation development: a case study of a therapeutic monoclonal antibody. Eur J Pharm Biopharm 75 (1):16–25
110. Herhut M, Brandenbusch C, Sadowski G (2016) Modelling and prediction of protein solubility using the second osmotic virial coefficient. Fluid Phase Equilib 411:32–42
111. Colandene JD, Maldonado LM, Creach AT, Vrettos JS, Goad KG, Spitznagel TM (2007) Lyophilizatin cycle development for a high-concentration monoclonal antibody formulation lacking a crystalline bulking agent. J Pharm Sci 96(6):1598–1608
112. Cao W, Krishnan S, Speed Ricci M, Shih LY, Liu D, Hua Gu J, Jameel F (2013) Rational design of lyophilised high concentration protein formulations-mitigating the challenge of slow reconstitutin with multidisciplinary strategies. Eur J Pharm Biopharm 85:287–293
113. Garidel P, Pevestorf B, Bahrenburg S (2015) Stability of buffer-free freeze-dried formulations: a feasibility study of a monoclonal antibody at high protein concentrations. Eur J Pharm Biopharm 97:125–139
114. Schersch K, Betz O, Garidel P, Muehlau S, Bassarab S, Winter G (2010) Systematic investigation of the effect of lyophilizate collapse on pharmaceutically relevant proteins 1: Stability after freeze-drying. J Pharm Sci 99 (5):2256–2278
115. Schersch K, Betz O, Garidel P, Muehlau S, Bassarab S, Winter G (2010) Systematic investigation of the effect of lyophilizate collapse on pharmaceutically relevant proteins 2: Stability during storage at elevated temperatures. J Pharm Sci 101(7):2288–2306
116. Schersch K, Betz O, Garidel P, Muehlau S, Bassarab S, Winter G (2010) Systematic investigation of the effect of lyophilizate collapse on pharmaceutically relevant proteins 3: Collapse during storage at elevated temperatures. Eur J Pharm Biopharm 85(2):240–252
117. Chang L, Shepherd D, Sun J, Tang X, Pikal MJ (2005) Effect of sorbitol and residual moisture on the stability of lyophilized antibodies: implications for the mechanism of protein stabilization in the solid state. J Pharm Sci 94(7):1445–1455
118. Kasper JC, Friess W (2011) The freezing step in lyophilization: physico-chemical fundamentals, freezing methods and consequences on process performance and quality attributes of biopharmaceuticals. Eur J Pharm Biopharm 78(2):248–263
119. Rambhatla S, Ramot R, Bhugra C, Pikal MJ (2004) Heat and mass transfer scale-up issues during freeze drying: II. Control and characterization of the degree of supercooling. AAPS PharmSciTech 5(4):54–62
120. Searles JA, Carpenter JF, Randolph TW (2001) The ice nucleation temperature determines the primary drying rate of lyophilization for samples frozen on a temperature-controlled shelf. J Pharm Sci 90(7):860–871
121. van den Berg L, Rose D (1959) Effect of freezing on the pH and composition of sodium and potassium phosphate solutions: the reciprocal system KH2PO4---Na2HPO4---H2O. Arch Biochem Biophys 81(2):319–329
122. Konstantinidis AK, Kuu W, Otten L, Nail SL, Sever RR (2011) Controlled nucleation in freeze-drying: effects on pore size in the dried product layer, mass transfer resistance, and primary drying rate. J Pharm Sci 100 (8):3453–3470
123. Geidobler R, Winter G (2013) Controlled ice nucleation in the field of freeze-drying: fundamentals and technology review. Eur J Pharm Biopharm 85:214–222

124. Gasteyer TH, Sever RR, Hunel B, Grinter N, Verdone ML (2007) Lyophilization system and method. US Patent 20070186437A1
125. Awotwe-Otoo D, Agarabi C, Read EK, Lute S, Brorson KA, Khan MA, Shah RB (2013) Impact of controlled ice nucleation on process performance and quality attributes of a lyophilized monoclonal antibody. Int J Pharm 450(1–2):70–78
126. Geidobler R, Konrad I, Winter G (2013) Can controlled ice nucleation improve freeze-drying of highly-concentrated protein formulations? J Pharm Sci 102:3915–3919

Chapter 13

Mechanical Behavior and Structure of Freeze-Dried Cakes

Sarah H. M. Hedberg, Sharmila Devi, Arnold Duralliu, and Daryl R. Williams

Abstract

Freeze-drying or the lyophilization of biopharmaceuticals is a standard method for product manufacture in order to increase product shelf-life and minimize the tendency of re-constituted products to aggregate. However, the physical and or mechanical stability of freeze-dried cakes can be problematic, which can directly result in financial losses due to unusable or damaged products. Currently, there is very limited systematic knowledge of the relationship between lyophilization process conditions and the cake-specific physical structure, mechanical performance, and stability. This Chapter reviews the detailed mechanical properties and structure of freeze-dried cakes formed from aqueous solutions with concentrations from 1 to 40% w/v of common excipients, mannitol, sucrose, and trehalose in some detail. In addition, the mechanical properties of commercial freeze-dried products as well as effects of moisture content and ingress into freeze-dried cakes are also reported. Both experimentally measured Young's moduli and yield stress data scale well with reduced cake density, in line with theoretical predictions from classical cellular solids theory. A novel compressive indentation method is reviewed which can accurately determine a cake's Young's modulus and yield stress within 1 min, allowing the potential future use of these mechanical cake attributes as Critical Quality Attributes (CQAs).

Key words Compressive mechanics, Young's modulus, Sucrose, Trehalose, Mannitol, Yield stress, Normal indentation

1 Introduction

1.1 Current QC Methods for Solid State Freeze-Dried Products

Freeze-drying or lyophilization is the most common method of preservation and the extension of shelf-life for biopharmaceutical products. It is widely used for preparing biopharmaceutical products for subsequent dissolution and delivery of bioactive therapeutic agents to patients in liquid-based formulations. Liquid formulations are the easiest to handle and the most cost-effective route to manufacture, but many of the products are at risk to physical (such as aggregation and precipitation) as well as chemical degradation (deamidation and oxidation) processes during storage and transport [1, 2]. These degradation processes can be avoided or

Kevin R. Ward and Paul Matejtschuk (eds.), *Lyophilization of Pharmaceuticals and Biologicals: New Technologies and Approaches*, Methods in Pharmacology and Toxicology, https://doi.org/10.1007/978-1-4939-8928-7_13,

at least slowed down by lyophilization with the resultant solid state products having a longer shelf-life and being stable for months or years under ambient conditions [3]. Freeze-drying has been used to preserve a wide range of biopharmaceuticals, viruses, biological specimens, food products, and archaeological artifacts. In 2004 freeze-drying accounted for 46% of all biologics approved by the Food and Drug Administration (FDA) [4] and 9 years later, in 2013, four out of the six top selling biologics were freeze-dried products.

Even though freeze-drying is a standard method used for the manufacture of solid state biopharmaceuticals, many final freeze-dried products are physically or mechanically fragile and can easily be damaged during processing or transportation [5]. Fracture, delamination, and crumbling of a freeze-dried cake is not an uncommon event. Such damaged freeze-dried products are no longer acceptable for re-constitution and subsequent delivery to patients, resulting in financial losses as well as a loss of confidence in the product. Therefore, it is of great interest to use experimental methods that are capable of quantifying changes in the mechanical and physical properties of these fragile freeze-dried cakes [6].

The general characterization of freeze-dried products has attracted significant research interest in the past 40 years and over 20 different characterization methods have been reported in the literature. However, out of these 20 methods, only around 6 methods are used regularly. Table 1 summarizes the type of information that can be obtained from the different tests, ease of operation, offline or online nature of test, and whether the test is destructive to the material.

1.2 Mechanical Characterization of Freeze-Dried Cakes

In addition to finding a fast and reliable method to measure the mechanical properties of the freeze-dried cake, it is important to gain a detailed understanding of the relationship between mechanical behavior of lyophilized biopharmaceutical cakes and the process conditions and product formulations involved. This knowledge could be used as a critical quality attribute (CQA) to enable the manufacture of robust lyophilized products at the first attempt using a quality by design approach, instead of trial and error based approaches. The understanding of the CQAs of final products, including the lyophilized products, is one of the main focuses in the biopharmaceutical industry to ensure the quality of new medicines.

The CQAs that are currently used for freeze-dried products include properties such as cake physical structure and physical appearance, residual moisture content, in process formulation stability, product reconstitution time and color, bio-activity, as well as shelf life [18]. In addition to these practically important CQAs, the relationship between these CQAs and lyophilization process conditions is equally important. By knowing how to obtain a certain

Table 1
Current characterization methods for freeze-dried biopharmaceuticals [7]

Method	Information or data determined	Ease of test	On-line/off line	Extent of use	Destructive/ nondestructive	References
Physical appearance	Color, finish, topography, shrinkage	Easy	Both	Regularly	Nondestructive	[8, 9]
Reconstitution	Reconstitution time	Easy	Offline	Regularly	Destructive	[10, 11]
Karl Fischer (KF) titration	Residual moisture content	Easy	Offline	Regularly	Destructive	[12–14]
Frequency modulation spectroscopy (FMS)	Head space moisture or A_w	Easy	Offline	Hardly	Nondestructive	[15]
Bioassay	Potency/efficacy/bioactivity	Complex	Offline	Regularly	Destructive	[16–18]
Differential scanning calorimetry (DSC)	T_g, T'_g, Eutectic temperature Possibility of phase change during freeze-drying Molecular mobility Phase separation	Easy	Offline	Regularly	Destructive	[19–21] [22] [23] [24]
Differential thermal analysis (DTA)	Occurrence of crystallization	Easy	Offline	Regularly	Destructive	[25]
Freeze-drying microscopy (FDM)	Collapse temperature (T_c), morphology of ice crystals	Easy	Offline	Regularly	Destructive	[26, 27]
Freeze-drying X-ray diffraction (FD-XRD)	Crystallization of components	Complex	On line	Rarely	Nondestructive	[28, 29]
Cryo environmental SEM	Ice crystal morphological changes during process	Complex	On line	Rarely	Nondestructive	[30]
Thermoelectric analysis (TEA)	T_g, T'_g, T_m and Eutectic temperature	Complex	Online	Rarely	Nondestructive	[25, 31]
(Dynamic) thermal mechanical analysis (DMTA, TMA)	T_g, T'_g, T_m and Eutectic temperature	Medium	Offline	Hardly	Destructive	[21, 32–34]
Dielectric Analysis (DEA)	T_c	Medium	Offline	Hardly	Destructive	[35]

(continued)

Table 1 (continued)

Method	Information or data determined	Ease of test	On-line/off line	Extent of use	Destructive/ nondestructive	References
Nuclear magnetic resonance (NMR)	Mobility	Medium	On-line and off-line	Hardly	Nondestructive	[36, 37]
Near infrared reflectance spectroscopy (NIR)	Sublimation rate or residual moisture	Easy	On-line and off-line	Hardly	Nondestructive	[38–40]
Dynamic vapour sorption (DVS)	Residual moisture content and water sorption isotherms	Easy	Offline	Rarely	Nondestructive	[41–43]
X-ray powder diffraction (XRPD)	Crystallinity/amorphicity	Easy	offline	Regularly	Nondestructive	[44]
Polarized light microscopy (PLM)		Easy	Offline	Regularly	Nondestructive	[45]
Scanning electron microscopy (SEM)	Structure/morphology	Medium	Offline	Hardly	Destructive	[46]
Isothermal micro-calorimetry (IMC)	Storage stability /mobility	Easy	Offline	Hardly	Destructive	[47]
Thermally stimulated current spectroscopy (TSC)	Storage stability/mobility	Easy	Offline	Hardly	Destructive	[48]
Surface area (BET)	Surface area	Medium	Offline	Hardly	Destructive	[49, 50]
X-ray tomography	Structure of cake	Complex	Offline	Rarely	Nondestructive	[13]
Compressive indentation	Young's modulus and crushing yield stress/strength	Easy	Offline	Rarely	Destructive	[51–54]

CQA, and how it can be measured easily and reliably, improvements and refinements in process conditions can be implemented with likely favorable outcomes.

Currently, a commonly used CQA for freeze-dried cakes is their physical appearance, which is derived from the color, finish, and/or shrinkage of the final dried cake. All of these properties are reported qualitatively, or at best semi-quantitatively, therefore it is very difficult to make comparisons between different researchers measuring the properties and the materials produced by the same laboratory. Having at most semi-quantitative properties causes a problem for developing favorable conditions and parameters for optimum product formulation and process optimization, leading most experiments to be trial and error. These are some of the crucial developments for freeze-dried biopharmaceuticals in order to ensure product safety and quality, without incurring significant financial losses due to batch failures and rejections.

1.3 Excipients in Freeze-Dried Cakes

Excipients are classified as stabilizers, buffers, bulking agents, preservatives, surfactants, and tonicifiers and they can help in maintaining stability during the lyophilization process, handling, shipping, and storage. They are generally added to biopharmaceutical formulations to provide physical or chemical stability to freeze-dried cakes. Typical formulations contain one or more excipients. Apart from enhancing stability, excipients also help to provide the cakes with increased density and additional rigidity, which are both a contributing factor in improving the mechanical properties of the cakes.

Excipient buffers are required in pharmaceutical formulations to stabilize pH, therefore their choices are critical. Phosphate buffers, especially sodium phosphate, can undergo drastic pH changes during freezing [55, 56], so the best choices are Tris, histidine, and citrate which, at low concentrations, only undergo minor pH changes [2]. Bulking agents provide the majority of the formulation and are especially important when formulations have a low concentration of the active ingredient. Bulking agents that are crystalline help provide an elegant structure of the cake and good mechanical properties but are generally less effective in stabilizing proteins [55]. The most effective excipient stabilizers for proteins are disaccharides as they form sugar-based amorphous glasses. Sucrose and trehalose are two of the most common inert disaccharide stabilizers used. Tonicifiers or tonicity adjusters are critical for providing isotonic solutions, meaning that the osmotic pressure needs to be equal with respect to a membrane, i.e., the blood cells or cardiovascular tissue for intravenous formulations, with no movement between either side of the membrane. In order to adjust this factor, which could be necessary for formulations with high drug concentrations, low injection volumes, or stability issues, a tonicifier might be needed in the formulation [57].

Kang et al. [58] summarized the most common liquid and solid formulation conditions for one of the largest classes of biopharmaceuticals, monoclonal antibodies (mAbs). Out of 37 commercial mAb formulations, 12 were lyophilized formulations. Out of these 12 formulations the most common stabilizing excipients were sucrose and trehalose, sucrose being the most prevalent one. Mannitol was another common stabilizing excipient for commercial formulations.

1.4 Mechanics of Cellular Solids and Foams

Freeze-dried cakes are an example of cellular materials which are commonly referred to as foams, and consist of a number of cells that can have solid faces and solid edges. These cellular solid structures have often been described as solid struts and plates that together form the different units of cells [59]. There are many applications for cellular materials, often lightweight organic polymer based, such as packaging, thermal insulation and for structural uses including bone replacement therapies and light weight structures for buoyancy applications [60]. In the last two decades there has been an increase in the number of industrial and commercial applications in sectors like the automotive and aerospace industry that has driven research toward a better understanding of their mechanical behavior.

If the structures within the cellular materials have no directionality they are considered isotropic while if their cellular structures are axisymmetric (like cork) or orthotropic (like wood) they are considered anisotropic. The mechanical properties of foams also reflects these isotropic or anisotropic structures [61]. Cellular materials can both have open cells and closed cells; open cells are when the material structure is divided into small columns or beams that form the edges of the cells whereas closed cells when the material is distributed into small plates that form the faces of the cells. The mechanical properties of these materials are also dependent on the open versus closed cell structures (Fig. 1). The most important property of any foam structure is the relative density, which is defined as the density of the solid foam over the density of the solid that that foam is made from. This ratio can vary between 0.01 and 1 and the mechanical properties of the foams are shown to relate directly to their relative density [61].

The different types of cell structures are critical for understanding the mechanical properties of foams. It is believed that the relative density followed by the anisotropy are the most important factors that can describe the mechanical performance of a foam. Other topological aspects that can have a significant impact on the mechanical properties include the cell shape, the edge connectivity, and the number of contact neighbors. As cellular materials do not exist with a single relative density, isotropicity or topological aspect and instead have statistical distribution of these properties, it is almost impossible to be able to give direct guidelines for mechanical property prediction *a priori* [7].

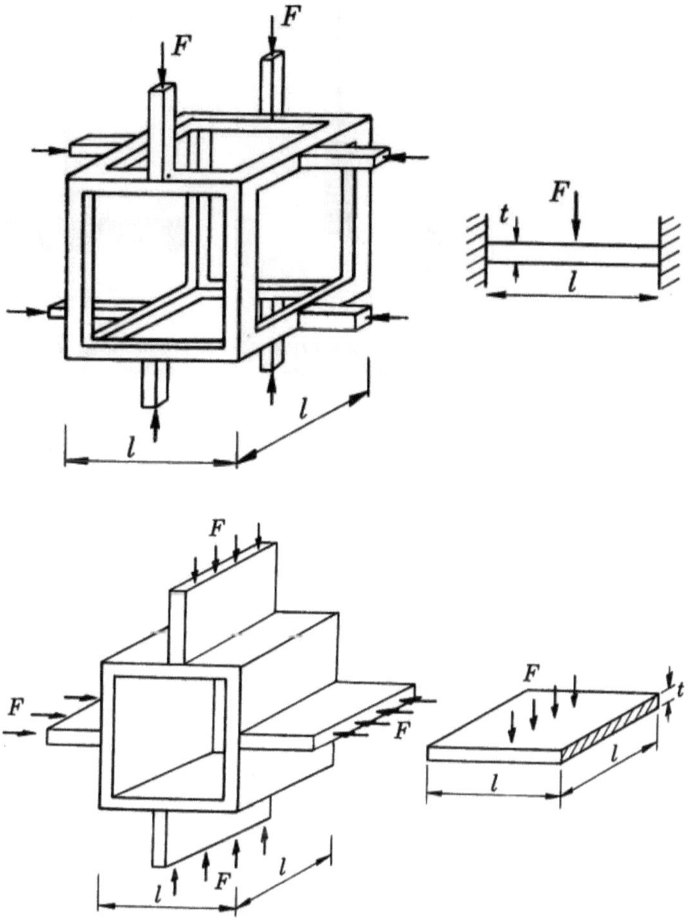

Fig. 1 Open (left) and closed (right) cellular structures [62]

All materials will deform when stress is applied, but the deformational behavior will depend on material composition and structure. Brittle materials will deform elastically until a critical stress is reached when the material will start to fracture. Ductile materials will instead yield plastically with increasing strain before failing.

There are three modes of compressional deformation: confined compression, unconfined compression, and indentation (Fig. 2). In confined compression, the sample is placed into a container that confines the sample at the bottom and on the sides and this represents an idealized deformation. In unconfined compression, the sample is placed between two rigid, flat plates letting the sample expand laterally. Indentation is when the sample is indented by a frictionless probe often with a cylindrical, spherical, or pyramidal shape. Foams are divided into two broad categories based on their structural uniformity, where the performance of the isotropic material is identical regardless of the direction of the test, whereas for anisotropic material, this depends on the direction of the test.

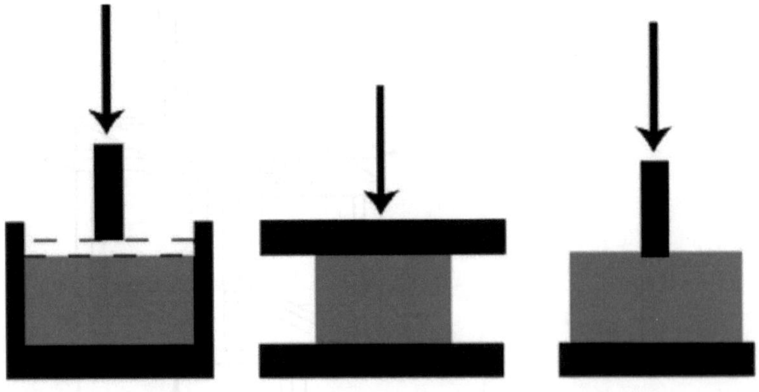

Fig. 2 Modes of compressive deformation

Honeycombs are regular two-dimensional cellular materials that enable the development of closed-form expressions for describing the mechanical performance of macroscopic in-plane properties of foams. Even though cells in honeycombs are most often hexagonal, they can take three basic lattice structures: the hexagonal structure, the square structure, and the fully triangulated structure [59].

1.5 Mechanical Attributes of Freeze-Dried Products

As reported previously, some of the challenges with freeze-drying are the poor understanding of how process conditions affect cake structure and mechanical properties. Along with the process conditions, the choice of excipients, buffer, and solution composition are carefully chosen for the specific material to be freeze-dried. In the biopharmaceutical industry, a better understanding of how these changes in formulation affect the mechanical properties of the final freeze-dried protein would be highly desirable. This understanding would allow us to map out process conditions and solution formulation required to produce good quality cakes that do not break easily on handling or storage.

Devi [7] has provided a thorough literature review on the different steps in the freeze-drying process and how different process parameters can be adjusted to achieve a desirable product. However, acceptable CQAs chosen vary between researchers, e.g., De Beer et al. [63] used attributes like onset and duration of crystallization process steps, duration of primary drying, and residual moisture content, while other researchers used dry layer flow resistance, hence primary drying time, as the key measurable attributes against the process variables of shelf temperature and pressure [64–66]. Cannon and Shemeley [67] measured the ice sublimation rates for various vial types to better understand the relationship between vial glass types, vial diameter and base concavity, and the ice sublimation rates. The effect of excipients on freezing temperature and sublimation rate has also previously been studied [68]. Sunderland proposed suitable but practical CQAs for freeze-drying, which included physical appearance, reconstitution time, residual moisture content, and protein assay [69]. In terms of the physical appearance this mainly included quality descriptors such as color in hue, tint and tone, shade and intensity. The visual inspection also included the cake structure such as coarseness of the cake, signs of pockets, voids, or collapse.

Many of these descriptors may be good for process understanding but they may not be suitable as CQAs and provide no insight to improve our understanding between process conditions and properties—including mechanical—of the freeze-dried cakes. Furthermore, the explicit relationship between the processing conditions and the mechanical characteristics of the final freeze-dried cakes is not clear as the literature reports few studies on this topic [7].

Today, there is a clear understanding of how to control the internal structure of the cake by varying the freezing conditions and excipients used in the formulation. Examples include the use of faster cooling rates that will produce smaller ice crystals because there is insufficient time for Ostwald ripening to occur or to enlarge the size of the crystal. Thus, smaller ice crystals create smaller pore cavities in the cakes. Slower cooling rates on the other hand will allow the ice crystals to become larger because of the Ostwald ripening and therefore create larger cavities in the cakes. Very low freezing temperatures (e.g., −80 °C) will create smaller pores while higher temperatures (−20 °C) will create larger pores because of the larger ice crystals formed [51]. If the ice nucleation is spontaneous then a larger variability in the cake properties between the vials will be observed. In such cases, ice crystal formation will not be uniform, and an irregular distribution of pore sizes is created. On the other hand, controlled nucleation will produce ice crystals with more uniform sizes which will in turn lead to the formation of pores that will have much narrower size distributions [7].

2 Experimental Studies

2.1 Freeze-Drying of Sucrose, Trehalose, and Mannitol

Sucrose (Sigma Aldrich, Dorset UK) and trehalose (Cargill 1640 Minneapolis, MN, USA) were used to make 1.0%, 2.5%, 5.0%, 20.0%, 30.0%, and 40.0% w/w solutions with purified, deionized water (>18.2 MΩ cm at 25 °C). D-Mannitol (Sigma Aldrich, Dorset UK) was only prepared in 5.0% w/w solutions with purified, deionized water. 2 mL aliquots of solution from each concentration were dispensed into 6 mL borosilicate glass vials (VCDIN6R, Schott, Germany) and placed on the trays in a hexagonal pattern which maximizes the number of vials that can fit on the tray. In total 168 vials were placed on each of the two trays in the freeze-dryer in a semi-stoppered position. Solutions were freeze-dried (FD) using a VirTis Advantage Plus freeze-dryer (SP Scientific, Warminster, PA, USA). The freeze-drying runs were performed according to two protocols, the first one consisting of a freezing rate of 0.3 °C/min until reaching the primary drying temperature of −40 °C where the product was held for 190 h. Afterward the temperature was ramped up at 0.3 °C/min until reaching the secondary drying temperature of 20 °C where the sample was held for 24 h. However, after seeing cracks in the SEM images [7], the run was performed according to a second protocol with a primary drying temperature of −50 °C and a hold time of 160 h. Afterward the sample was only held for 12 h at the secondary drying temperature of 20 °C. After freeze-drying all the vials were sealed under a 50 mTorr vacuum and stored at around 18 °C until used.

For the moisture exposure study sucrose (Sigma: S5016-1 kg, Dorset, UK) and trehalose (Cargill 1640 Minneapolis, MN, USA) were used to make the 5%, 10%, and 20% (w/w) solutions with purified deionized water. All concentration solutions were freeze-dried using a Telstar Lyobeta 15 (Azbil-Telstar SpA, Terressa, Spain). The freeze-drying cycle run consisted of a freezing rate of 0.2 °C/min and a primary drying temperature of −35 °C/min held for 20 h. Secondary drying temperature was at 25 °C where the sample was held for 16 h. After the cycle had finished the vials were backfilled with nitrogen gas before stoppering.

2.2 IgG Freeze-Drying Cycles

Screw capped vials with 5 mL nominal volume, height of 41.5 mm × internal diameter 18 mm (Adelphi Tubes, Haywards Heath, UK) were filled with IgG at varying concentrations (10, 50, 100, and 200 mg/mL) to a fill-depth of 1 mL using an automated Multipette stream repeater pipette (Eppendorf, UK). For each separate run, 200 vials were loaded onto a stainless steel tray and placed on top shelf of the LyoBeta 15 freeze dryer. Two runs were completed where vials for 10, 50, 100, and 200 mg/mL IgG underwent lyophilization using the low moisture run and the other second batch of 50 mg/mL w/v IgG using the high moisture run cycle (Table 2). After the cycle had finished, the vials were backfilled with nitrogen gas before stoppering the 13 mm diameter igloo halobutyl stoppers (Adelphi Group, Haywards Heath, UK). Afterward, the vials were capped by hand and labeled. The process conditions and timings were varied slightly for the samples containing IgG. The protocol is summarized in Table 2.

2.3 Scanning Electron Microscopy

Samples for Scanning Electron Microscopy (SEM) were prepared by carefully separating the cake vertically, into halves using a sharp scalpel. One half of the cake was then divided into quarters vertically. The second half of the cake was first separated into quarters and each quarter was divided horizontally into two portions. Approximately 0.4 cm^3 samples, with the freshly separated surface

Table 2
Freeze-drying cycle for each material

Material	Freezing temperature (°C)	Freezing ramp rate (°C/min)	Freezing hold time (min)	Primary drying temperature (°C)	Primary hold time (min)	Secondary drying temperature (°C)	Secondary hold time (min)
IgG (10–200 mg/mL) "Low Moisture" Run	−40	1.00	120	−15	1200	30	600
IgG (50 mg/mL) "High Moisture" Run	−40	1.00	120	−40	900	15	60

orientated upwards, were mounted on the SEM stub covered with a drop of conducting silver paint and allowed to dry. The sample was sputter coated with Au for 120 s in an Ar atmosphere (Emitech K550). A TM-1000 (Hitachi, Japan) table-top SEM (15 kV accelerating voltage and solid state backscattered electron detector) was used to scan the morphology of the freeze-dried cakes at magnifications of up to 5000×. The dimensions of cell height and length were measured from the micrographs (×500 and ×1000) using a graduated ruler (inserted in the image) and the thickness from the ×5000 micrographs, using computer-based software (Image J, National Institute of Health, USA). Using the length scale of the image, the cell area was measured. On average, at least 50 cell dimensions ($n \geq 50$) were measured for each sample and mean dimensions determined and reported.

2.4 Relative Density Determination

The relative density, ρ_{rel}, of freeze-dried cakes that is referred to here is obtained by dividing apparent density, ρ_{app}, by true or absolute density, ρ_{true}, if the porosity is zero and follows the full procedure outlined in Devi and Williams [54].

ρ_{rel} is determined by the mass and the volume that is occupied by the cake. The volume is calculated using the dimensions of the cake that is often cylindrical.

ρ_{app} was determined using a helium pycnometer (AccuPyc 1330, Micromeritics Instrument Corp., Norcross, GA, USA) and the accuracy of the instrument was checked using AccuPyc 1330 calibration standard (AccuPyc 1330, Micromeritics) of known volume. Before measurements, the excipient samples and compact powder discs were purged with helium for at least 15 h to remove any sorbed moisture. During measurements, the samples and compacts were purged with dry helium ten times in the instrument test chamber to effectively remove any residual moisture prior to final data collection. The reported results are averages of ten consecutive measurements ($n = 10$). The true material densities for the different excipient samples were estimated by plotting the absolute density of the compacts as a function of compaction force and extrapolating the linear line to the *y*-axis to read the true density where porosity is expected to be zero.

2.5 Mechanical Tests

The mechanical tests followed what was outlined in Devi and Williams [54]. The indenter probe, a flat-faced 5 or 10 mm diameter punch, was directly attached to a load cell (Futek, UK). The load cell was connected to computer via a strain bridge amplifier (Fylde, UK) and attached to a *z* direction motion stage (Zaber, Canada). The load cell performance was validated using a series of calibrations weights and the system was controlled by Labview style software. The sealed vials containing the cakes were equilibrated at 22 °C before testing. A compression indentation test was carried out on the cake immediately after removing the stopper from the vial using a loading velocity 10 μm/s, recording force data every 50 μm. The cakes were approximately 6.0 mm thick and 19.6 mm in diameter. The force measured (g) versus displacement (μm) was recorded during the compression into the central zone of the dried cakes. Time of the experiment took typically 0.5 min and was conducted at 22 °C and 40%RH.

The global compressive strain ε was calculated using:

$$\varepsilon = \frac{h_0 - h}{h_0} \tag{1}$$

where h is the height of the sample after movement of the indenter, and h_0 is the original cake height. It was assumed that there is no lateral spreading of the cake as it is contained in the vial. h_0 was measured by lowering the indenter into an empty vial and determining the height at which the indenter touched the vial base; h_1. Afterward the indenter was lowered into a vial containing a sample. The height at which the indenter makes contact with the cake is noted as h_2. The original height of cake h_0 can be obtained from the difference between h_2 and h_1. The global compressive strain ε is limited to the range between 0 and 1. The compressive indentation stress, σ_i, was calculated using:

$$\sigma_i = \frac{F}{A_0} \tag{2}$$

where F is the measured force, and A_0 is the contact surface area in m^2 of the flat faced indenter. As there is a variation in the force data obtained due to cracking/fracturing of the brittle cakes as the indenter pushes through the cake, the maximum force data points were taken from each experimental set and used in the maximum stress-strain curves.

Young's modulus, E, can be determined from indentation compression data using the previously established formula from Sneddon [70]:

$$E = \frac{\mu}{2(1 + \nu)} \tag{3}$$

where μ is the rigidity modulus ($\mu = F(1 - \nu)/4rh$), r is the cylindrical indenter radius, h is the displacement, F is the force applied, and ν is the Poisson's ratio from:

$$F = \frac{4\mu rh}{1 - \nu} = 4\left[\frac{E}{2(1 + \nu)}\right]\frac{rh}{(1 - \nu)} \tag{4}$$

The indenter used is a flat faced cylindrical probe with 5 mm radius (Fig. 3). It is assumed that the Poisson's ratio for all freeze-dried, brittle, cellular cakes of sucrose, trehalose, and mannitol used in this study is 0.2. The Young's modulus for freeze-dried foams,

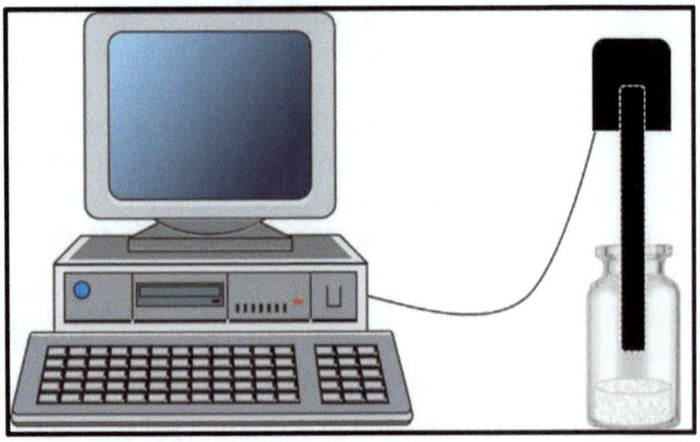

Fig. 3 Schematic of mechanical indentation instrument (not to scale)

E_f, (where the subscript denotes that the material is a foam) can be calculated using

$$E_{\mathrm{f}} = F\frac{1 - v^2}{h2r} \tag{5}$$

3 Mechanical Performance and Structure of Freeze-Dried Cakes

3.1 Compressive Indentation Stress-Strain Behavior of Excipient Cakes

Figure 4 shows sets of mean stress-strain curves for freeze-dried mannitol, sucrose, and trehalose for $n = 3$ [53]. Mannitol cakes were observed to exhibit the lowest crushing stress of 11 kPa, while both sucrose and trehalose exhibited much higher crushing strengths of 25 kPa and 31 kPa respectively. The apparent Young's modulus values were also significantly different between mannitol, sucrose, and trehalose, measuring 25 kPa, 150 kPa, and 210 kPa, respectively.

In order to compare the two best stabilizers, solutions of sucrose and trehalose at a range of concentrations between 1 and 40% w/v were studied and the mechanical behavior of the freeze-dried cakes measured. They have previously been reported in the concentrations of 1.0%, 2.5%, 5.0%, 20.0%, 30.0%, and 40.0% w/v for sucrose [54] and trehalose [7].

3.2 SEM Images of Excipient Freeze-Dried Cakes

SEM images were obtained for samples of mannitol, sucrose and trehalose freeze-dried from 5% w/w solutions [53].

The images displayed in Fig. 5 show typical honey-comb-shaped cells of different sizes. The SEM images confirmed the approximate same sizes of the cells for all three excipients: 120 μm × 60 μm × 60 μm. Changes in the excipient did not significantly impact the cell size or the cell wall thickness, for the

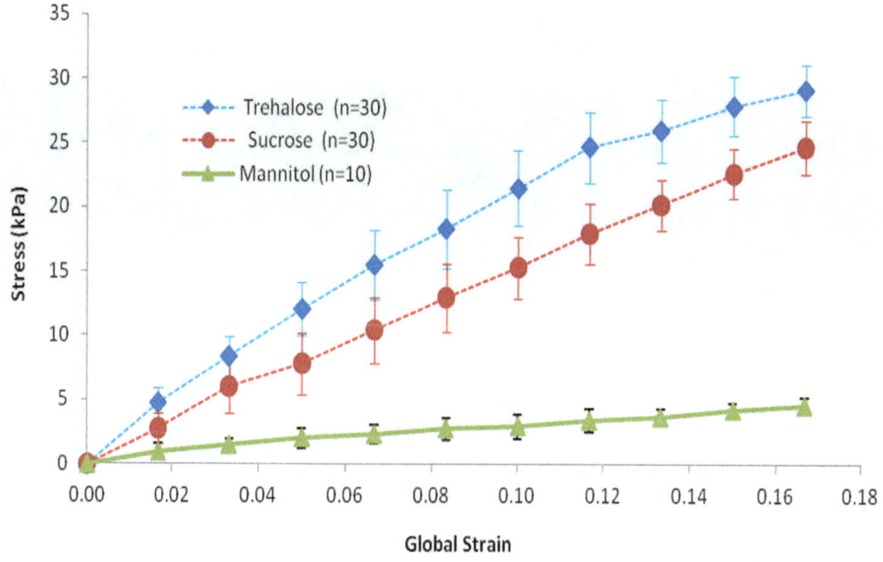

Fig. 4 Mean maximum stress-strain curves for 5% w/v freeze-dried mannitol, sucrose and trehalose cakes. The formulations had been frozen at −50 °C

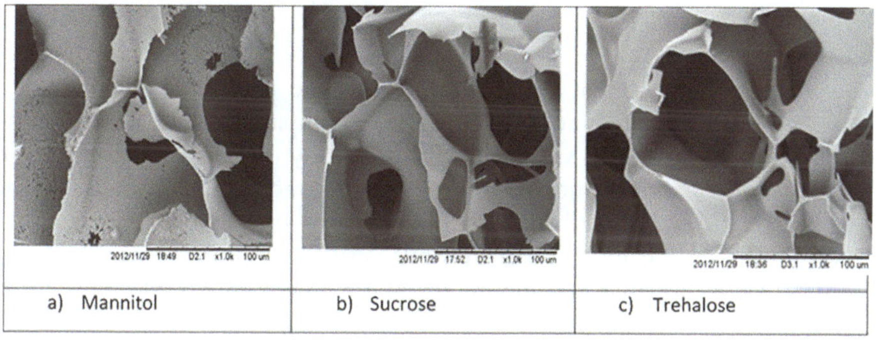

Fig. 5 SEM images of 5% w/v concentrations of freeze-dried mannitol, sucrose and trehalose

same concentration and same processing conditions. As the excipient choice does not play an important part of determining the pore shape and structure, the mechanical performance of the cake will mainly be primarily determined by the intrinsic mechanical properties of the pure excipient material [53].

The structure of the freeze dried cakes of sucrose and trehalose resembles a cork-like, cellular structure with the size of the cellular dimensions varying with the different concentrations (Fig. 6). The structures become more "closed" and continuous as the concentration is increased until the open cells become fully independent closed celled structures. Both sucrose and trehalose exhibit a similar structural arrangement for 20% and 40% w/w but where it can be

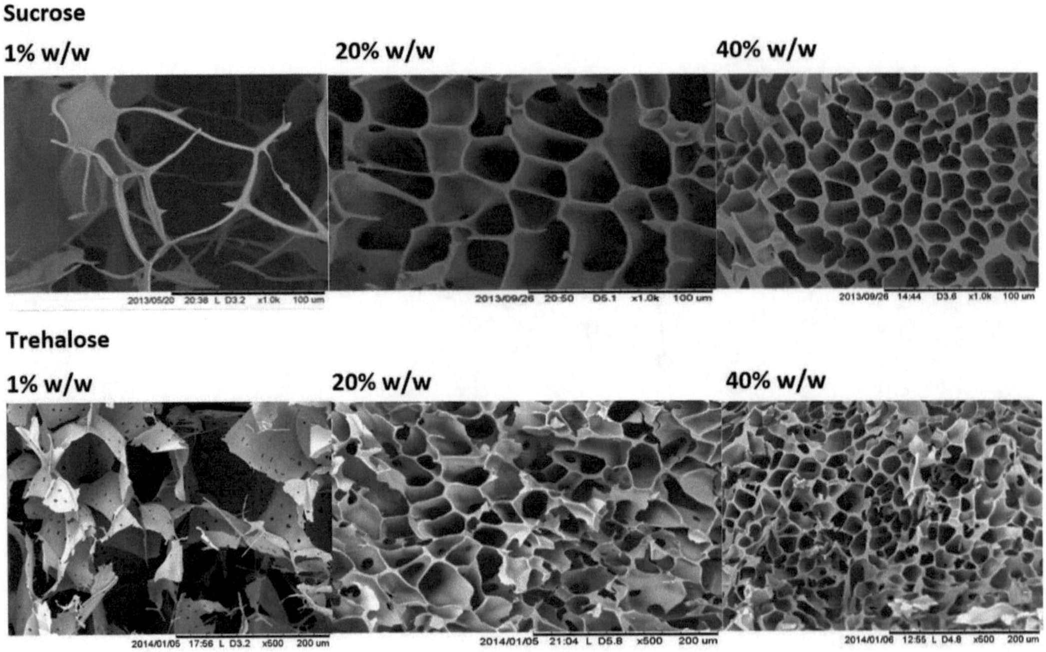

Fig. 6 SEM images of freeze-dried sucrose and trehalose from solutions with concentrations 1%, 20% and 40% w/w

seen that the cell walls and the individual cells appear slightly thicker and larger in sucrose compared to trehalose. Cakes formed from 1% sucrose exhibit a slightly more open-cell structure that is interconnected by mostly struts and a few thin walls. Trehalose has considerably thinner walls than sucrose and the cake has already started to form thin but very fragile-looking irregular walls. The relative densities reported for 1% w/w are 0.008 for sucrose, 0.005 for trehalose, and for 40% w/v 0.302 for sucrose and 0.187 for trehalose.

The reason why trehalose form cells already at a lower concentration than sucrose could be because trehalose is known to decrease the surface tension of water by a larger degree than sucrose [71]. This will allow trehalose to interact with water in a different way than sucrose does, particularly during ice formation, and possibly explains the differences seen in the structures where the edges become rounder as density increases [7].

The behavior of sucrose and trehalose with higher concentrations has been reported for other freeze-dried products too, e.g., graphene [72] and collagen-glycosaminoglycan [73]. These materials both displayed higher densities and more complete and continuous wall structures at higher freeze-dried concentrations. Previous reported freeze-dried products have shown for both chitosan-gelatin [74] and collagen-glycosaminoglycan [73] that when the density increased the pore sizes decreased.

3.3 Mechanical Properties and Cake Density

Relating the relative density to direct mechanical properties such as Young's modulus and maximum stress at failure, it is possible to derive explicit property correlations:

$$\frac{E_{\rm f}}{E_{\rm s}} = C\left(\frac{\rho_{\rm f}}{\rho_{\rm s}}\right)^n \tag{6}$$

where E_f is the Young's modulus for the freeze-dried cake, E_s is the Young's modulus of the pure non-porous solid used for the cakes and $\frac{\rho_f}{\rho_s}$ is the relative density. C and n are constants that depend on the morphology and microstructure of the cellular network and the material being tested, where n can be found in the range of $1 < n < 4$ [59, 75].

Figure 7 shows for the relative Young's modulus as a function of relative density for sucrose and trehalose. It can be seen that there is a linear increase of the relative Young's modulus with an increasing relative density. The line of best fit of the experimental data shows an excellent R^2 value using $n = 1$. This means that the structures of the cells mainly stress stretch when exposed to load and any bending of the struts or walls inside the cake has a negligible contribution to compressive loading [7, 59]. The k value for sucrose (k_s) for the line of best fit is 0.0034 ± 0.0001 and the k value for trehalose (k_T) is 0.0107 ± 0.0003. Comparing these two materials, trehalose has a steeper slope than sucrose, meaning it has a significantly higher Young's modulus even at lower relative densities. Based on the k value for the two equations it can be seen that E_f/E_s is three times as high for trehalose for the same ρ_f/ρ_s. A freeze-dried trehalose cake with the same relative density can therefore withstand approximately three times higher mechanical stresses.

It was also investigated how the freeze-dried cakes with different densities responded to stress, where the maximum compressive load bearing ability before fracturing was recorded. The maximum stress at failure can directly correlate to density by

$$\sigma_{\max} = k\left(\frac{\rho_{\rm f}}{\rho_{\rm s}}\right)^b \tag{7}$$

where σ_{max} is the maximum stress at failure in kPa while k and b are materials constants.

Figure 8a and b show the maximum failure stresses of sucrose and trehalose as a function of relative densities. At a trehalose concentration of 20% w/w or higher, relative density of 0.093, the maximum stress was outside the load cell range. As can be seen by the equations predicted from the best fit, the k_s is 3800 ± 220 and the k_T is 7700 ± 220, while the b values are 1.48 and 1.46 respectively. This means that the increase in the maximum stress at failure for trehalose is increasing approximately twice as fast with increasing relative density. The power index of

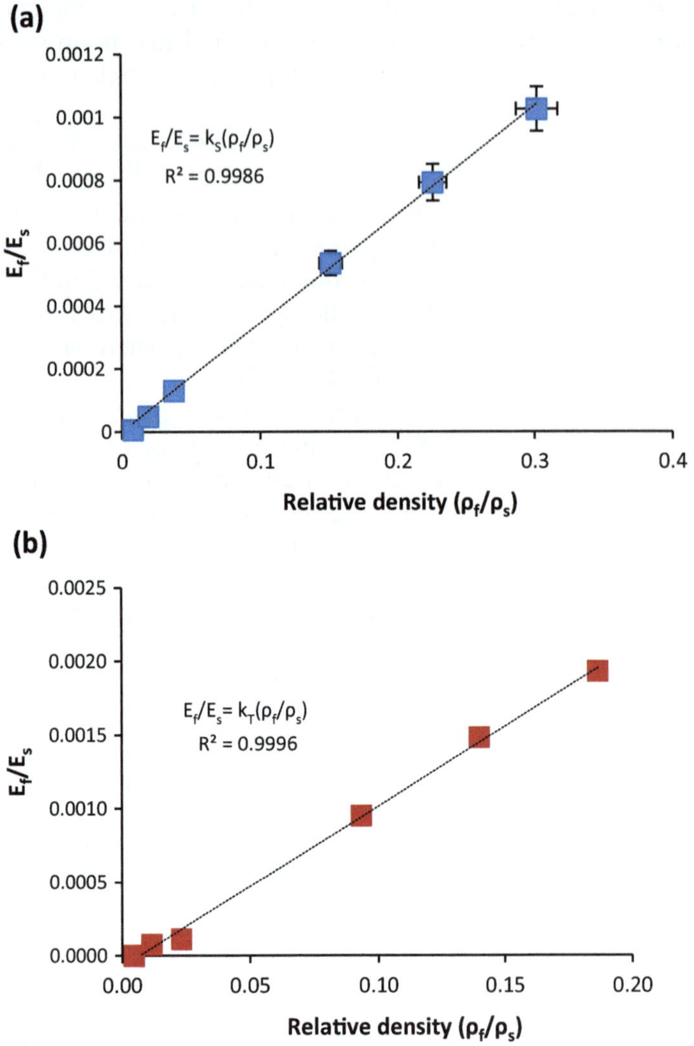

Fig. 7 Relative Young's modulus and relative density of freeze-dried (**a**) sucrose and (**b**) trehalose

both materials is close to 1.4 which describes an open celled behavior according to Gibson and Ashby [59].

Figures 7 and 8 both confirm that trehalose exhibits superior mechanical properties than sucrose, giving higher values of Young's modulus and being able to withstand significantly more stress before fracturing.

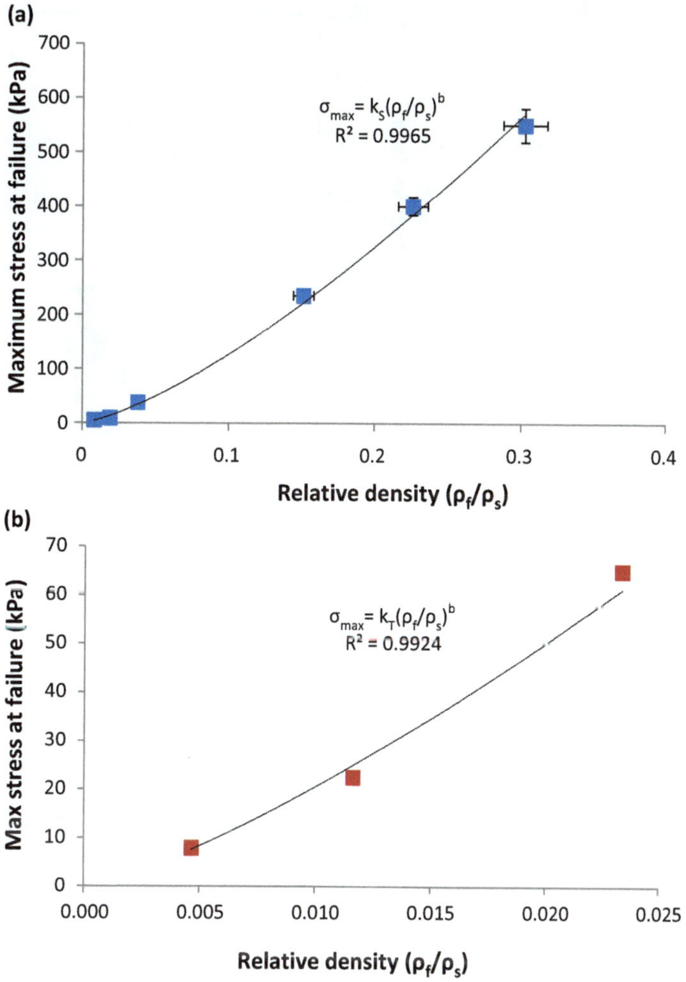

Fig. 8 Maximum stress at initial failure and relative density of freeze-dried (**a**) sucrose and (**b**) trehalose

3.4 Mechanical Properties for Freeze-Dried IgG

In Fig. 9 the mechanical compression data is shown for an IgG formulation at various concentrations stored at −20 °C and tested at 25 °C ($n = 3$). The y-axis represents the Young's modulus (kPa) and the x-axis represents the concentrations of IgG at 10, 50, 100, and 200 mg/mL. With increasing concentration an anticipated increase of Young's modulus and thus cake stiffness is observed. The highest concentration at 200 mg/mL has almost 16× greater Young's modulus than the lowest concentration at 10 mg/mL. Over time, aggregation, chemical degradation, and moisture ingress can all potentially affect the mechanical properties of the cake. However, the use of this compressive indentation technique could help to detect any minor changes in cake properties over time and in storage, which may in turn then be used to correlate to product stability.

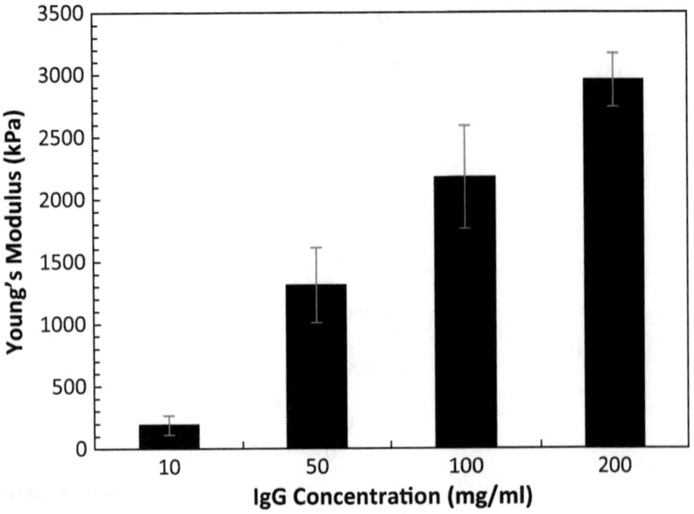

Fig. 9 Young's Modulus of freeze-dried IgG at various concentrations stored at −20 °C

3.5 Mechanical Properties of Freeze-Dried Cakes Exposed to Moisture

Most freeze-dried materials are highly hygroscopic. Over time they will exhibit moisture uptake in storage. Figure 10 shows the Young's modulus of IgG at 50 mg/mL at two different moisture contents. The same IgG formulation for the two freeze-drying cycles was used to obtain two different moisture contents (1 day cycle with short secondary drying step for high moisture and 2 day cycle with a longer secondary drying step for low moisture cakes). This figure shows that the cake with the lowest amount of moisture is stiffer and has a ~2 times greater Young's modulus than the higher moisture content sample. High moisture contents sees the cake beginning to exhibit a loss in mechanical properties. With increasing moisture content there will be a reduction of glass transition temperature (T_g) due to moisture-induced plasticization which explains the significant decrease in Young's modulus. Further decreases in Young's modulus will eventually herald cake collapse. Such behavior has recently been reported in detail by Duralliu et al. [43].

In Fig. 11a, b, Young's modulus is plotted against three concentrations (5%, 10%, and 20% w/w) for two common industrial excipients, sucrose and trehalose. The freeze-dried vials were opened and exposed to a room atmosphere of 25 °C and 40%RH at three time-points. At time $t = 0$ the samples were tested immediately after opening, taking not more than 15 s to complete the experiment. Open vials were then left to stand and the time was followed with a stopwatch, with measurements then being made after an additional 1 and 60 min. Both trehalose and sucrose at 5% and 10% w/w showed no significant differences in Young's

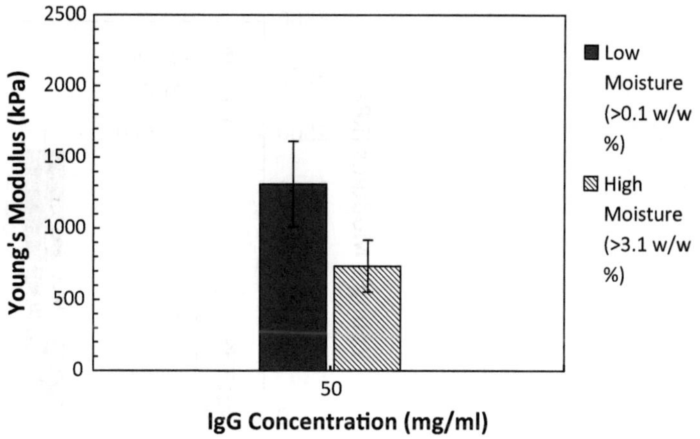

Fig. 10 Young's Modulus of freeze-dried IgG 5% w/v with high and low moisture contents

modulus after a 1 min exposure. However at 20% w/w concentrations there is a significant drop in Young's modulus for both excipients, which indicates that the higher concentration cakes are more susceptible to moisture uptake and hence loss in mechanical properties over shorter times. After 60 min both sucrose (5%, 10%, and 20% w/w) and trehalose (5% w/w) samples exhibit significantly large decreases in Young's modulus. However, trehalose at 10% and 20% w/w exhibited no significant change from any of the times exposed. This may indicate trehalose's greater resistance to moisture uptake over such times over sucrose at those concentrations. The large error bars for all experiments indicate that not all the cakes might be completely homogenous even though they come from the same batch. This mechanical characterization technique clearly demonstrates the ability to differentiate between very high and low moisture containing cakes whether the moisture arrives during the process or after manufacture.

4 Conclusion

This Chapter has reviewed a relatively new topic in lyophilization—the mechanical properties of freeze-dried cakes. An experimental technique for the compressive mechanical indentation of a cake while still in the vial has been shown to be a fast and reliable method for characterizing freeze-dried cakes. It is sensitive to excipient type and excipient concentration, consistent with the SEM observed cake structures, as well as being sensitive to moisture content in the cake. Both experimentally measured Young's modulus and yield stress data scale well with reduced cake density, in line with theoretical predictions from classical cellular solids theory. It is feasible that these mechanical properties could be used in the industry to determine material property-based freeze cake attributes which in turn could be

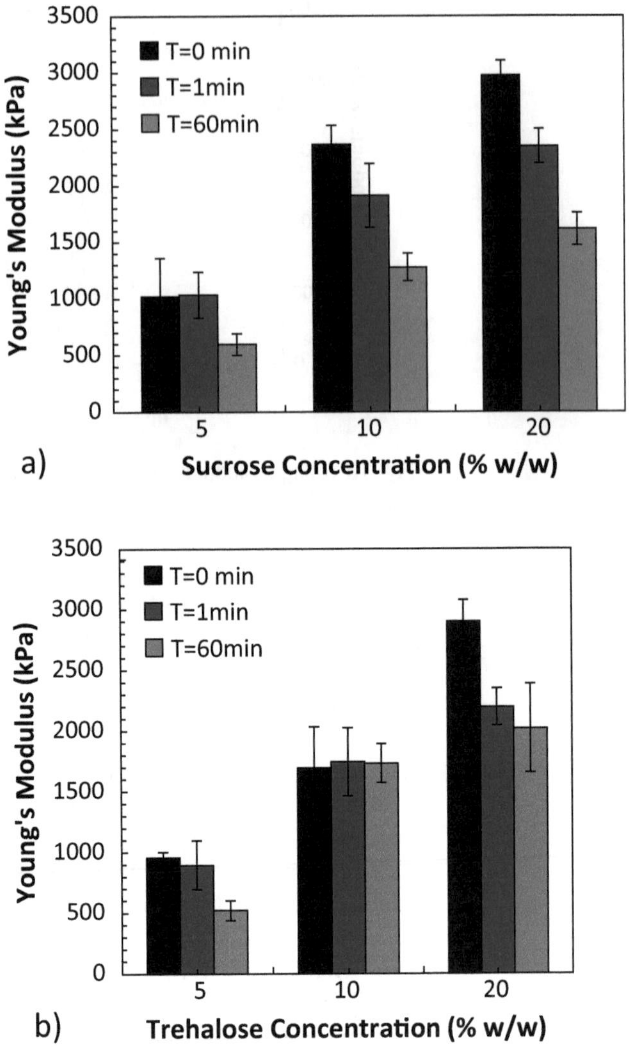

Fig. 11 The effect of vial opening with exposure to moist atmospheric air over time on the Young's Modulus for freeze-dried (**a**) sucrose and (**b**) trehalose

used as a quality metric for a freeze-dried batch control. Mechanical properties offer excellent scope as a future CQA for measuring the stiffness and strength of any freeze-dried product.

Acknowledgments

A.D. acknowledges the support of the EPSRC Centre for Doctoral Training in Emergent Macromolecular Therapies (CDT) at University College London in collaboration with National Institute for Biological Standards and Control (NIBSC, UK). S.H.M.H. acknowledges the financial support of the EPSRC Impact Acceleration Account at Imperial College.

References

1. Arakawa T, Prestrelski SJ, Kenney WC, Carpenter JF (2001) Factors affecting short-term and long-term stabilities of proteins. Adv Drug Deliv Rev 46:307–326
2. Carpenter JF, Pikal MJ, Chang BS, Randolph TW (1997) Rational design of stable lyophilized protein formulations: some practical advice. Pharm Res 14:969–975
3. Pikal MJ (1994) Freeze-drying of proteins: process, formulation, and stability. ACS Publications, Washington, DC
4. Costantino HR (2004) Excipients for use in lyophilized pharmaceutical peptide, protein and other bioproducts. In: Constantino HR, Pikal MJ (eds) Lyophilization of biopharmaceuticals. AAPS Press, Arlington, VA
5. Telikepalli S, Kumru OS, Kim JH, Joshi SB, O'Berry KB, Blake-Haskins AW, Perkins MD, Middaugh CR, Volkin DB (2015) Characterization of the physical stability of a lyophilized IgG1 mAb after accelerated shipping-like stress. J Pharm Sci 104:495–507
6. Patel SM, Nail SL, Pikal MJ, Geidobler R, Winter G, Hawe A, Davagnino J, Rambhatla Gupta S (2017) Lyophilized drug product cake appearance: what is acceptable? J Pharm Sci 106:1706–1721
7. Devi S (2014) Mechanical characterisation of freeze-dried biopharmaceuticals. Ph.D. Thesis, Imperial College London
8. Suzuki Y, Takeda T, Inazu K, Sakamoto T (1990) Influences of physical stress given to supersaturated cephalothin sodium solution upon the freeze-dried product quality, 1. Yakugaku Zasshi 110:849–857
9. DeLuca P (1976) Research and development of phamaceutical dosage forms. Dev Biol Stand 36:41–50
10. Di Tommaso C, Como C, Gurny R, Möller M (2010) Investigations on the lyophilisation of MPEG–hexPLA micelle based pharmaceutical formulations. Eur J Pharm Sci 40:38–47
11. Schersch K, Betz O, Garidel P, Muehlau S, Bassarab S, Winter G (2012) Systematic investigation of the effect of lyophilizate collapse on pharmaceutically relevant proteins, Part 2: Stability during storage at elevated temperatures. J Pharm Sci 101:2288–2306
12. Wekx J, De Kleijn J (1990) The determination of water in freeze dried pharmaceutical products by performing the Karl Fischer titration in the glass container itself. Drug Dev Ind Pharm 16:1465–1472
13. Parker A, Rigby-Singleton S, Perkins M, Bates D, Le Roux D, Roberts CJ, Madden-Smith C, Lewis L, Teagarden DL, Johnson RE (2010) Determination of the influence of primary drying rates on the microscale structural attributes and physicochemical properties of protein containing lyophilized products. J Pharm Sci 99:4616–4629
14. May JC, Wheeler RM, Etz N, Del Grosso A (1992) Measurement of final container residual moisture in freeze-dried biological products. Dev Biol Stand 74:153–164
15. Duncan DI, Veale JR, Cook I, Ward K (2010) Using laser-based headspace moisture analysis for rapid nondestructive moisture determination of sterile freeze-dried product. Lighthouse Instruments White Paper, 1–10
16. Schneid SC, Stärtzel PM, Lettner P, Gieseler H (2011) Robustness testing in pharmaceutical freeze-drying: inter-relation of process conditions and product quality attributes studied for a vaccine formulation. Pharm Dev Technol 16:583–590
17. Jovanović N, Bouchard A, Hofland GW, Witkamp G-J, Crommelin DJ, Jiskoot W (2006) Distinct effects of sucrose and trehalose on protein stability during supercritical fluid drying and freeze-drying. Eur J Pharm Sci 27:336–345
18. FDA (2009) Inspection guide lyophilization of parenterals 7/93. US FDA
19. Hatley R, Franks F (1991) Applications of DSC in the development of improved freeze-drying processes for labile biologicals. J Therm Anal Calorim 37:1905–1914
20. Pikal M (1995) Modulated DSC studies on proteins in the solid state: relaxation enthalpy, glass transitions and denaturation. Pharm Res 135:13–29
21. Chang BS, Randall CS (1992) Use of subambient thermal analysis to optimize protein lyophilization. Cryobiology 29:632–656
22. Overcashier DE, Patapoff TW, Hsu CC (1999) Lyophilization of protein formulations in vials: investigation of the relationship between resistance to vapor flow during primary drying and small-scale product collapse. J Pharm Sci 88:688–695
23. Shamblin SL, Tang X, Chang L, Hancock BC, Pikal MJ (1999) Characterization of the time scales of molecular motion in pharmaceutically important glasses. J Phys Chem B 103:4113–4121
24. Chongprasert S, Knopp SA, Nail SL (2001) Characterization of frozen solutions of glycine. J Pharm Sci 90:1720–1728

25. Ma X, Wang D, Bouffard R, MacKenzie A (2001) Characterization of murine monoclonal antibody to tumor necrosis factor (TNF-MAb) formulation for freeze-drying cycle development. Pharm Res 18:196–202
26. Pikal M, Shah S, Senior D, Lang J (1983) Physical chemistry of freeze-drying: measurement of sublimation rates for frozen aqueous solutions by a microbalance technique. J Pharm Sci 72:635–650
27. Nail SL, Her L-M, Proffitt CP, Nail LL (1994) An improved microscope stage for direct observation of freezing and freeze drying. Pharm Res 11:1098–1100
28. Cavatur RK, Suryanarayanan R (1998) Characterization of frozen aqueous solutions by low temperature X-ray powder diffractometry. Pharm Res 15:194–199
29. Chatterjee K, Shalaev EY, Suryanarayanan R (2005) Raffinose crystallization during freeze-drying and its impact on recovery of protein activity. Pharm Res 22:303–309
30. Meredith P, Donald AM, Payne RS (1996) Freeze-drying: in situ observations using cryoenvironmental scanning electron microscopy and differential scanning calorimetry. J Pharm Sci 85:631–637
31. Her L-M, Jefferis RP, Gatlin LA, Braxton B, Nail SL (1994) Measurement of glass transition temperatures in freeze concentrated solutions of non-electrolytes by electrical thermal analysis. Pharm Res 11:1023–1029
32. Le Meste M, Huang V (1992) Thermomechanical properties of frozen sucrose solutions. J Food Sci 57:1230–1233
33. Kararli TT, Hurlbut JB, Needham TE (1990) Glass–rubber transitions of cellulosic polymers by dynamic mechanical analysis. J Pharm Sci 79:845–848
34. Blond G (1994) Mechanical properties of frozen model solutions. In: Fito P, Mulet A, Mckenna B (eds) Water in foods. Pergamon, Amsterdam
35. Morris KR, Evans SA, Mackenzie AP, Scheule D, Lordi NG (1994) Prediction of lyophile collapse temperature by dielectric analysis. PDA J Pharm Sci Technol 48:318–329
36. Marques JM, Loch C, Wolff E, Rutledge D (1991) Monitoring freeze-drying by low resolution pulse NMR: determination of sublimation endpoint. J Food Sci 56:1707–1710
37. Izutsu K, Yoshioka S, Kojima S (1995) Effect of cryoprotectants on the eutectic crystallization of NaCl in frozen solutions studied by differential scanning calorimetry (DSC) and broad-line pulsed NMR. Chem Pharm Bull 43:1804–1806
38. Lin TP, Hsu CC (2002) Determination of residual moisture in lyophilized protein pharmaceuticals using a rapid and non-invasive method: near infrared spectroscopy. PDA J Pharm Sci Technol 56:196–205
39. Kamat MS, Lodder RA, DeLuca PP (1989) Near-infrared spectroscopic determination of residual moisture in lyophilized sucrose through intact glass vials. Pharm Res 6:961–965
40. Brülls M, Folestad S, Sparén A, Rasmuson A (2003) In-situ near-infrared spectroscopy monitoring of the lyophilization process. Pharm Res 20:494–499
41. Chan H-K, Au-Yeung K-L, Gonda I (1999) Development of a mathematical model for the water distribution in freeze-dried solids. Pharm Res 16:660–665
42. Costantino HR, Curley JG, Wu S, Hsu CC (1998) Water sorption behavior of lyophilized protein–sugar systems and implications for solid-state interactions. Int J Pharm 166:211–221
43. Duralliu A, Matejtschuk P, Williams DR (2018) Humidity induced collapse in freeze dried cakes: a direct visualization study using DVS. Eur J Pharm Biopharm 127:29–36
44. Suryanarayanan R, Rastogi S (1995) X-ray powder diffractometry. In: Brittain HG, Bogdanowich SJ, Bugay DE, DeVincentis J, Lewen G, Newman AW (eds) Physical characterization of pharmaceutical solids, Drugs and the pharmaceutical sciences. Marcel Dekker, Inc., New York
45. Guo Y, Byrn SR, Zografi G (2000) Effects of lyophilization on the physical characteristics and chemical stability of amorphous quinapril hydrochloride. Pharm Res 17:930–936
46. Overcashier DE (2004) Microscopy of lyophilized proteins. In: Costantino HR, Pikal MJ (eds) Lyophilization of biopharmaceuticals. AAPS press, Arlington, VA
47. Mosharraf M (2004) Assessment of degree of disorder (Amorphicity) of lyophilized formulations of growth hormone using isothermal microcalorimetry. Drug Dev Ind Pharm 30:461–472
48. Reddy R, Chang LL, Luthra S, Collins G, Lopez C, Shamblin SL, Pikal MJ, Gatlin LA, Shalaev EY (2009) The glass transition and sub-Tg-relaxation in pharmaceutical powders and dried proteins by thermally stimulated current. J Pharm Sci 98:81–93
49. Pikal MJ, Shah S (1990) The collapse temperature in freeze drying: dependence on measurement methodology and rate of water removal from the glassy phase. Int J Pharm 62:165–186

50. Konstantinidis AK, Kuu W, Otten L, Nail SL, Sever RR (2011) Controlled nucleation in freeze-drying: effects on pore size in the dried product layer, mass transfer resistance, and primary drying rate. J Pharm Sci 100:3453–3470
51. Harnkarnsujarit N, Charoenrein S, Roos YH (2012) Microstructure formation of maltodextrin and sugar matrices in freeze-dried systems. Carbohydr Polym 88:734–742
52. Bashir JA, Avis K (1973) Evaluation of excipients in freeze-dried products for injection. Bull Parenter Drug Assoc 27:68–83
53. Devi S, Williams D (2013) Morphological and compressional mechanical properties of freeze-dried mannitol, sucrose, and trehalose cakes. J Pharm Sci 102:4246–4255
54. Devi S, Williams DR (2014) Density dependent mechanical properties and structures of a freeze dried biopharmaceutical excipient–Sucrose. Eur J Pharm Biopharm 88:492–501
55. Bedu-Addo FK (2004) Understanding lyophilization formulation development. Pharm Technol 20:10–19
56. Pikal-Cleland KA, Rodríguez-Hornedo N, Amidon GL, Carpenter JF (2000) Protein denaturation during freezing and thawing in phosphate buffer systems: monomeric and tetrameric β-galactosidase. Arch Biochem Biophys 384:398–406
57. Williams RO, Watts AB, Miller DA (2016) Formulating poorly water soluble drugs. Springer International Publishing, New York
58. Kang J, Lin X, Penera J (2016) Rapid formulation development for monoclonal antibodies BioProcess Int 14(4):40
59. Gibson LJ, Ashby MF (1999) Cellular solids: structure and properties. Cambridge University Press, Cambridge
60. Deville S, Saiz E, Nalla RK, Tomsia AP (2006) Freezing as a path to build complex composites. Science 311:515–518
61. Ashby MF, Medalist RM (1983) The mechanical properties of cellular solids. Metall Trans A 14:1755–1769
62. Gibson LJ, Ashby MF (1982) The mechanics of three-dimensional cellular materials. Proc R Soc Lond A 382:43–59
63. De Beer T, Wiggenhorn M, Hawe A, Kasper J, Almeida A, Quinten T, Friess W, Winter G, Vervaet C, Remon JP (2011) Optimization of a pharmaceutical freeze-dried product and its process using an experimental design approach and innovative process analyzers. Talanta 83:1623–1633
64. Koganti VR, Shalaev EY, Berry MR, Osterberg T, Youssef M, Hiebert DN, Kanka FA, Nolan M, Barrett R, Scalzo G (2011) Investigation of design space for freeze-drying: use of modeling for primary drying segment of a freeze-drying cycle. AAPS PharmSciTech 12:854–861
65. Mockus L, LeBlond D, Basu PK, Shah RB, Khan MA (2011) A QbD case study: Bayesian prediction of lyophilization cycle parameters. AAPS PharmSciTech 12:442–448
66. Kremer D, Pikal M, Petre W, Shalaev E, Gatlin L, Kramer T (2009) A procedure to optimize scale-up for the primary drying phase of lyophilization. J Pharm Sci 98:307–318
67. Cannon A, Shemeley K (2004) Statistical evaluation of vial design features that influence sublimation rates during primary drying. Pharm Res 21:536–542
68. Grant Y, Matejtschuk P, Dalby PA (2009) Rapid optimization of protein freeze-drying formulations using ultra scale-down and factorial design of experiment in microplates. Biotechnol Bioeng 104:957–964
69. Sunderland W (2012) 5th International conference on lyophilisation and freeze drying, Bologna, Italy
70. Sneddon IN (1965) The relation between load and penetration in the axisymmetric boussinesq problem for a punch of arbitrary profile. Int J Eng Sci 3:47–57
71. Chen J, Kimura Y, Adachi S (2007) Surface activities of monoacyl trehaloses in aqueous solution. LWT Food Sci Technol 40:412–417
72. Qiu L, Liu JZ, Chang SL, Wu Y, Li D (2012) Biomimetic superelastic graphene-based cellular monoliths. Nat Commun 3:1241
73. Kanungo BP, Gibson LJ (2010) Density–property relationships in collagen–glycosaminoglycan scaffolds. Acta Biomater 6:344–353
74. Mao JS, Zhao LG, Yin YJ, De Yao K (2003) Structure and properties of bilayer chitosan--gelatin scaffolds. Biomaterials 24:1067–1074
75. Roberts AP, Garboczi EJ (2001) Elastic moduli of model random three-dimensional closed-cell cellular solids. Acta Mater 49:189–197

Chapter 14

High-Resolution Mass Spectrometric Methods for Proteins in Lyophilized Solids

Karthik Balakrishna Chandrababu, Rajashekar Kammari, Yuan Chen, and Elizabeth M. Topp

Abstract

Lyophilization (freeze-drying) is used to produce amorphous solid powders of protein drugs. Though lyophilization is usually used in an attempt to stabilize the protein, degradation processes can still occur in the solid state, and are often poorly correlated with measurable properties of the protein and the powder. This chapter describes two novel, high-resolution mass-spectrometry-based methods for assessing protein structure and interactions in solid powders: solid-state hydrogen-deuterium exchange (ssHDX) and solid-state photolytic labeling (ssPLL) with mass spectrometric analysis (ssHDX-MS, ssPLL-MS). ssHDX-MS measures the rate of deuterium incorporation in the protein on exposure of the solid powder to D_2O vapor. ssHDX-MS is thought to provide information regarding the network of inter- and intramolecular hydrogen bonds experienced by the protein in the solid state, and recent studies have shown that ssHDX metrics are highly correlated with stability on storage. ssPLL-MS provides complementary information on the protein's side chain environment. The chapter summarizes the methods and recent results both ssHDX-MS and ssPLL-MS, and suggests directions for future research.

Key words Mass spectrometry, Hydrogen-deuterium exchange (HDX), Solid-state HDX, Photolytic labeling, Peptides, Proteins

1 Introduction

Lyophilization (freeze-drying) is a manufacturing process used to produce solid powders of therapeutic protein drugs [1]. These powders may be used as the final drug product, or to store the protein between manufacturing steps, and must be reconstituted prior to subsequent manufacturing or administration to a patient. Despite the added cost of producing a dried powder and the inconvenience of reconstitution, the lyophilized form is often chosen to preserve chemical composition, native structure, and activity during shelf storage when solution forms are not sufficiently stable [2, 3]. The selection of appropriate excipients and the design of suitable drying cycles are critical to achieving this goal [4]. Due to

Kevin R. Ward and Paul Matejtschuk (eds.), *Lyophilization of Pharmaceuticals and Biologicals: New Technologies and Approaches*, Methods in Pharmacology and Toxicology, https://doi.org/10.1007/978-1-4939-8928-7_14,

the nature of the lyophilization process and the properties of the proteins themselves, lyophilized protein formulations are generally amorphous rather than crystalline, and interactions with excipients are thought to stabilize and protect proteins in the solid state [5, 6].

In lyophilized solids, protein stability on storage is evaluated by measuring the concentration of protein that retains its native physical structure, chemical structure, and activity over a period of months to years [2]. Stability studies are used not only to ensure the quality of the finished product, but also to optimize the lyophilization cycle and the composition of the formulation. This reliance on stability studies slows the development of formulation and process. Analytical techniques such as solid-state nuclear magnetic resonance spectroscopy (ssNMR), Fourier transform infrared spectroscopy (FTIR), near infrared spectroscopy (NIR), and Raman spectroscopy have long been used to characterize lyophilized protein formulations and to probe protein structure in the solid state. Though useful for characterization, these measurements are often poorly correlated with stability on storage and provide only low resolution information on protein structure in the solid matrix. Currently, no analytical method or combination of methods can be used as a reliable surrogate for time-consuming stability studies in formulation and process development.

Hydrogen deuterium exchange coupled with mass spectrometry (HDX-MS) has been used to analyze protein conformation and dynamics in solution for many years [7] and has been adapted by our group to study proteins in the solid state. Solid-state hydrogen deuterium exchange coupled with mass spectrometry (ssHDX-MS) (Fig. 1) provides information on protein structure and matrix interactions in amorphous solid powders, and has been shown to be highly correlated with protein aggregation and chemical degradation on storage [8, 9]. More recently, we have also developed solid-state photolytic labeling with mass spectrometric analysis (ssPLL-MS) (Fig. 2) to probe protein-protein, protein-water, and protein excipient interactions in lyophilized powders [10–12]. This chapter describes the two methods, summarizes our findings to date, and suggests directions for additional research.

2 Solid-State Hydrogen Deuterium Exchange with Mass Spectrometric Analysis (ssHDX-MS)

Labile amide hydrogen atoms in a protein undergo exchange with deuterium in the presence of a deuterium donor (e.g., D_2O). Analytical methods that can distinguish deuterium from hydrogen can be used to measure the rate and extent of the exchange reaction. In particular, mass spectrometry can be used to measure the mass increase in deuterated proteins relative to the native

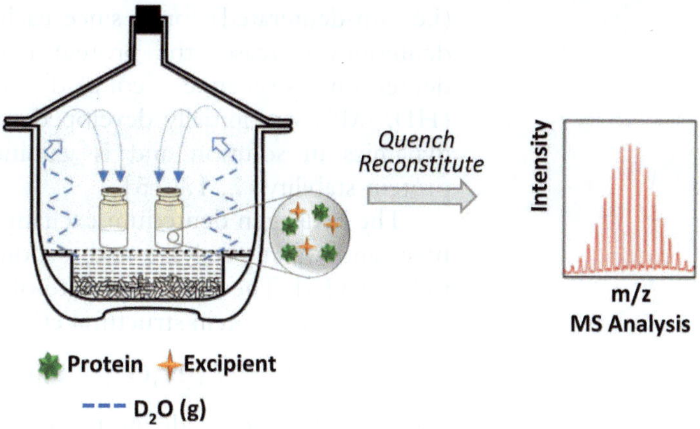

Fig. 1 Methods for solid-state hydrogen deuterium exchange with mass spectrometric analysis (ssHDX-MS). Uncapped vials containing a lyophilized protein are placed in a sealed desiccator at constant temperature. The desiccator contains a saturated salt solution of D_2O, which maintains constant D_2O vapor phase activity. Samples are removed at various times, stored at −80 °C until analysis, reconstituted under quench conditions, and analyzed by tandem liquid chromatography mass spectrometry (LC/MS) to determine deuterium incorporation. Proteolytic digestion using pepsin (in-line or off-line; not shown) allows deuterium incorporation to be measured for both the intact protein and its proteolytic fragments, so that sites of deuteration can be identified and mapped

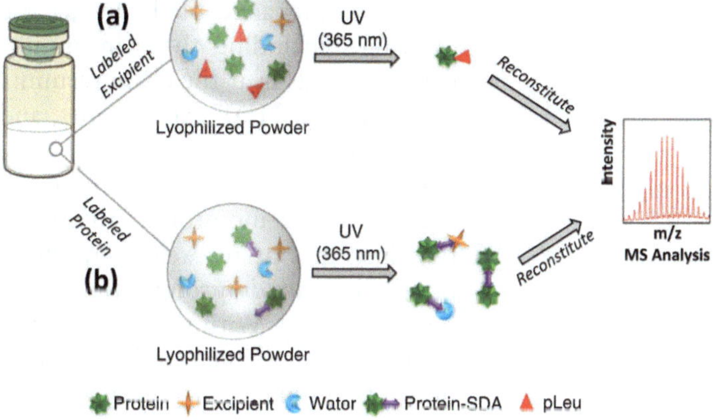

Fig. 2 Methods for solid-state photolytic labeling with mass spectrometric analysis (ssPLL-MS). Vials containing a lyophilized protein formulation with photolytically labeled excipient (**a**) and/or photolytically labeled protein (**b**) are exposed to UV light, activating the label. Exposure to UV light at 365 nm (shown) activates diazirine groups. Reaction products include covalent protein-protein, protein-excipient and protein-water adducts (**a**, **b**), as well as "dead-end" or intramolecular reactions (not shown). Samples are removed at various times, reconstituted, and analyzed by tandem liquid chromatography mass spectrometry (LC/MS) to determine the extent of labeling. Proteolytic digestion (in-line or off-line; not shown) allows sites of labeling to be identified and mapped

(i.e., un-deuterated) form, since each exchange of hydrogen for deuterium increases the protein mass by +1 amu. Hydrogen deuterium exchange coupled with mass spectrometry (HDX-MS) was initially developed to study protein folding and dynamics in solution and is gaining attention for studies of protein stability [7, 13–15].

The hydrogen deuterium exchange reaction is subject to acid, base, and water catalysis, and is dominated by base catalysis at pH > 3 [16]. The "intrinsic" rate of exchange (k_{int}), observed in the absence of protein structural effects, is given by:

$$k_{int} = k_A[H_3O^+] + k_B[OH^-] + k_w[H_2O]$$

where k_A, k_B, and k_w define the contributions of acid, base, and water catalysis, respectively [16]. The intrinsic rate of exchange is typically at a minimum near pH 2.7. In an HDX experiment, exchange is usually quenched using low pH and low temperature, with the goal of minimizing the loss of the deuterium label by the reverse reaction ("back exchange") during analysis. The back-exchange rate for backbone amide groups typically is several orders of magnitude slower than that of exchangeable side chain groups [7, 16].

The hydrogen atoms in a protein can be categorized into three groups with respect to their ability to undergo hydrogen-deuterium exchange: (1) un-exchangeable hydrogen atoms, such as those in methylene groups, for which the reaction does not occur, (2) exchangeable hydrogen atoms that undergo rapid back exchange, including those in amino acid side chains and in the peptide bonds near the chain termini, which thus cannot be monitored in most HDX experiments, and (3) exchangeable hydrogen atoms for which back exchange is slow enough, under quenched conditions of low pH and temperature, to allow the exchange reaction to be monitored. Interestingly, the hydrogen atoms in the third group are exclusively those associated with the peptide bonds (i.e., amide groups) that link amino acids to form the primary sequence. With the exception of the two N- and C-terminal peptide bonds (which undergo rapid back exchange) and peptide bonds to proline (which have no exchangeable hydrogen), it is the peptide bonds along the protein sequence that are monitored by hydrogen deuterium exchange.

In solution, HDX of peptide-bond hydrogen atoms depends not only on the intrinsic chemical rate of exchange, but also on solvent accessibility. Solvent accessibility, in turn, is influenced by protein dynamics; opening and closing events transiently increase and decrease the number of solvent accessible peptide bonds. Solvent accessible peptide bond hydrogen atoms typically exchange rapidly, while those that are shielded from the solvent and buried inside the core of a protein, or that participate in the intramolecular hydrogen bonds that contribute to protein structure, often exchange more slowly.

Using proteolytic digestion, deuterium incorporation can be monitored at the peptide level in an HDX experiment, as well as for the intact protein. Pepsin is typically used for proteolytic ("bottom up") digestion and analysis, since the enzyme is active at the low pH conditions used to minimize back exchange. MS-MS fragmentation ("top down") is not used for peptide level analysis in electrospray ionization mass spectrometry (ESI-MS) instruments because the site of deuterium labeling changes ("scrambles") during analysis. Because the masses and sequences of the peptides produced by pepsin digestion are usually unique, deuterium incorporation measured in the peptides can be mapped back onto the protein structure. In this way, the kinetics of exchange can be monitored with peptide level resolution.

2.1 Information Content of ssHDX-MS

Over the past decade, our group has developed ssHDX-MS as a novel analytical method for proteins in amorphous solids [8, 9, 12, 17–23]. We have demonstrated that the method is feasible for solid samples [17, 18, 24, 25] and have shown that the rate of exchange is much slower than the rate of water (or D_2O) vapor sorption, indicating that ssHDX is not simply a measure of mass transport processes [19, 20]. We have also shown that ssHDX is sensitive to changes in formulation [8, 9, 18, 24], moisture content [19, 20], and processing method [12, 23] that go undetected by conventional methods (e.g., FTIR, Raman). Using proteolytic digestion, we have shown that ssHDX provides information on the solid-state environment of the protein with peptide level resolution, resolution not achievable with conventional methods for assessing protein structure in the solid state [8, 19, 20, 26].

More recently, we have shown that ssHDX-MS metrics are highly correlated with storage stability [8, 9]. In a study of five different lyophilized myoglobin formulations, the extent of aggregation on storage for up to 1 year was correlated with ssHDX-MS kinetic parameters measured immediately after lyophilization, but showed poor correlation with ssFTIR α-helix band position or band intensity [9]. Similar studies have been conducted for lyophilized mAb formulations. In these studies, a leading biopharmaceutical company provided four different lyophilized mAb formulations, for which 2.5 years of storage stability data had already been acquired [8]. In a blinded study, ssHDX-MS correctly rank-ordered the stability of the four formulations in ~3 weeks. In subsequent un-blinded studies, aggregation and chemical degradation were strongly correlated with deuterium incorporation on ssHDX. In contrast, commonly-used physical and biophysical metrics (e.g., FTIR peak position, intensity, moisture content, glass transition temperature) were poorly correlated with aggregation, incorrectly predicted rank-order and often conflicted with one another [8].

Since the effect of the lyophilization process on the protein is also of interest [27–30], ssHDX studies have also been conducted on solid mAb formulations prepared by different processing methods. Solid powders containing a mAb with different excipients were prepared by: (1) spray drying, (2) lyophilization without controlled ice-nucleation, (3) lyophilization with controlled ice-nucleation, and (4) lyophilization with extended annealing during freezing [23]. ssHDX-MS detected changes in the protein structure and matrix interactions not observed using ssFTIR or solid-state fluorescence spectroscopies. In ssHDX-MS studies, the deconvoluted mass spectra for some spray dried samples showed greater peak broadening than samples prepared by other methods; bimodal peaks ("peak splitting") were also observed for some spray dried samples [23]. Peak broadening may reflect a wider distribution of protein conformations or solid environments, while peak splitting may reflect the existence of subpopulations of the protein in different conformations or environments.

These results strongly suggest that ssHDX-MS may be useful in formulation development, process scale-up and tech transfer for lyophilized protein drugs. The method accurately predicts relative stability in far less time than the storage stability studies in current use, and with far greater accuracy than conventional solids characterization methods. With appropriate additional validation, ssHDX-MS may ultimately become a surrogate for stability studies, greatly reducing the time needed for formulation and process development.

2.2 Experimental Methods for ssHDX-MS

A solution HDX-MS experiment involves exposing the protein to D_2O in solution, sampling and quenching the solution at various times, and analyzing the intact protein and its digests using mass spectrometry. The reader is referred to several excellent reviews that describe solution HDX-MS methods in greater detail [31–33]. Here, we focus on methods for ssHDX-MS studies and the analysis of the resulting data.

In an ssHDX-MS experiment, vials containing a lyophilized protein, in a formulation together with various excipients, are placed uncapped in a sealed desiccator and exposed to D_2O in the vapor phase (i.e., $D_2O_{(g)}$) (Fig. 1). The dessicator is maintained at constant temperature and $D_2O_{(g)}$ activity, i.e., constant relative humidity in D_2O rather than H_2O, which can be achieved using saturated solutions of various salts in D_2O. Vials are removed at time intervals ranging from a few hours to weeks, flash frozen in liquid nitrogen to slow the reaction and minimize back exchange, and stored at −80 °C prior to analysis. To determine the overall deuterium incorporation, the vials are reconstituted using ice-cold 0.1% formic acid solution with or without methanol and quickly injected into a tandem liquid chromatography/mass spectrometry system. Electrospray ionization mass spectrometry (ESI-MS) is well suited to ssHDX-MS studies due to its high mass range and mass accuracy, though other systems also offer advantages [31, 34]. To the extent possible, the time for re-constitution and injection is minimized and maintained constant, and manual handling errors are quantified by performing replicate analyses. Refrigeration (~2 °C) during desalting and LC separation also helps to minimize back exchange. Prior to injection, the sample is passed through a protein/peptide microtrap for desalting and to remove excipients before entering the mass spectrometer. In ESI-MS, the mass-to-charge ratio in the instrument is set according to the size of the protein. The number of deuterium atoms incorporated is calculated from the deconvoluted *m/z* spectra by subtracting the mass value at each time point from the native (non-deuterated) mass of the protein. As an example, our previous ssHDX-MS studies of myoglobin formulations (Fig. 3) illustrate that the rate and extent of deuterium incorporation are highly influenced by excipient type and the relative humidity of $D_2O_{(g)}$ to which the samples are exposed [20].

For peptide level quantification, sample handling is identical to that for the intact protein, except that the protein is digested prior to LC/MS analysis. For in-line digestion, an immobilized pepsin column is placed inside an oven that maintains a constant temperature of 23 °C, optimal for pepsin activity. The digested peptides are desalted using a peptide microtrap and then passed through a C18 reverse phase LC column to separate the peptides, using gradient elution with acetonitrile. The peptides are analyzed by mass spectrometry by setting a *m/z* window, typically 100–1700. This process is repeated thrice for each protein and only peptide fragments seen in all three runs are used in determining deuterium incorporation. The identity of the peptide fragments is confirmed by MS/MS analysis. The deconvoluted masses of peptic fragments from the native (un-deuterated) protein are then subtracted from the deconvoluted masses of the corresponding deuterated fragments to determine the extent of deuterium incorporation for each fragment. Deuterium incorporation for the fragments can be mapped onto a three-dimensional structure or a homology model of the protein using commercially available software to provide a visual representation of deuterium incorporation. As an example, global deuterium incorporation was measured by ssHDX-MS for four different mAb-IgG_1 formulations (Fig. 4). Using pepsin digestion, the local deuterium uptake of various peptic fragments was then identified (Fig. 5) and the degree of deuterium incorporation mapped on to a homology model of the mAb structure (Fig. 6) [8].

2.3 Data Analysis for HDX-MS and ssHDX-MS

In solution HDX-MS experiments, deuterium uptake kinetics often shows mono-exponential (Eq. 1) or bi-exponential (Eq. 2) behavior:

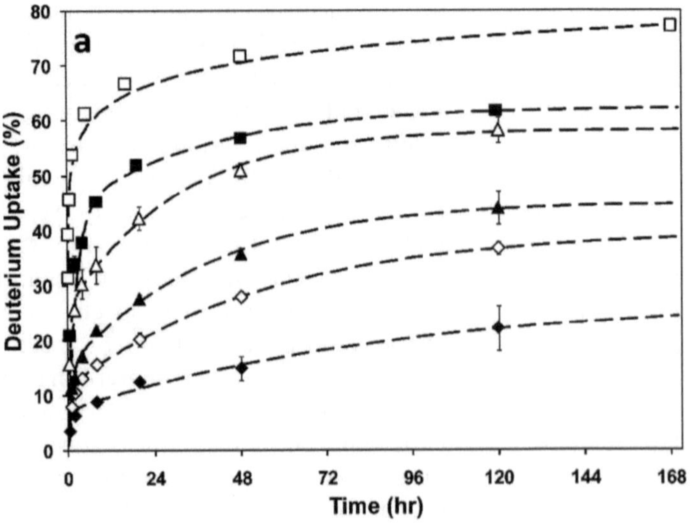

Fig. 3 Deuterium uptake kinetics for lyophilized myoglobin formulated with (**a**) mannitol or (**b**) sucrose and incubated in $D_2O_{(g)}$ vapor at various RH: 11% (closed diamond), 23% (open diamond), 33% (closed triangle) 43% (open triangle), or 75% (closed square). Results were compared with a solution HDX sample (open square) and fitted to a biexponential model (see Eq. 2). Reproduced with permission from reference [20]; copyright © 2012, American Chemical Society

$$D(t) = D_{\max}\left(1 - e^{-k_{\text{obs}}t}\right) \tag{1}$$

$$D(t) = N_{\text{fast}}\left(1 - e^{-k_{\text{fast}}t}\right) + N_{\text{slow}}\left(1 - e^{-k_{\text{slow}}t}\right) \tag{2}$$

These relationships are often used to fit kinetic data and to determine regression parameters. In Eq. 1, $D(t)$ is the number of deuterons taken up at time t, $D_{\max}$ is the maximum number of

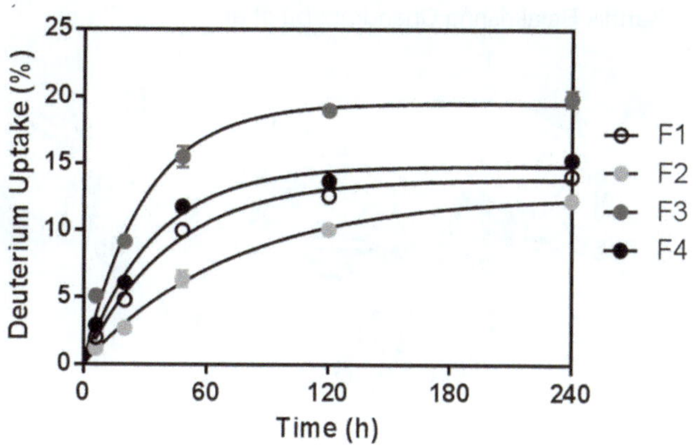

Fig. 4 Deuterium uptake kinetics for a lyophilized monoclonal antibody (mAb-IgG1) in four formulations (F1, F2, F3, F4) containing different excipients. ssHDX-MS was performed 11% RH in $D_2O_{(g)}$ and was fitted using a monoexponential model (see Eq. 1). Reproduced with permission from reference [8]; copyright © 2018, American Chemical Society

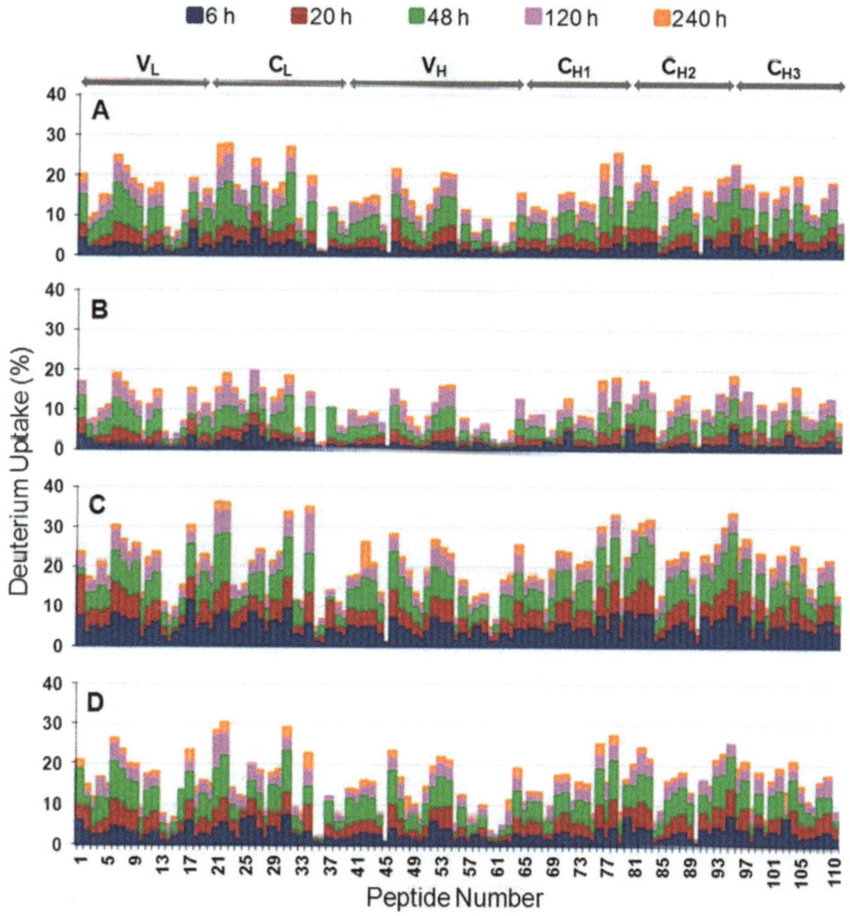

Fig. 5 Deuterium uptake in peptic fragments for the mAb-IgG1 formulations of Fig. 4: (**A**) F1, (**B**) F2, (**C**) F3, and (**D**) F4. Pepsin digestion of both heavy chain (HC) and light chain (LC) led to 110 overlapping peptides, represented sequentially on the *x*-axis by peptide number. Time points for ssHDX and the domain locations are shown at the top of the figure. Values are averages of three independent experiments. Reproduced with permission from reference [8]; copyright © 2018, American Chemical Society

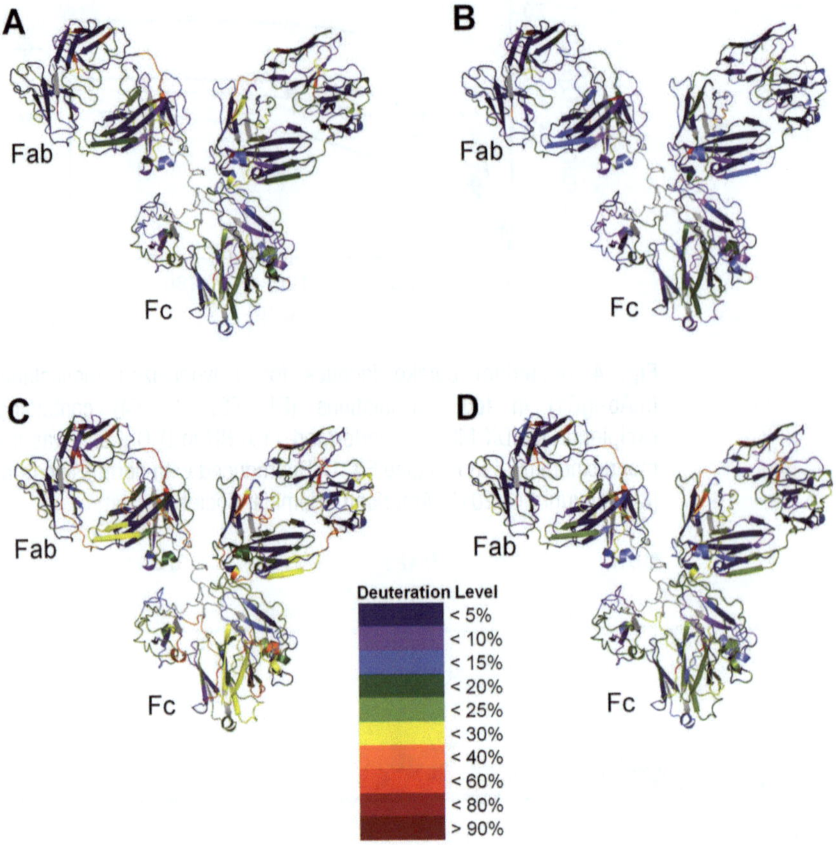

Fig. 6 Deuterium uptake mapped onto a homology model of the mAb structure for the four formulations of Figs. 4 and 5: (**A**) F1, (**B**) F2, (**C**) F3, and (**D**) F4. The maximum deuterium incorporation (D_{max}) for each formulation is shown. Reproduced with permission from reference [8]; copyright © 2018, American Chemical Society

deuterium incorporated at large t, and k_{obs} is the observed apparent first-order rate constant. In Eq. 2, exchangeable amide groups are assumed to belong to rapidly and slowly exchanging pools, so that N_{fast} is the number of amide hydrogens in the rapidly exchanging pool, N_{slow} is the number of amide hydrogens in the slowly exchanging pool, and k_{fast} and k_{slow} are the apparent first-order rate constants for the rapidly and slowly exchanging pools, respectively [19, 20, 31]. The designation of rapidly and slowly exchanging pools is consistent with the solvent exposure of some portion of amide hydrogen atoms in the molecule, and the "protection" of other amide hydrogen atoms by higher order structure.

At a phenomenological level, deuterium uptake in solid-state HDX-MS experiments often shows mono- or bi-exponential kinetics similar to that observed in solution. However, a number of observations suggest that the mechanistic interpretations applied to solution state HDX-MS may not apply in ssHDX, and that a different interpretation is needed.

2.4 Mechanistic Interpretation of Solution HDX-MS Data: Limitations for ssHDX-MS

Solution HDX data are often interpreted mechanistically using the Linderstrom-Lang model, which asserts that exchange is the result of reversible protein unfolding (i.e., "opening" and "closing" events), which may be global or local, followed by an irreversible "chemical" exchange reaction at free amide groups [31, 34].

$$N_H \underset{k_{cl}}{\overset{k_{op}}{\rightleftharpoons}} U_H \xrightarrow{k_{ch}} U_D \underset{k_{op}}{\overset{k_{cl}}{\rightleftharpoons}} N_D \tag{3}$$

Here, N_H represents the native protein in its protonated form, U_H represents the unfolded protein in its protonated form, and U_D and N_D are the corresponding deuterated versions of these species. The model relates the observed rate of exchange (k_{obs}, Eq. 1) to rate constants for opening (k_{op}), closing (k_{cl}), and chemical exchange (k_{ch}). Two limiting cases have been identified. In the EX1 limit, $k_{ch} \gg k_{cl}$ and $k_{obs} = k_{op}$, while in the more common EX2 limit, $k_{cl} \gg k_{ch}$ and $k_{obs} = K_{op}k_{ch}$, where K_{op} is the equilibrium constant for opening and closing ($K_{op} = k_{op}/k_{cl}$) [31, 34]. Thus, the Linderstrom-Lang model relates experimentally observed rates of exchange (k_{obs}) in solution to protein structural dynamics (k_{cl}, k_{op}, K_{op}).

A number of observations suggest that the Linderstrom-Lang model does not adequately describe ssHDX at a mechanistic level. Both the rate and extent of ssHDX are strongly affected by stabilizing excipients [8, 9, 17, 18, 25]; protein-excipient interactions are not described by the Linderstrom-Lang model. Similarly, ssHDX is affected by $D_2O_{(g)}$ activity [19, 20], a parameter not included in Linderstrom-Lang. An ssHDX experiment takes days to weeks to complete, far longer than solution HDX experiments [8, 9, 19, 20]. This suggests that rate processes much slower than those identified by the Linderstrom-Lang model (k_{cl}, k_{op}, k_{ch}) dominate ssHDX, or at the very least that the Linderstrom-Lang rate constants are greatly reduced in solids. Finally, applying the Linderstrom-Lang model requires an independent measure of k_{ch}, which depends on pH and temperature [31]; pH is not defined in the solid state and glass transitions may complicate interpretation of observed temperature dependences.

In solution HDX, both protein structure and opening/closing events are related to hydrogen bonds. These include the intramolecular hydrogen bonds that contribute to higher order structure as well as the intermolecular hydrogen bonds between the protein and water. The Linderstrom-Lang model regards opening and exchange as sequential rather than concerted events, so that an intramolecular hydrogen bond must break before exchange can occur at that site. Intra- and intermolecular hydrogen bonds are likely to govern ssHDX as well, though in different ways, as discussed below.

2.5 Hydrogen Bonds of Proteins in Solution and Amorphous Solids

Hydrogen bonds can form when an electronegative atom such as oxygen (O) is covalently bound to hydrogen (H), leading to partial negative charge on O and partial positive charge on H. These partial charges, also occurring on nearby molecules or groups, lead to the formation of weak electrostatic interactions between the electronegative atoms and hydrogen, termed hydrogen bonds [35]. The hydrogen atom is effectively shared between the electronegative donor and acceptor atoms [35]. Hydrogen bonds have been categorized as "weak," "moderate," or "strong." Hydrogen bonds are considered "moderate" if they are associated with energies in the range of 4–15 kcal mol^{-1} and resemble hydrogen bonds between water molecules. Strong hydrogen bonds have bond energies greater than 15 kcal mol^{-1}, while weak hydrogen has bond energies less than 4 kcal mol^{-1} [36].

Proteins are large biomolecules with many hydrogen bond donors and acceptors. The backbone amide groups (peptide bonds) can form intramolecular hydrogen bonds, leading to stable secondary structures such as α-helices and β-sheets with well-known hydrogen bonding patterns [37, 38]. On average, each residue in a protein forms 1.1 hydrogen bonds in the native folded state. The side chain functional groups of a protein (e.g., -OH, $-NH_2$, -COOH) are also capable of forming hydrogen bonds, both inter- and intra-molecularly. In general, the stability of a protein increases with the number of intramolecular hydrogen bonds [39]. In aqueous solution, the native structure is also determined by intermolecular hydrogen bonds to water. These interactions are a relatively constant feature of the aqueous environment, but become more limited and more variable as water is removed to form solids.

For proteins in amorphous solids, the intramolecular hydrogen bonds of the native form are present if structure is maintained. In addition, there may be intermolecular hydrogen bonds between the protein and excipients, residual water, and/or other protein molecules in the surrounding matrix. According to the water replacement hypothesis, proteins are stabilized in the amorphous solid state by the formation of hydrogen bonds to excipients. These hydrogen bonds are said to "replace" the hydrogen bonds to water that help to stabilize the structure in solution, and are thought to involve, for example, the hydroxyl groups on sugars. The number and strength of the hydrogen bonds formed between protein and excipient depend on factors such as excipient structure, molecular weight, and glass transition temperature (T_g). Excipients with lower T_g are thought to stabilize proteins by forming more hydrogen bonds than those with high T_g. Formulations with high T_g excipients are thought to have greater intermolecular interactions between excipient molecules than those with low T_g excipients, so that the disruption of excipient-excipient interactions is difficult and fewer hydrogen bonds between excipient protein are formed. Conversely, low T_g excipients may have weaker excipient-excipient interactions, allowing greater protein-excipient hydrogen bonding.

Residual moisture in amorphous solids containing proteins is also important, since the water forms hydrogen bonds with the protein and also acts as a plasticizer, lowering T_g. Both protein-excipient and protein-water hydrogen bonds are thought to be important in determining protein stability in the amorphous state, and completely dry amorphous protein formulations often show poorer storage stability than those containing modest (2–5% w/w) residual moisture content [40].

2.6 Toward a Mechanistic Interpretation of ssHDX-MS

We propose that the rate and extent of deuterium incorporation in an ssHDX-MS experiment provide information about the hydrogen bond network experienced by the protein in the amorphous solid state. As described above, this network includes both the intramolecular hydrogen bonds that contribute to protein structure and the intermolecular hydrogen bonds between the protein and the surrounding matrix. We envision that the rapidly exchanging pool in ssHDX (N_{fast}, k_{fast}; Eq. 1) includes amide hydrogen atoms that do not participate in hydrogen bonds, and thus can exchange readily with D_2O adsorbed from the vapor phase. The rapidly exchanging pool may also include amide hydrogen atoms that participate in relatively weak hydrogen bonds to residual water or excipient. We envision that the slowly exchanging pool (N_{slow}, k_{slow}; Eq. 1) includes amide hydrogen atoms engaged in stronger hydrogen bonds, whether structural hydrogen bonds within the protein or intramolecular hydrogen bonds to excipients. In a typical ssHDX experiment, some of the theoretically exchangeable backbone amide hydrogen atoms do not undergo exchange. We envision that this "un-exchangeable" pool represents strong structural hydrogen bonds in the core of the folded protein.

While the model outlined above is consistent with ssHDX results to date, it also raises additional questions. First, while chemical exchange is assumed to be irreversible in the Linderstrom-Lang model, this assumption is unlikely to be valid on the much longer time scale of an ssHDX experiment. Whether or not exchange is reversible in ssHDX is unclear at this point. Similarly, it is unclear whether ssHDX is the result of sequential hydrogen bond breaking and chemical exchange, as in the Linderstrom-Lang model, or whether the two processes occur in a concerted fashion. The extent to which D_2O mass transport affects ssHDX kinetics also is not fully understood. In studies reported to date, $D_2O_{(g)}$ sorption typically is complete in several hours, while ssHDX experiments continue for hundreds of hours or more. While D_2O mass transport thus is unlikely to influence exchange kinetics past the first few hours, mass transport effects may mask rapid exchange events, complicating the interpretation of ssHDX kinetics. Finally, the relative contributions of protein structure (intramolecular hydrogen bonds) and matrix interactions (intermolecular hydrogen bonds) to ssHDX results have not been explored, though ongoing studies of unstructured model peptides may shed light on these effects.

2.7 Further Development of ssHDX-MS

ssHDX-MS shows promise as a surrogate for stability studies in formulation development, process scale-up, and tech transfer for lyophilized proteins. Establishing its validity will require broader evaluation for a range of proteins and processes, with the goal of establishing the predictive ability and limitations of the method. For example, in recent studies of a lyophilized mAb, adding histidine enhanced storage stability but did not affect ssHDX metrics [22]. This suggests that histidine stabilizes the mAb by a mechanism not detected by ssHDX, which requires further investigation. Many of the studies relating ssHDX to storage stability have focused on protein aggregation. While there is some indication that ssHDX may be correlated with chemical instability in solids as well, this too requires further study. As described above, there is evidence that the Linderstrom-Lang model does not adequately describe ssHDX, and an alternative is needed. Such a model would not only enable better interpretation of ssHDX-MS data, but would also improve our understanding of the amorphous solid state and the factors that control protein stability therein. Finally, automation of $D_2O_{(g)}$ exposure and sample analysis would facilitate broader adoption of the method and its application in the biopharmaceutical industry.

3 Solid-State Photolytic Labeling with Mass Spectrometric Analysis (ssPLL-MS)

In solution-state studies of protein conformation and interactions, covalent labeling approaches have been developed to complement HDX [41, 42]. One such approach introduces photolytically activatable functional groups (e.g., diazirine) into a protein of interest [42]. On exposure to UV light of the appropriate wavelength, the activated functional group reacts with neighboring molecules, allowing the protein's interactions with them to be interrogated. Amino acid analogs with photoactive functional groups have been developed and are commercially available. These "photo-amino acids" can be incorporated into a peptide or protein sequence site-specifically, either by expression or chemical synthesis. Photolytic labeling has been used to study protein structure and protein-protein interactions in vitro and in vivo [43–48]. For example, the photoactive amino acid *p*-benzoyl-L-phenylalanine (pBpA) was site specifically incorporated into the adaptor protein Grb2. After UV exposure at 365 nm, protein variants with pBpA near the ligand-binding pocket were cross-linked with the epidermal growth factor receptor, showing the protein-protein interactions involved in the cell signaling pathway [44]. To provide additional information on protein interactions in lyophilized powders, we have adapted photolytic labeling for use in the amorphous solid state.

The use of photo reactive reagents in lyophilized protein formulations can be classified into two groups: (1) photo-reactive excipients, in which the label is included in a component of the solid matrix other than the protein and (2) photo-reactive peptides/proteins, in which the label is introduced into one or more amino acid side chains during synthesis or expression, or through post-translational modification (Fig. 2). Since photolytic labeling products are covalent and the reactions are irreversible, the products are not susceptible to back exchange and are considered to be stable during analysis procedures, an advantage over ssHDX. In addition, solid-state photolytic labeling approaches are complementary to ssHDX in that they probe side-chain interactions with the matrix, rather than addressing the hydrogen bond network of the protein backbone.

3.1 Information Content of ssPLL-MS

3.1.1 Results with Photolytically Labeled Excipients

Photo-reactive excipients can be co-lyophilized with the protein formulation and used to probe formulation and process effects on interactions with the protein. For example, photo-leucine (pLeu), a commercially available diazirine-containing analog of leucine, was co-lyophilized with apomyoglobin and sucrose at different compositions [10]. The molar ratio of apomyoglobin to pLeu was increased from 0 to 1:100, while the protein to sucrose ratio was kept at 1:2 (w/w). The labeling products were analyzed with MS at the intact protein level and the kinetics of labeling were also studied. MS and MS/MS were used to analyze apomyoglobin digests to identify and map the sites of labeling. To evaluate formulation effects, apomyogloblin was lyophilized with sucrose or guanidine hydrochloride with 100-fold molar excess of pLeu incorporated in the formulation.

The results demonstrated that pLeu labeling occurs in lyophilized solids on exposure to light. In sucrose-based formulations with increasing concentrations of pLeu, apomyoglobin acquired up to 6 pLeu labels. A kinetic profile of the labeling reaction was established at 1:100 molar ratio of apomyoglobin to pLeu (Fig. 7). The rate of labeling was rapid and reached a plateau in around 30 min with ~20% of protein remaining unlabeled. Labeling was observed across helices ABCDG and H with increasing concentrations of pLeu (Fig. 8). No labeling was observed for residues A57–K96, which form helices E and F.

As a photo-reactive excipient, pLeu was also used to investigate the effects of formulation and controlled nucleation on lyophilized myoglobin [12]. pLeu was incorporated in the formulation at a molar ratio of 100:1 to myoglobin, with or without the presence of sucrose. The formulations were lyophilized using uncontrolled or controlled nucleation. For the formulation without sucrose, uncontrolled and controlled nucleation showed similar pLeu

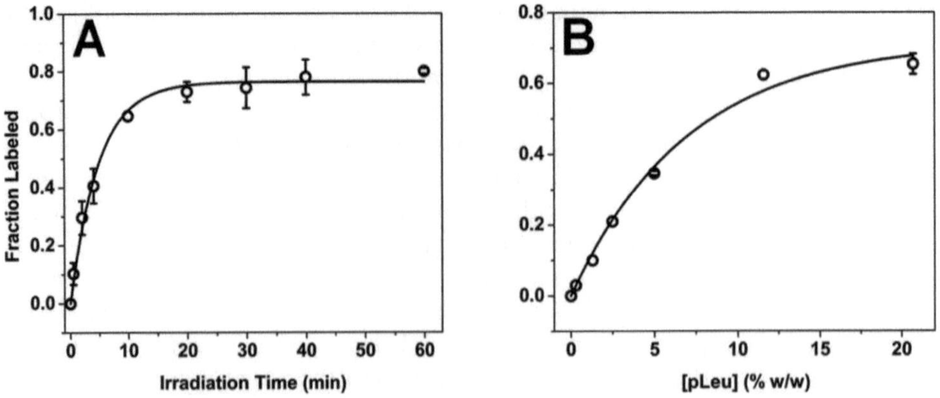

Fig. 7 (**A**) Kinetics of photolytic labeling of apomyoglobin (apoMb) in lyophilized solids containing 20.7% (w/w) pLeu (apoMb:pLeu molar ratio = 1:100). (**B**) Dependence of apoMb photolytic labeling on the concentration of pLeu after 40 min UV exposure. In both (**A**) and (**B**), $n = 3 \pm$ SD. The solid lines are fit to an exponential model $F_L(C, t) = A(1 - e^{-k_1 t})(1 - e^{-k_2 C})$. $F_L(C, t)$ is the fraction of labeled protein as a function of pLeu concentration (C) and irradiation time (t), k_1 and k_2 are apparent first-order rate constants, and A is the fraction of protein labeled at the plateau. Reproduced with permission from reference [10]; copyright © 2013, American Chemical Society

labeling fraction of myoglobin, which was 6 (±1)% and 7 (±1)% respectively. In contrast, myoglobin lyophilized with sucrose using controlled nucleation showed the largest fraction of labeled protein (11±1%). The sucrose-free and sucrose-containing formulations lyophilized with controlled nucleation showed different labeling in the myoglobin structure at peptide Leu^{32}-Lys^{42}.

3.1.2 Results with Photolytically Labeled Peptides and Proteins

When a photo-reactive functional group is incorporated into the protein sequence at an amino acid side chain, it can form cross-linked products with molecules near the side chain, and thus can provide information about the local environment of the protein in the solid matrix. Information regarding these nearest neighbors and the effects of excipients on the local environment can be deduced from the cross-linked products. A peptide or protein with a photo-reactive amino acid side chain can be produced by: (1) incorporating the photo-reactive amino acid into the sequence during peptide synthesis or cell expression or (2) labeling amino acid side chains, post-translationally or following synthesis, using a bifunctional reagent with a photo-reactive moiety.

As an example the first approach, a photo-reactive amino acid was incorporated into the sequence of a model peptide through peptide synthesis [10]. The peptide sequence 1-HSQGTFTS-8 (GCG (1–8)) was derived from human glucagon. The photo-reactive amino acid analog pBpA was substituted for phenylalanine (F6) in solid phase synthesis, producing a site-specifically labeled peptide designated GCG (1–8)*. GCG (1–8)* was then co-lyophilized with the individual excipients sucrose,

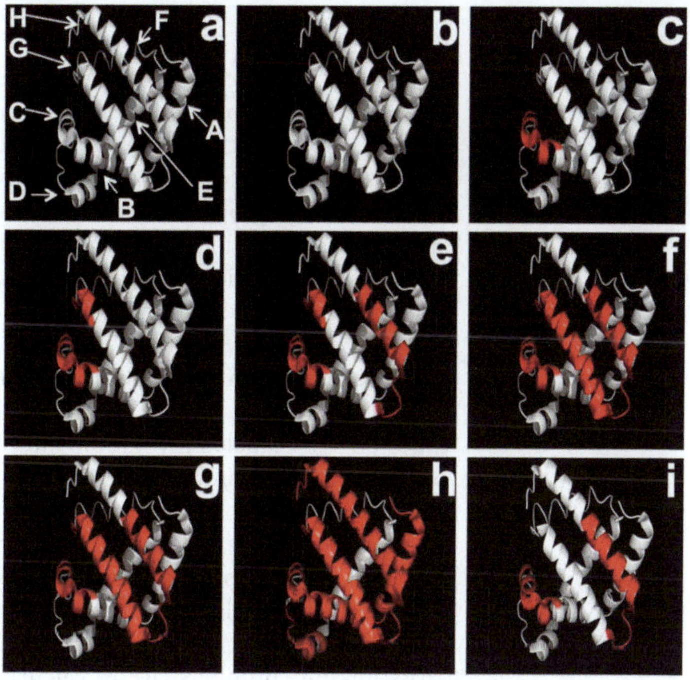

Fig. 8 Sites of photolytic labeling in red of apomyoglobin in lyophilized solids containing photoleucine (pLeu). (**a**) Ribbon diagram of unlabeled apoMb showing helices A–E, G, and H. (**b–h**) Ribbon diagram of apoMb showing sites of labeling with increasing pLeu in solids containing sucrose: (**b**) 0%, (**c**) 0.3%, (**d**) 1.3%, (**e**) 2.5%, (**f**) 5.0%, (**g**) 11.6%, and (**h**) 20.7% w/w pLeu. (**i**) Ribbon diagram of apoMb showing covalent labeling with 20.7% w/w pLeu in the presence of guanidine hydrochloride (1.5 M). The ribbon diagrams were generated using PyMOL (PyMOL Molecular Graphics System, Version 1.4.1, Schrödinger, LLC) and the crystal structure of myoglobin (PDB ID 1WLA; www.rcsb.org). Helix F (H82–H97) in the myoglobin structure was modified to an unstructured region, as observed for native apoMb at neutral pH [53]. Reproduced with permission from reference [10]; copyright © 2013, American Chemical Society

trehalose, L-methionine, L-leucine, urea or pLeu, and with a combination of pLeu and sucrose. Solution controls consisted of solutions of the peptide with each excipient or excipient mixture prior to lyophilization. After UV exposure at 365 nm, peptide-peptide adducts were formed in both solution and solid samples, and included dimers and trimers of GCG (1–8)*. Peptide-excipient adducts were observed in formulations containing L-methionine or L-leucine formulations in solution and in lyophilized solids, but were not observed in sucrose, trehalose, or urea formulations. In formulations containing GCG (1–8)* and pLeu with and without sucrose, peptide excipient adducts were detected with or without loss of N_2. The loss of N_2 indicated that labeling occurred through the activation of pLeu rather than through the labeled peptide.

As an example of the second approach, myoglobin was derivatized with succinimidyl 4,4′-azipentanoate (SDA) in solution, and protein-protein and protein-matrix interactions were probed using photolytic activation in lyophilized solids [11]. No significant secondary structural changes were detected by CD spectroscopy and solid-state FTIR for SDA-labeled myoglobin compared to the unlabeled myoglobin. Derivatized myoglobin was lyophilized alone or using raffinose or guanidine hydrochloride as excipients. As above, photolytic labeling in the solid samples was activated with UV exposure at 365 nm and samples were analyzed by LC-MS.

Following SDA derivatization, a heterogenous mixture was produced in which myglobin carried up to five SDA labels. While SDA reacts preferentially with lysine side chains, LC-MS analysis of digested SDA-labeled myoglobin indicated that SDA derivatization occurred at other amino acids as well, with serine and tyrosine side chains as likely secondary sites. After UV exposure, peptide-peptide adducts, peptide-water adduct, and peptide-excipient adducts were detected and mapped semi-quantitatively by showing the number of times a particular product was detected in triplicate analyses. Peptides forming cross-linked products were grouped and peptide cross-linking numbers were calculated to analyze differences among the formulations. Peptide cross-linking numbers were used to show how many adducts the peptide had formed. Together, the results indicated the heterogeneous nature of lyophilized protein formulations and demonstrated that protein-matrix interactions can be mapped with peptide level resolution using ssPLL-MS.

3.2 Experimental Methods for ssPLL-MS

In ssPLL-MS studies using photolytically labeled excipients (Fig. 2a), the photo-excipient is first co-lyophilized with the protein and formulation of interest. To date, commercially available photo-labeled amino acid analogs have been used for this purpose, including photo-leucine (L-2-amino-4,4′-azipentanoic acid; pLeu), photo-methionine (L-2-amino-5,5-azi-hexanoic acid; pMet), and *p*-benzoyl-L-phenylalanine (pBpA). The solid samples are then exposed to UV light at an activating wavelength to produce the activated species and initiate the labeling reactions. Both pLeu and pMet contain a photoactive diazirine group, which loses a molecule of $N_{2(g)}$ and forms a reactive carbene after exposure to UV light at 350–365 nm. The reactive carbene can insert into any X-H bond ($X = C, O, N, S$), add to a C=C double bond, or undergo internal conversion. Formation of the carbene allows pLeu and pMet to label the protein and other components of the matrix. Photolytic reactions are not limited to diazirine chemistry; pBpA forms a reactive ketyl radical on the benzophenone group after UV exposure, which reacts preferentially with C-H bonds. The reaction time and photo-excipient:protein ratio must be optimized to ensure sufficient labeling without undue heating of the solid sample during UV exposure. To monitor the rate and extent of the labeling reaction, samples are removed at various times, reconstituted with an appropriate buffer, and analyzed using LC/MS. Spectra are selected in the expected mass range of the protein, with an increased upper limit to allow detection of the high mass photo-excipient adducts. Typically, a heterogeneous mixture of adducts is produced, showing a distribution in the number of photo-excipient species added to the protein. The sites of labeling on the protein can be identified using proteolytic digestion (e.g., with trypsin/chymotrypsin) or in MS/MS analysis. The peptide fragments may differ in native and labeled forms of the protein, however, complicating data analysis.

For ssPLL-MS studies using photolytically labeled protein, the label must first be introduced into the protein of interest. As noted above, this can be accomplished during peptide synthesis or cell expression (1) or post-translational modification (2). The introduction of non-native amino acids, including photo-amino acids, into a peptide sequence (1) is well established in solid-phase peptide synthesis [49], and commercial peptide synthesis companies offer this service at a cost comparable to that of native peptides of similar molecular weight. For larger proteins, methods for expressing mutant forms of proteins that contain photo-amino acids (1) have been established [43, 50–52]. For example, pBpA-containing mutants can be expressed using an orthogonal aminoacyl tRNA synthetase-tRNA$_{CUA}$ pair that incorporates pBpA at the position encoded by the amber codon TAG. The TAG codon can be introduced into the protein cDNA sequence by site directed mutagenesis PCR, then transfected into an appropriate cell line for expression of the mutant [43, 50]. Both custom peptide synthesis and the expression of mutant proteins allow the photolytic label to be introduced in a site-specific manner, but require significant time and/or resources. Alternatively, the label may be introduced post-translationally (2). For example, proteins may be labeled post-translationally using the bifunctional reagent SDA (succinimidyl 4,4′-azipentanoate; NHS-diazirine). At neutral pH, SDA reacts preferentially with lysine side chains, creating an amide bond that links the diazirine group to the protein. In larger proteins with multiple lysine groups, labeling is heterogeneous and a mixture of products is formed, and labeling can also occur at side chain with hydroxyl functional group of other amino acids (e.g., Ser). While it is possible to fractionate or purify the product mixture, this reduces yield. Thus, while post-translational labeling (2) is often faster and experimentally more straightforward than peptide synthesis and cell expression (1) approaches, this advantage is counterbalanced by the heterogeneity of the labeled protein.

Once the labeled protein has been produced, ssPLL-MS studies are conducted in a manner analogous to those with labeled excipient. Products of the photolytic reaction include protein-protein, protein-excipient, and protein-water adducts, as well as unproductive intramolecular and "dead-end" products. These differ from the products of ssPLL-MS using labeled excipient, where only protein-excipient adducts are detected. For ssPLL-MS using labeled protein, proteolytic digestion or MS/MS fragmentation can be used to identify the sites of protein-protein interactions in the solid state, which may be useful in identifying interactions that may lead to aggregation on storage or reconstitution. Similarly, sites of protein-excipient and protein-water interactions can also be mapped, providing information on the local environment near the label.

3.3 Data Analysis and Interpretation in ssPLL-MS

At the intact protein level, ssPLL-MS products can be quantified using extracted ion chromatograms (EIC) obtained in LC/MS analysis, with the assumption that ionization efficiency is not affected by the label. Using this approach, the kinetics of pLeu labeling of apomyoglobin in lyophilized powders were shown to depend exponentially on time and pLeu concentration [10]. For smaller photolytically peptides, it may be possible to generate synthetic standards of the expected reaction products, allowing more precise quantitation. At the digest level, heterogeneity of reaction products makes quantitation difficult, particularly for post-translationally labeled proteins. Semi-quantitative analysis of such digests is possible, however, e.g., by counting the number of times a particular product is detected on replicate MS injections, thus allowing the sites of protein-protein, protein-excipient, and protein-water interactions to be mapped [11]. The relationship of the rate and extent of ssPLL-MS to protein stability on storage in the solid state is not known.

3.4 Further Development of ssPLL-MS

ssPLL-MS is a promising method for mapping the local environment of proteins in solid formulations. The approach is considerably newer than ssHDX-MS and there is much to be learned. For example, unlike ssHDX-MS, the relationship of protein stability in the solid state to ssPLL-MS metrics is not known. While it is reasonable to expect that more extensive protein-protein interactions measured by ssPLL-MS would be correlated to increased aggregation on storage, this has not been tested. Studies to date have demonstrated that ssPLL-MS is feasible when the photolytic label is incorporated either in the protein or in an excipient, or both. The complexity of labeling during protein expression and the heterogeneity of post-translationally labeled protein suggest that photolytically labeled excipients will be more immediately useful in formulation applications. The development of new photolytically labeled excipients that better mimic the range of excipient structures used in pharmaceutical development would help to advance this approach. Finally, improved approaches to quantitation and data analysis are needed; bottom-up analysis of digests of ssPLL-

MS samples is hindered by the effects of labeling on the sites of digestion and by the lack of commercial software for identification of labeled fragments.

4 Summary

Lyophilization (freeze-drying) is used to produce amorphous solid powders of protein drugs. Though lyophilization is usually used in an attempt to stabilize the protein, degradation processes can still occur in the solid state, and the rate and extent of degradation are often poorly correlated with measurable properties of the protein and the powder. Solid-state hydrogen-deuterium exchange (ssHDX) and solid-state photolytic labeling (ssPLL) with mass spectrometric analysis (ssHDX-MS, ssPLL-MS) are novel, high-resolution methods for measuring protein structure and matrix interactions in solid powders. ssHDX-MS measures the rate and extent of deuterium incorporation on exposure of the powder to D_2O vapor. In limited studies, the extent of deuterium incorporation in ssHDX-MS has been shown to be highly correlated with aggregation on storage, suggesting that the method can serve as a surrogate for time-consuming stability studies in formulation and process development. Further development of ssHDX-MS will require broader evaluation to define the limits of the method and an alternative to the Linderstrom-Lang model to allow mechanistic interpretation of the results. ssPLL-MS identifies the covalent adducts formed when a solid powder containing photolytically labeled protein and/or excipient is exposed to light at an activating wavelength. ssPLL-MS allows the local solid-state environment of the label to be mapped with high resolution. Further development of ssPLL-MS will require an evaluation of its relationship to storage stability, the creation of novel photolytically labeled excipients, and improved approaches to quantitation and data analysis.

References

1. Manning MC, Chou DK, Murphy BM, Payne RW, Katayama DS (2010) Stability of protein pharmaceuticals: an update. Pharm Res 27 (4):544–575
2. Lowe D, Dudgeon K, Rouet R, Schofield P, Jermutus L, Christ D (2011) Aggregation, stability, and formulation of human antibody therapeutics. Adv Protein Chem Struct Biol 84:41–61
3. Forney-Stevens KM, Bogner RH, Pikal MJ (2016) Addition of amino acids to further stabilize lyophilized sucrose-based protein formulations: I. Screening of 15 amino acids in two model proteins. J Pharm Sci 105(2):697–704
4. Ohtake S, Kita Y, Arakawa T (2011) Interactions of formulation excipients with proteins in solution and in the dried state. Adv Drug Deliv Rev 63(13):1053–1073
5. Carpenter JF, Crowe JH (1989) An infrared spectroscopic study of the interactions of carbohydrates with dried proteins. Biochemistry 28(9):3916–3922
6. Duddu SP, Zhang G, Dal Monte PR (1997) The relationship between protein aggregation and molecular mobility below the glass transition temperature of lyophilized formulations containing a monoclonal antibody. Pharm Res 14(5):596–600

7. Zhang Z, Smith DL (1993) Determination of amide hydrogen exchange by mass spectrometry: a new tool for protein structure elucidation. Protein Sci 2(4):522–531
8. Moorthy BS, Zarraga IE, Kumar L, Walters BT, Goldbach P, Topp EM et al (2018) Solid-state hydrogen–deuterium exchange mass spectrometry: correlation of deuterium uptake and long-term stability of lyophilized monoclonal antibody formulations. Mol Pharm 15 (1):1–11
9. Moorthy BS, Schultz SG, Kim SG, Topp EM (2014) Predicting protein aggregation during storage in lyophilized solids using solid state amide hydrogen/deuterium exchange with mass spectrometric analysis (ssHDX-MS). Mol Pharm 11(6):1869–1879
10. Iyer LK, Moorthy BS, Topp EM (2013) Photolytic labeling to probe molecular interactions in lyophilized powders. Mol Pharm 10 (12):4629–4639
11. Iyer LK, Moorthy BS, Topp EM (2015) Photolytic cross-linking to probe protein–protein and protein–matrix interactions in lyophilized powders. Mol Pharm 12(9):3237–3249
12. Iyer LK, Sacha GA, Moorthy BS, Nail SL, Topp EM (2016) Process and formulation effects on protein structure in lyophilized solids using mass spectrometric methods. J Pharm Sci 105(5):1684–1692
13. Wales TE, Engen JR (2006) Hydrogen exchange mass spectrometry for the analysis of protein dynamics. Mass Spectrom Rev 25 (1):158–170
14. Tsutsui Y, Wintrode PL (2007) Hydrogen/deuterium exchange-mass spectrometry: a powerful tool for probing protein structure, dynamics and interactions. Curr Med Chem 14(22):2344–2358
15. Houde D, Berkowitz SA, Engen JR (2011) The utility of hydrogen/deuterium exchange mass spectrometry in biopharmaceutical comparability studies. J Pharm Sci 100 (6):2071–2086
16. Majumdar R, Middaugh CR, Weis DD, Volkin DB (2015) Hydrogen-deuterium exchange mass spectrometry as an emerging analytical tool for stabilization and formulation development of therapeutic monoclonal antibodies. J Pharm Sci 104(2):327–345
17. Li Y, Williams TD, Schowen RL, Topp EM (2007) Trehalose and calcium exert site-specific effects on calmodulin conformation in amorphous solids. Biotechnol Bioeng 97 (6):1650–1653
18. Sinha S, Li Y, Williams TD, Topp EM (2008) Protein conformation in amorphous solids by FTIR and by hydrogen/deuterium exchange with mass spectrometry. Biophys J 95 (12):5951–5961
19. Sophocleous AM, Topp EM (2012) Localized hydration in lyophilized myoglobin by hydrogen-deuterium exchange mass spectrometry. 2. Exchange kinetics. Mol Pharm 9 (4):727–733
20. Sophocleous AM, Zhang J, Topp EM (2012) Localized hydration in lyophilized myoglobin by hydrogen–deuterium exchange mass spectrometry. 1. Exchange mapping. Mol Pharm 9 (4):718–726
21. Moorthy BS, Iyer LK, Topp EM (2015) Characterizing protein structure, dynamics and conformation in lyophilized solids. Curr Pharm Des 21(40):5845–5853
22. Moussa EM, Singh SK, Kimmel M, Nema S, Topp EM (2018) Probing the conformation of an IgG1 monoclonal antibody in lyophilized solids using solid-state hydrogen–deuterium exchange with mass spectrometric analysis (ssHDX-MS). Mol Pharm 15(2):356–368
23. Moussa EM, Wilson NE, Zhou QT, Singh SK, Nema S, Topp EM (2018) Effects of drying process on an IgG1 monoclonal antibody using solid-state hydrogen deuterium exchange with mass spectrometric analysis (ssHDX-MS). Pharm Res 35(1):12
24. Li Y, Williams TD, Schowen RL, Topp EM (2007) Characterizing protein structure in amorphous solids using hydrogen/deuterium exchange with mass spectrometry. Anal Biochem 366(1):18–28
25. Li Y, Williams TD, Topp EM (2008) Effects of excipients on protein conformation in lyophilized solids by hydrogen/deuterium exchange mass spectrometry. Pharm Res 25(2):259–267
26. Moorthy BS, Iyer LK, Topp EM (2015) Mass spectrometric approaches to study protein structure and interactions in lyophilized powders. J Vis Exp (98):52503
27. Sane SU, Wong R, Hsu CC (2004) Raman spectroscopic characterization of drying-induced structural changes in a therapeutic antibody: correlating structural changes with long-term stability. J Pharm Sci 93 (4):1005–1018
28. Chang LL, Shepherd D, Sun J, Ouellette D, Grant KL, Tang XC et al (2005) Mechanism of protein stabilization by sugars during freeze-drying and storage: native structure preservation, specific interaction, and/or immobilization in a glassy matrix? J Pharm Sci 94 (7):1427–1444
29. Schüle S, Frieß W, Bechtold-Peters K, Garidel P (2007) Conformational analysis of protein

secondary structure during spray-drying of antibody/mannitol formulations. Eur J Pharm Biopharm 65(1):1–9

30. Park J, Nagapudi K, Vergara C, Ramachander R, Laurence JS, Krishnan S (2013) Effect of pH and excipients on structure, dynamics, and long-term stability of a model IgG1 monoclonal antibody upon freeze-drying. Pharm Res 30(4):968–984
31. Brown KA, Wilson DJ (2017) Bottom-up hydrogen deuterium exchange mass spectrometry: data analysis and interpretation. Analyst 142(16):2874–2886
32. Konermann L, Pan J, Liu Y-H (2011) Hydrogen exchange mass spectrometry for studying protein structure and dynamics. Chem Soc Rev 40(3):1224–1234
33. Deng B, Lento C, Wilson DJ (2016) Hydrogen deuterium exchange mass spectrometry in biopharmaceutical discovery and development–a review. Anal Chim Acta 940:8–20
34. Huang RY-C, Chen G (2014) Higher order structure characterization of protein therapeutics by hydrogen/deuterium exchange mass spectrometry. Anal Bioanal Chem 406 (26):6541–6558
35. Hubbard RE, Kamran HM (2001) Hydrogen bonds in proteins: role and strength. In: eLS. Wiley, Chichester
36. Steiner T (2002) The hydrogen bond in the solid state. Angew Chem Int Ed 41 (1):48–76
37. Koehl P (2006) Protein structure classification. In: Lipkowitz KB, Cundari TR, Gillet VJ, Boyd DB (eds) Reviews in computational chemistry. Wiley, Chichester, pp 1–55
38. Crommelin DJA, Sindelar RD, Meibohm B (2013) Pharmaceutical biotechnology: fundamentals and applications. Springer Science & Business Media, New York
39. Pearl FMG, Sillitoe I, Orengo CA (2001) Protein structure classification. In: eLS. Wiley, Chichester
40. Breen ED, Curley JG, Overcashier DE, Hsu CC, Shire SJ (2001) Effect of moisture on the stability of a lyophilized humanized monoclonal antibody formulation. Pharm Res 18 (9):1345–1353
41. Fitzgerald MC, West GM (2009) Painting proteins with covalent labels: what's in the picture? J Am Soc Mass Spectrom 20(6):1193–1206
42. Dubinsky L, Krom BP, Meijler MM (2012) Diazirine based photoaffinity labeling. Bioorg Med Chem 20(2):554–570
43. Chin JW, Martin AB, King DS, Wang L, Schultz PG (2002) Addition of a photocrosslinking amino acid to the genetic code of Escherichia coli. Proc Natl Acad Sci U S A 99 (17):11020–11024
44. Hino N, Okazaki Y, Kobayashi T, Hayashi A, Sakamoto K, Yokoyama S (2005) Protein photo-cross-linking in mammalian cells by site-specific incorporation of a photoreactive amino acid. Nat Methods 2(3):201
45. Suchanek M, Radzikowska A, Thiele C (2005) Photo-leucine and photo-methionine allow identification of protein-protein interactions in living cells. Nat Methods 2(4):261
46. Jumper CC, Schriemer DC (2011) Mass spectrometry of laser-initiated carbene reactions for protein topographic analysis. Anal Chem 83 (8):2913–2920
47. Kölbel K, Ihling CH, Sinz A (2012) Analysis of peptide secondary structures by photoactivatable amino acid analogues. Angew Chem Int Ed 51(50):12602–12605
48. Brodie NI, Makepeace KAT, Petrotchenko EV, Borchers CH (2015) Isotopically-coded short-range hetero-bifunctional photo-reactive cross-linkers for studying protein structure. J Proteome 118:12–20
49. Hansen PR, Oddo A (2015) Fmoc solid-phase peptide synthesis. In: Houen G (ed) Peptide antibodies. Springer, New York, pp 33–50
50. Farrell IS, Toroney R, Hazen JL, Mehl RA, Chin JW (2005) Photo-cross-linking interacting proteins with a genetically encoded benzophenone. Nat Methods 2(5):377
51. Venditti V, Fawzi NL, Clore GM (2012) An efficient protocol for incorporation of an unnatural amino acid in perdeuterated recombinant proteins using glucose-based media. J Biomol NMR 52(3):191–195
52. Young TS, Ahmad I, Yin JA, Schultz PG (2010) An enhanced system for unnatural amino acid mutagenesis in E. coli. J Mol Biol 395(2):361–374
53. Janz JM, Ren Y, Looby R, Kazmi MA, Sachdev P, Grunbeck A et al (2011) Direct interaction between an allosteric agonist pepducin and the chemokine receptor CXCR4. J Am Chem Soc 133(40):15878–15881

Index

Kevin R. Ward and Paul Matejtschuk (eds.), *Lyophilization of Pharmaceuticals and Biologicals: New Technologies and Approaches*, Methods in Pharmacology and Toxicology, https://doi.org/10.1007/978-1-4939-8928-7,

D

E

F

K

L

M

N

O

P

MIX
Papier aus verantwortungsvollen Quellen
Paper from responsible sources
FSC® C105338

If you have any concerns about our products,
you can contact us on
ProductSafety@springernature.com

In case Publisher is established outside the EU,
the EU authorized representative is:
Springer Nature Customer Service Center GmbH
Europaplatz 3, 69115 Heidelberg, Germany

Printed by Libri Plureos GmbH
in Hamburg, Germany